Problems in GI Surgery

A. Velasco   1991

COMMON PROBLEMS IN
GASTROINTESTINAL SURGERY

COMMON PROBLEMS IN
GASTROINTESTINAL SURGERY

JOSEF E. FISCHER, M.D., F.A.C.S.
Christian R. Holmes Professor of Surgery
Chairman, Department of Surgery
University of Cincinnati College of Medicine
Surgeon-in-Chief
University Hospital and Holmes Division
Children's Hospital Medical Center
Cincinnati, Ohio

YEAR BOOK MEDICAL PUBLISHERS, INC.
CHICAGO • LONDON • BOCA RATON

Copyright © 1989 by Year Book Medical Publishers, Inc. All rights reserved. No part of this publication may be reproduced, stored in a retrieval system, or transmitted, in any form or by any means—electronic, mechanical, photocopying, recording, or otherwise—without prior written permission from the publisher. Printed in the United States of America.

1 2 3 4 5 6 7 8 9 0   PR   93 92 91 90 89

Library of Congress Cataloging-in-Publication Data

Common problems in gastrointestinal surgery / [edited by] Josef E. Fischer.
    p.   cm.
Includes bibliographies and index.
ISBN 0-8151-3237-9
    1. Gastrointestinal system—Surgery—Case studies. I. Fischer, Josef E., 1937–
    [DNLM: 1. Gastrointestinal Diseases—therapy—case studies.
2. Gastrointestinal System—surgery—case studies. WI 900 C734]
RD540.C624   1989   88-20656
617'.43—dc 19   CIP
DNLM/DLC
for Library of Congress

Sponsoring Editor: Nancy E. Chorpenning
Assistant Director, Manuscript Services: Fran Perveiler
Production Project Manager: Gayle Paprocki
Proofroom Manager: Shirley E. Taylor

COMMON PROBLEMS IN SURGERY SERIES

SERIES EDITOR

RICHARD F. KEMPCZINSKI, M.D.
Professor of Surgery
University of Cincinnati
Chief, Vascular Surgery
University Hospital
Cincinnati, Ohio

van Heerden/**Common Problems in Endocrine Surgery**
Fischer/**Common Problems in Gastrointestinal Surgery**
Wanebo/**Common Problems in Surgical Oncology**
Hurst/**Common Problems in Trauma**
Brewster/**Common Problems in Vascular Surgery**

Additional volumes under development.

To Karen, Erich, and Alexandra

CONTRIBUTORS

JOHN ALEXANDER-WILLIAMS, M.D.
Consultant Surgeon, The General Hospital, Birmingham, England

STANLEY W. ASHLEY, M.D.
Fellow in General Surgery, Washington University School of Medicine, St. Louis, Missouri

ROBERT J. BAKER, M.D., F.A.C.S.
Chairman, Department of Surgery, Medical Center of Delaware, Wilmington, Delaware

CHRIS S. BALL, M.D.
Surgical Research Fellow, Department of Surgery, Creighton University, Omaha, Nebraska

ROBERT W. BEART, JR., M.D., F.A.C.S.
Frank and Shari Caywood Professor of Surgery, Mayo Clinic, Scottsdale, Arizona

GEORGE E. BLOCK, M.D., F.A.C.S.
Thomas D. Jones Professor of Surgery, University of Chicago, Chicago, Illinois

EDWARD L. BRADLEY, III, M.D., F.A.C.S.
Piedmont Professor of Surgery, Emory University, Atlanta, Georgia

JOHN L. CAMERON, M.D., F.A.C.S.
Professor and Chairman, Department of Surgery, The Johns Hopkins University School of Medicine, Baltimore, Maryland

DAVID C. CARTER, M.D.
St. Mungo Professor of Surgery, University of Glasgow, Royal Infirmary, Glasgow, Scotland

JOEL D. COOPER, M.D., F.R.C.S.(C.), F.A.C.S.
Head, Section of Thoracic Surgery, Barnes Hospital at Washington University, St. Louis, Missouri

KENNETH DAVIS, JR., M.D., F.A.C.S.
Assistant Professor of Surgery, University of Cincinnati College of Medicine, Cincinnati, Ohio

TOM R. DeMEESTER, M.D., F.A.C.S.
Professor and Chairman, Department of Surgery, Creighton University School of Medicine, Omaha, Nebraska

RICHARD M. DEVINE, M.D.
Associate Professor of Surgery, Mayo Clinic, Rochester, Minnesota

WARREN E. ENKER, M.D., F.A.C.S.
Associate Professor of Surgery, Cornell University Medical College; Attending Surgeon, Rectal and Colon Service, Memorial Sloan-Kettering Cancer Center, New York City, New York

VICTOR W. FAZIO, M.D., F.R.A.C.S., F.A.C.S.
Chairman, Department of Colorectal Surgery, The Cleveland Clinic, Cleveland, Ohio

DAVID V. FELICIANO, M.D., F.A.C.S.
Associate Professor of Surgery, Baylor College of Medicine; Director, Surgical Intensive Care Unit, Ben Taub General Hospital, Houston, Texas

JOSEF E. FISCHER, M.D., F.A.C.S.
Christian R. Holmes Professor and Chairman, Department of Surgery, University of Cincinnati College of Medicine; Surgeon-in-Chief, University Hospital and Holmes Division, Children's Hospital Medical Center, Cincinnati, Ohio

BERNARD FISHER, M.D., F.A.C.S.
Distinguished Service Professor of Surgery, University of Pittsburgh School of Medicine; Project Chairman, National Surgical Adjuvant Project for Breast and Bowel Cancers, Pittsburgh, Pennsylvania

JAMES H. FOSTER, M.D., F.A.C.S.
Professor of Surgery, University of Connecticut School of Medicine, Farmington, Connecticut

CHARLES F. FREY, M.D., F.A.C.S.
Professor and Vice Chairman, Department of Surgery, University of California at Davis, Sacramento, California

DONALD S. GANN, M.D., F.A.C.S.
J. Murray Beardsley Professor of Surgery, Chairman, Department of Surgery, Brown University Division of Biology and Medicine; Surgeon-in-Chief, Rhode Island Hospital, Providence, Rhode Island

STANLEY M. GOLDBERG, M.D., F.A.C.S.
Clinical Professor of Surgery, Director, Division of Colon and Rectal Surgery, University of Minnesota, Minneapolis, Minnesota

PHILIP H. GORDON, M.D., F.R.C.S.(C.), F.A.C.S.
Senior Surgeon, Sir Mortimer B. Davis Jewish General Hospital; Associate Professor of Surgery, McGill University, Montreal, Quebec, Canada

FRANK E. GUMP, M.D., F.A.C.S.
Professor of Surgery, Columbia University College of Physicians and Surgeons, Columbia-Presbyterian Medical Center, New York City, New York

ROBERT E. HERMANN, M.D., F.A.C.S.
Chairman, Department of General Surgery, The Cleveland Clinic, Cleveland, Ohio

BERNARD M. JAFFE, M.D., F.A.C.S.
Professor and Chairman, Department of Surgery, State University of New York, Health Sciences Center at Brooklyn, Brooklyn, New York

RAYFORD SCOTT JONES, M.D., F.A.C.S.
Professor and Chairman, Department of Surgery, University of Virginia School of Medicine, Charlottesville, Virginia

PAUL H. JORDAN, JR., M.D., F.A.C.S.
Professor of Surgery, Baylor College of Medicine, Houston, Texas

KEITH A. KELLY, M.D., F.A.C.S.
Professor and Chairman, Department of Surgery, Mayo Medical School, Rochester, Minnesota

RICHARD F. KEMPCZINSKI, M.D., F.A.C.S.
Professor of Surgery, University of Cincinnati, Chief, Vascular Surgery, University Hospital, Cincinnati, Ohio

INDRU T. KHUBCHANDANI, M.D., F.A.C.S.
Chief, Colon and Rectal Surgery, Allentown Affiliated Hospitals, Allentown, Pennsylvania; Professor of Clinical Surgery, Hahnemann University Hospital, Philadelphia, Pennsylvania

ALEX G. LITTLE, M.D., F.A.C.S.
Associate Professor of Surgery; Chief, Section of Thoracic Surgery, University of Chicago Medical Center, Chicago, Illinois

ANN C. LOWRY, M.D.
Clinical Instructor of Surgery, Division of Colon and Rectal Surgery, University of Minnesota Medical School, Minneapolis, Minnesota

LEONARD MAKOWKA, M.D., Ph.D.
Associate Professor of Surgery, University of Pittsburgh Health Center, Veterans Administration Medical Center, Pittsburgh, Pennsylvania

LESTER W. MARTIN, M.D., F.A.C.S.
Professor of Surgery and Pediatrics, University of Cincinnati College of Medicine; Director of Pediatric Surgery, Children's Hospital Medical Center, Cincinnati, Ohio

CHARLES K. McSHERRY, M.D., F.A.C.S.
Director of Surgery, Beth Israel Medical Center; Professor of Surgery, Mount Sinai School of Medicine, New York City, New York

WILLIAM J. MILLIKAN, JR., M.D., F.A.C.S.
Professor of Surgery, Emory University School of Medicine, Atlanta, Georgia

ASHBY C. MONCURE, M.D., F.A.C.S.
Associate Clinical Professor of Surgery, Harvard Medical School; Visiting Surgeon, Massachusetts General Hospital, Boston, Massachusetts

DAVID L. NAHRWOLD, M.D., F.A.C.S.
Loyal and Edith Davis Professor and Chairman, Department of Surgery, Northwestern University Medical School, Chicago, Illinois

GEORGE L. NARDI, M.D., F.A.C.S.
Professor of Surgery, Harvard Medical School; Visiting Surgeon, Massachusetts General Hospital, Boston, Massachusetts

MICHAEL S. NUSSBAUM, M.D.
Assistant Professor of Surgery, University of Cincinnati College of Medicine; Attending Surgeon and Director of Surgical Education, The Jewish Hospital, Cincinnati, Ohio

LLOYD M. NYHUS, M.D., F.A.C.S., F.R.C.S.
Warren H. Cole Professor and Head, Department of Surgery, University of Illinois at Chicago, Chicago, Illinois

MARK B. ORRINGER, M.D., F.A.C.S.
Professor and Head, Section of Thoracic Surgery, University of Michigan, Ann Arbor, Michigan

W. SPENCER PAYNE, M.D., F.A.C.S.
James C. Masson Professor of Surgery, Mayo Clinic, Rochester, Minnesota

RAYMOND POLLAK, M.B., F.A.C.S., F.R.C.S.
Assistant Professor of Surgery, University of Illinois College of Medicine at Chicago, Chicago, Illinois

JOHN H. C. RANSON, M.D., F.A.C.S.
Professor of Surgery, New York University Medical Center, New York City, New York

WALLACE P. RITCHIE, JR., M.D., Ph.D., F.A.C.S.
Professor and Chairman, Department of Surgery, Temple University School of Medicine, Philadelphia, Pennsylvania

JACK A. ROTH, M.D., F.A.C.S.
Professor and Chairman, Department of Thoracic Surgery, University of Texas System Cancer Center, M. D. Anderson Hospital and Tumor Institute, Houston, Texas

ROBB H. RUTLEDGE, M.D., F.A.C.S.
Clinical Associate Professor of Surgery, University of Texas Health Science Center, Dallas, Texas

JOHN L. SAWYERS, M.D., F.A.C.S.
Professor and Chairman, Department of Surgery, Vanderbilt University, Nashville, Tennessee

GERALD W. SHAFTAN, M.D., F.A.C.S.
Director of Surgical Services, Bookdale Hospital Medical Center; Professor of Surgery, State University of New York, Health Science Center at Brooklyn, Brooklyn, New York

GEORGE F. SHELDON, M.D., F.A.C.S.
Zack D. Owens Professor and Chairman, Department of Surgery, University of North Carolina at Chapel Hill, Chapel Hill, North Carolina

WILLIAM SILEN, M.D., F.A.C.S.
Johnson and Johnson Professor of Surgery, Harvard Medical School; Surgeon-in-Chief, Beth Israel Hospital, Boston, Massachusetts

DAVID B. SKINNER, M.D., F.A.C.S.
President, The New York Hospital; Professor of Surgery, The New York Hospital-Cornell Medical Center, New York City, New York

DONNA L. STAHL, M.D., F.A.C.S.
Associate Clinical Professor of Surgery, University of Cincinnati College of Medicine, Cincinnati, Ohio

THOMAS E. STARZL, M.D., Ph.D., F.A.C.S.
Professor of Surgery, University of Pittsburgh Health Center, Veterans Administration Medical Center, Pittsburgh, Pennsylvania

DONALD D. TRUNKEY, M.D., F.A.C.S.
Professor and Chairman, Department of Surgery, Oregon Health Sciences University, Portland, Oregon

CHIU-AN WANG, M.D., F.A.C.S.
Clinical Professor of Surgery Emeritus, Harvard Medical School; Chief, Endocrine Surgery, Massachusetts General Hospital, Boston, Massachusetts

KENNETH W. WARREN, M.D., F.A.C.S.
Surgeon, New England Baptist Hospital; Former Chairman, Department of Surgery, Lahey Clinic; Former Surgeon-in-Chief, New England Baptist Hospital, Boston, Massachusetts

W. DEAN WARREN, M.D., F.A.C.S.
Chairman, Department of Surgery, Emory University School of Medicine, Emory University Hospital, Atlanta, Georgia

CLAUDE E. WELCH, M.D., F.A.C.S.
Senior Surgeon, Massachusetts General Hospital; Clinical Professor of Surgery Emeritus, Harvard Medical School, Boston, Massachusetts

JOHN P. WELCH, M.D., F.A.C.S.
Associate Surgeon, Hartford Hospital; Associate Professor of Surgery, University of Connecticut School of Medicine, Hartford, Connecticut

SAMUEL A. WELLS, JR., M.D., F.A.C.S.
Professor and Chairman, Department of Surgery, Washington University School of Medicine, St. Louis, Missouri

D. LAWRENCE WICKERHAM, M.D.
Assistant Professor of Surgery, University of Pittsburgh School of Medicine; Assistant Director, National Surgical Adjuvant Project for Breast and Bowel Cancers, Pittsburgh, Pennsylvania

CHARLES J. YEO, M.D.
Assistant Professor of Surgery, The Johns Hopkins University School of Medicine, Baltimore, Maryland

ROBERT M. ZOLLINGER, M.D., F.A.C.S.
Professor Emeritus of Surgery, Former Chairman, Department of Surgery, Ohio State University College of Medicine, Columbus, Ohio

SERIES INTRODUCTION

With the proliferation of medical and surgical monographs on every conceivable subject, it is difficult to embark on yet another publishing venture in the belief that such a contribution can be fresh and original. However, I believe this series, **COMMON PROBLEMS IN SURGERY,** achieves this unique goal. It departs from the traditional formula of assigning topics within a given area to recognized experts who then exhaustively review the medical literature and assemble a comprehensive, and, hopefully, definitive exposition of their subject. Rather, this series which is intended for busy, practicing surgeons and surgeons-in-training is designed to convey a maximum amount of *practical* information as succinctly as possible. The subject material of each volume is limited to those problems which are encountered in any active surgical practice and all discussions are built around illustrative clinical cases. More importantly, the management of each case is approached entirely from the perspective of each consultant's personal experience. Accordingly, emphasis is on the transmission of useful, clinical information and literature citations are kept to a minimum.

Gastrointestinal surgery continues to represent a major component of the practice of most general surgeons and appropriately deserves a separate volume in any series devoted to common problems in surgery. Dr. Fischer has assembled a "star studded" list of contributors who are internationally recognized experts in this field. He has also compiled a comprehensive list of challenging clinical presentations of gastrointestinal disease which run the gamut of problems likely to be encountered by most busy practicing surgeons. These are grouped under the broad categories of esophagus and thorax; gastric; liver, biliary and pancreas; endocrine; small and large intestine; and trauma. The discussion of each of these cases clearly reflects the author's extensive personal experience and offers numerous practical suggestions in the management of these challenging problems.

Clearly, this volume is an outstanding addition to the series and promises to be a valuable and frequently consulted addition to the library of most surgeons and trainees.

>RICHARD F. KEMPCZINSKI, M.D.
>Professor of Surgery
>University of Cincinnati
>Chief, Vascular Surgery
>University Hospital
>Cincinnati, OH

PREFACE

When most authors (myself included) finish a book, they experience a sense of relief as if the weight of the world is lifted from their shoulders. They usually share another sensation, and that is to swear that they will never do another book.

I must confess that my response on finishing the editing of this book is somewhat different. I rather enjoyed it, and more than that, I learned something. I am greatly indebted to Daniel J. Doody, Senior Vice President and General Manager of Year Book Medical Publishers, and Dr. Richard F. Kempczinski, the Series Editor who also serves as the Chief of Vascular Surgery and is an important person in the Department of Surgery at the University of Cincinnati, for coming up with this concept, namely a different type of book—a "How I Do It" book, with a description of how an expert deals with a given clinical problem. I feel very fortunate to have had the participation of the "Who's Who" of American surgery, who are the authors of this book.

The chapters are by and large authoritative, direct, and representative of the cumulative experience of some of the most experienced surgeons in the United States. Happily, this was all accomplished without a great deal of stress and strain, and with a magnificent contribution on their part. To them, I am indebted. I am also indebted to Steve Wiesner, our indefatigable manuscript typist and editorial assistant, to Jean Loos (graphics) and Roger West (photography), and to my office staff—Pat Walk, my administrative assistant; Judith Braun; and Mary Wiseman—for putting up with me during this period. Last, but not least, I am indebted to my wife, Karen, who has provided incredible support and an anchor to windward during what continues to be a full (to say the least) academic career. She and my children have put up with sharing me with the books, papers, and immense load of paperwork I usually take home. My career simply would not have been possible without them.

JOSEF E. FISCHER, M.D., F.A.C.S.

CONTENTS

Series Introduction xv

Preface xvii

PART I ESOPHAGUS AND THORAX 1

1 / ESOPHAGEAL STRICTURE
  Joel D. Cooper.. 2

2 / ESOPHAGEAL STRICTURE WITH PERFORATION FOLLOWING DILATATION
  Alex G. Little.. 10

3 / PHARYNGOESOPHAGEAL (ZENKER'S) DIVERTICULUM
  W. Spencer Payne.. 16

4 / DYSPLASIA IN A BARRETT'S ESOPHAGUS WITH REFLUX
  David B. Skinner.. 23

5 / HIATUS HERNIA WITH REFLUX ESOPHAGITIS
  Chris S. Ball and Tom R. DeMeester..................................... 29

6 / SYMPTOMATIC PARAESOPHAGEAL HERNIA
  Mark B. Orringer... 37

7 / MYASTHENIA GRAVIS
  Josef E. Fischer... 46

8 / SOLITARY PULMONARY NODULE
  Jack A. Roth... 53

9 / BREAST MASS
  D. Lawrence Wickerham and Bernard Fisher............................... 59

10 / BILATERAL CARCINOMAS IN SITU
  Donna L. Stahl... 67

PART II GASTRIC 77

11 / PERFORATED DUODENAL ULCER
  Paul H. Jordan, Jr... 78

XIX

12 / ADENOCARCINOMA OF THE STOMACH
Robb H. Rutledge 86

13 / BENIGN GASTRIC ULCER
Raymond Pollak and Lloyd M. Nyhus 93

14 / BLEEDING DUODENAL ULCER
Ashby C. Moncure 104

15 / MANAGEMENT OF OBSTRUCTING DUODENAL ULCER
William Silen 112

16 / PYLORIC CHANNEL ULCER
John L. Sawyers 117

17 / RECURRENT MARGINAL ULCER
David C. Carter 124

18 / GIANT DUODENAL ULCER
Michael S. Nussbaum 130

19 / ALKALINE REFLUX GASTRITIS
Wallace P. Ritchie, Jr. 136

PART III LIVER, BILIARY, PANCREAS 143

20 / SCLEROSING CHOLANGITIS
Kenneth W. Warren 145

21 / KLATSKIN TUMOR
Charles J. Yeo and John L. Cameron 159

22 / ASYMPTOMATIC GALLSTONES
Charles K. McSherry 167

23 / ACUTE CHOLECYSTITIS
Robert E. Hermann 171

24 / POSTCHOLECYSTECTOMY SYNDROME
George L. Nardi 179

25 / CANCER OF THE GALLBLADDER
James H. Foster 184

26 / ALCOHOLIC PANCREATITIS WITH A CHAIN OF LAKES
Charles F. Frey 189

27 / GALLSTONE PANCREATITIS
John P. Welch 200

28 / PSEUDOCYSTS
Edward L. Bradley, III 207

29 / ACUTE PANCREATITIS
John H. C. Ranson 217

30 / VARICEAL BLEEDING
W. Dean Warren and William J. Millikan, Jr. 226

31 / DIVIDED COMMON BILE DUCT
    Rayford Scott Jones 233
32 / HEPATIC TRANSPLANT
    Leonard Makowka and Thomas E. Starzl 239

PART IV ENDOCRINE 251

33 / MEDULLARY CARCINOMA OF THE THYROID
    Stanley W. Ashley and Samuel A. Wells, Jr. 253
34 / ASYMPTOMATIC HYPERPARATHYROIDISM
    Chiu-an Wang 261
35 / ZOLLINGER-ELLISON SYNDROME
    Robert M. Zollinger 265
36 / ADRENAL CORTICAL TUMOR
    Donald S. Gann 271

PART V SMALL AND LARGE INTESTINE 279

37 / ACUTE MESENTERIC ARTERY THROMBOSIS
    Richard F. Kempczinski 281
38 / ILEAL FISTULA
    Josef E. Fischer 289
39 / ACUTE ILEITIS
    Frank E. Gump 298
40 / CROHN'S DISEASE
    George E. Block 303
41 / CARCINOID
    Bernard M. Jaffe 311
42 / OBSTRUCTION OF SPLENIC FLEXURE
    Claude E. Welch 318
43 / EXTENSIVE VILLOUS ADENOMA OF THE RECTUM
    Warren E. Enker 328
44 / SIGMOID VESICAL FISTULA (DIVERTICULITIS)
    Richard M. Devine and Robert W. Beart, Jr. 336
45 / ULCERATIVE COLITIS
    Lester W. Martin 342
46 / FAMILIAL POLYPOSIS COLI
    Keith A. Kelly 346
47 / ACUTE DIVERTICULITIS WITH INTRAMESENTERIC (PERICOLIC) PERFORATION
    Robert J. Baker 353

48 / DIVERTICULAR BLEEDING
David L. Nahrwold 363

49 / RECTAL PROLAPSE
Ann Lowry and Stanley M. Goldberg 371

50 / HIGH FISTULA-IN-ANO
Philip H. Gordon 379

51 / ACUTE PERFORATED DIVERTICULITIS
Victor W. Fazio 386

52 / REGIONAL ENTERITIS WITH STRICTURE
John Alexander-Williams 394

53 / CHRONIC FISSURE-IN-ANO
Indru T. Khubchandani 400

54 / IDIOPATHIC THROMBOCYTOPENIC PURPURA
George F. Sheldon 407

PART VI TRAUMA AND INTENSIVE CARE UNIT 413

55 / DUODENAL LACERATION
Donald D. Trunkey 414

56 / INFERIOR VENA CAVAL LACERATION
Kenneth Davis, Jr. 421

57 / CENTRAL HEPATIC LACERATION
David V. Feliciano 427

58 / STAB WOUND
Gerald W. Shaftan 436

INDEX 441

PART I

Esophagus and Thorax

1

Esophageal Stricture

A 56-year-old man presents with dysphagia and a ten-year history of heartburn relieved by antacids. Over the past several years the heartburn has become more symptomatic and occasionally not relieved by antacids. No melena is reported. Approximately six months ago the heartburn disappeared, but within the past several months progressive dysphagia occurred. Upper GI series shows a smooth tapering stricture at approximately 39 cm, and biopsies reveal only acute inflammation and scar tissue. No malignancy is identified.

Consultant: Joel D. Cooper, M.D.

The case involves a 56-year-old man with a long history of reflux symptoms who presents with progressive dysphagia and radiologic documentation of a stricture in the distal esophagus. The history and radiologic findings appear quite consistent with the diagnosis of chronic gastroesophageal reflux with subsequent development of a peptic esophageal stricture. The disappearance of heartburn six months prior to presentation with dysphagia is not uncommon and suggests decreased reflux as the stricture becomes tighter. (*Editor's note:* Rather than a desired response to therapy, this change in symptoms may presage a difficult complication. Should a dramatic improvement in symptoms occur in a patient who is being followed up for reflux, it is probably worthwhile to repeat endoscopy and/or barium swallow.)

DIAGNOSIS

For purposes of discussion, the differential diagnosis can be limited to peptic esophageal stricture vs. carcinoma of the esophagus. Certainly the development of distal esophageal carcinoma following years of reflux symptoms is not rare, and it may represent malignant degeneration in a columnar-lined esophagus. Although the development of an adenocarcinoma in a columnar-lined esophagus is being increasingly recognized, the exact incidence of this condition remains a subject for controversy.

Dx: multiple biopsies
cytologic brushings

No mention of weight loss is given in the history. The degree of weight loss as well as the pattern of weight loss are both important. Progressive weight loss is more likely to be seen with carcinoma, whereas more gradual weight loss, often with stabilization at a lower level, is the more frequent pattern seen with benign peptic stricture.

Biopsies in this case revealed acute inflammation and scar tissue, with no evidence of malignancy. However, carcinoma in the distal esophagus can be notoriously difficult to diagnose, often because there is intramural extension without much mucosal involvement. Brushings for cytologic examination as well as biopsy should be obtained, since cytologic material may yield a diagnosis in the face of multiple negative biopsies. Biopsies should be obtained not only from the diseased segment, but also from the segment of esophagus immediately proximal and distal to the narrowing. The presence of a segment of columnar-lined esophagus above the strictured area should increase the suspicion of carcinoma, as peptic strictures invariably develop at the squamocolumnar junction. Similarly, the presence of squamous epithelium lining the esophagus distal to the narrowed segment strongly suggests the possibility that the stricture is a malignant one, since the presence of squamous epithelium distal to a peptic stricture would be a most unusual finding. (*Editor's note:* An excellent diagnostic point, not often mentioned.)

The essential diagnostic maneuvers in this case include a carefully obtained history, a barium swallow and upper gastrointestinal (GI) series, and careful endoscopy. Preliminary endoscopy may be carried out using the flexible endoscope with the patient under local anesthesia. However, if the radiologic picture suggests that the endoscope will not pass through the stricture, I prefer using a general anesthetic to facilitate employment of the various endoscopic maneuvers and dilation techniques that may be required to properly assess the lesion. If the endoscope can be passed through the lesion without dilatation, then dilatation is not mandatory except to improve symptoms temporarily. If the endoscope cannot be passed through the stricture and a diagnosis of carcinoma cannot be verified, then dilatation must be carried out to assess the rigidity and true length of the stricture and to permit appropriate biopsies and brushing of the lesion as well as of the esophagus distal to the lesion. Furthermore, in the case of peptic stricture, complete endoscopic examination of the esophagus, stomach, and duodenum is advisable to rule out other upper GI pathology that might be contributing to the development of gastroesophageal reflux, such as bile reflux, duodenal ulcer, etc.

I will assume, for the balance of this discussion, that the diagnosis in this case is peptic esophageal stricture on the basis of chronic gastroesophageal reflux, without additional upper GI pathology. If the radiologic appearance of the stricture is relatively short and not too tight, initial dilatation may be carried out indirectly using the tapered mercury-filled Maloney bougies. I prefer the technique of gradual dilatation, using successively larger sizes, rather than an initial attempt at using a large bougie. The goal would be to dilate the stricture to a 50 F size. Should this stricture be a tight one, endoscopy would be carried out using the rigid esophagoscope with the patient under general anesthesia. Through this, the gum-tipped bougies can be passed using successive sizes up to a 30 F. With these bougies passed through the rigid esophagoscope, it is easier to control the exact force being applied to the stricture. Once the stricture has been initially dilated with gum-tipped bougies, the rigid esophagoscope can be removed and indirect Maloney bougies can normally be passed. If not, one may choose to use a guidewire under fluoroscopic control, over which are passed the Savary tapered dilators. It is well to remember, however, that perforation of an esophageal stricture at the time of dilatation is generally not due to penetration of the wall by the tip of the bougie, but rather to splitting of the esophagus because of the lateral force of the bougie.

From a practical standpoint, the only additional diagnostic studies I would utilize in this case would be esophageal manometric studies and esophageal pH monitoring. The manometric studies are useful to rule out an unsuspected motor disorder, such as scleroderma, that predisposes to gastroesophageal reflux and the development of peptic stricture. Furthermore, the tone of the lower esophageal sphincter and the degree of motor disorder (poor peristalsis) in the body of the esophagus may influence both medical and surgical management. A very hypotensive sphincter (less than 10 mm Hg) suggests that conservative medical management is not likely to succeed. A high frequency of poorly propagated, low-amplitude motor waves in the body of the esophagus may influence the type of surgical procedure carried out if an antireflux procedure is to be performed; an overcompetent fundoplication may lead to postoperative dysphagia in the face of poor esophageal function. (*Editor's note:* This point is receiving increased emphasis. A substantial number of poor operative results can be ascribed to an overly aggressive 360-degree fundoplication in the face of poor esophageal motor function. Better results can usually be obtained with a 270-degree or 180-degree wrap.)

In this particular case, typical symptoms of gastroesophageal reflux have been present for many years; thus, objective evidence and quantitation of reflux is not necessary. In the absence of typical reflux symptoms, diagnosis and quantitation of reflux is best done with esophageal pH monitoring. We have found that outpatient, eight-hour pH monitoring serves as a useful tool, and we employ overnight 24-hour pH monitoring only in unusual circumstances, when symptoms are primarily nocturnal or when documentation of nocturnal reflux and related aspiration is required.

MEDICAL MANAGEMENT

If satisfactory dilatation can be performed without undue difficulty, initial management of the patient would be conservative. The patient would be told that most individuals with the same length of history and with the presence of a peptic stricture will require antireflux surgery ultimately, but a trial of carefully supervised medical management may be worthwhile. (*Editor's note:* If the patient has been under medical management or is not compliant, surgery should be advised early.) If there is extensive ulcerative esophagitis, if the stricture is rigid and difficult to dilate, or if the patient's symptoms are intolerable, then surgical management may be advised early on.

Contributory factors such as obesity, smoking, and alcoholic intake must be addressed. Medications such as aspirin or antiarthritic, anti-inflammatory drugs should be reduced or eliminated as much as possible. Elevation of the bed on 6-in. blocks is one of the most important therapeutic maneuvers, as nocturnal reflux usually is a major factor in the development of peptic esophageal stricture, even in the absence of nocturnal symptoms.

Gastric emptying will be promoted with the use of metaclopamide, 10 mg four times a day, prior to meals and at bedtime. Gastric acid secretion will be diminished with the use of ranitidine, 150 mg twice daily. Ideally, conservative management will be maintained for at least six months, unless the severity of reflux symptoms or the continuation or progression of dysphagia convinces both the patient and the physician that surgical intervention is appropriate. If the patient is obese, fails to lose weight, or fails to comply with the other aspects of the medical program, surgical intervention will not be entertained. Following initial dilatation, it is likely that the patient's reflux symptoms will return, since the barrier to esophageal reflux caused by the stricture has now been reduced. These reflux symptoms will hopefully be controlled by the therapeutic program outlined above.

In this particular case, it is quite likely that medical management will not sufficiently relieve symptoms or prevent the development of a recurrent stricture, and operative repair will be employed.

SURGICAL MANAGEMENT

A variety of surgical procedures are currently utilized to control reflux, but most have certain essential elements in common—adequate dilatation of the stricture, a fundoplication of stomach around the distal esophagus to restore competence, and restoration of an intra-abdominal segment of esophagus.

It was Allison who described the pathophysiology of reflux-induced peptic esophagitis and stricture and Hill who demonstrated that control of reflux could lead to reversal of a peptic esophageal stricture. Thus, while esophageal resection for stricture was not uncommon prior to 1960, such procedures are extremely rare today, and few strictures prove "irreversible" once adequate reflux control is established.

For our particular case involving long-standing reflux symptoms and the development of peptic stricture, I would utilize the transthoracic approach for an antireflux procedure. This allows maximum esophageal mobilization and permits a gastroplasty to be performed to give additional length (Figs 1–1 and 1–2). This procedure consists of creation of a tube out of the upper lesser curvature of the stomach, in continuity with the esophagus. This tube is of esophageal diameter and usually about 5 cm in length. During the subsequent fundoplication, this segment is treated as esophagus, thus effectively giving additional length to reduce tension on the repair and restore a segment of esophageal-like tube below the diaphragm. This Collis gastroplasty can be combined with either a complete (Nissen) fundoplication or a partial (Belsey) fundoplication.

In the presence of a peptic stricture, I would routinely utilize the Collis gastroplasty, since esophageal shortening is invariably present and previous experience at many centers suggests that successful operative control of reflux is more difficult to accomplish in this setting. I favor the Belsey partial fundoplication since it gives good reflux control when combined with the gastroplasty and is less likely to produce the overcompetence often associated with a Nissen fundoplication, which can result in dysphagia, gas bloat, and the inability to belch easily. With the combination of Collis gastroplasty and Belsey fundoplication, the chances of a good-to-excellent long-term result would be 85% to 90%.

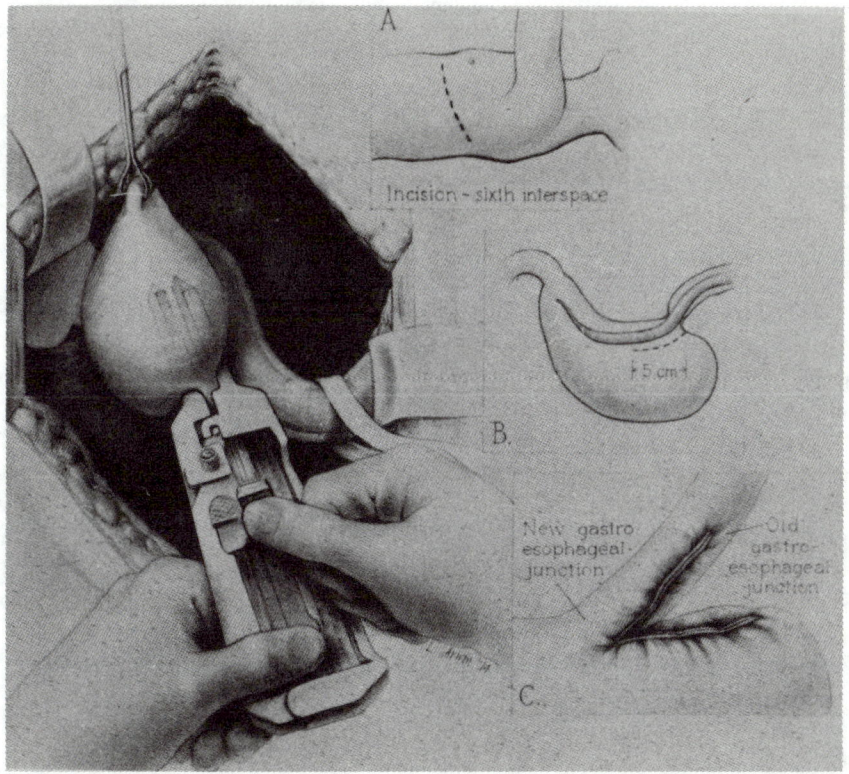

FIG 1–1.
Collis procedure using the GIA surgical stapler. *A*, mobilization of the esophagus and gastric fundus is performed through lateral thoracotomy in the sixth left intercostal space; *B*, a 60 F Hurst-Maloney dilator is passed through the esophagogastric junction and displaced against the lesser curvature of the stomach as the stapler is applied. The knife assembly is advanced (main illustration) and the stapler is removed; *C*, the result is a 5-cm long gastric tube extension of the esophagus. (From Orringer MB, Sloan H: *J Thorac Cardiovasc Surg* 1976; 71:295–303. Used by permission.)

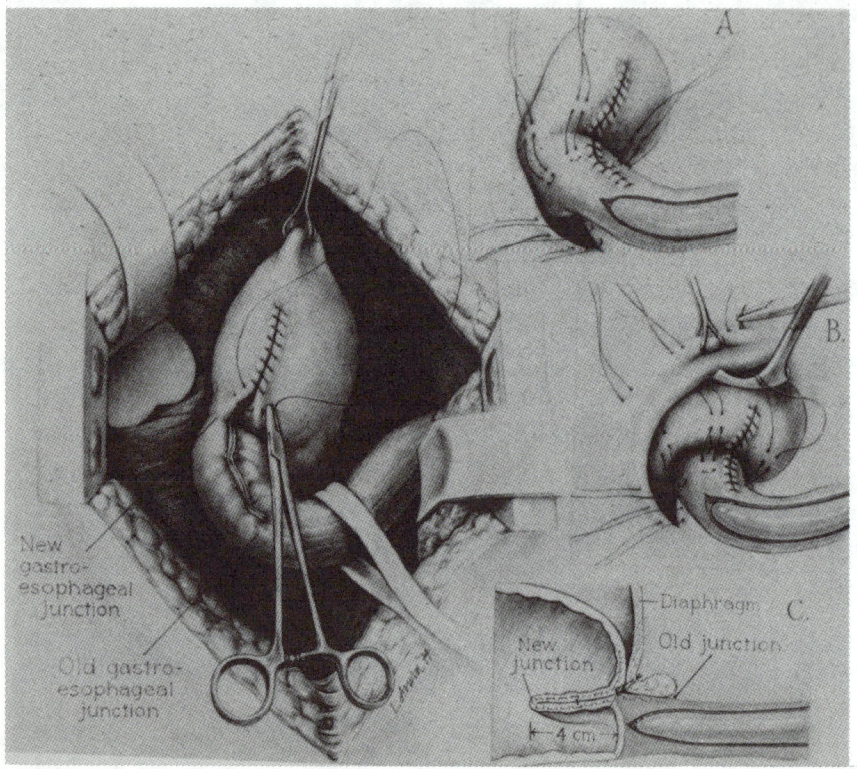

FIG 1-2.
Oversewing the staple suture line prior to performing esophagocardiomyotomy *(A)* that extends at least 1 cm beyond the esophagogastric junction onto stomach and is placed so as not to interfere with the suture line. The first *(A)* and the second *(B)* rows of sutures of the standard Belsey procedure are inserted. *(C)*, after reduction of the gastric fundus beneath diaphragm and tying of the posterior crural sutures, there are 4 cm of intra-abdominal distal "esophagus" beyond the end of the esophagocardiomyotomy. (From Orringer MB, Sloan H: *J Thorac Cardiovasc Surg* 1976; 71:295–303. Used by permission.)

BIBLIOGRAPHY

1. Allison PR: Reflux esophagitis, sliding hiatal hernia, and the anatomy of repair. *Surg Gynecol Obstet* 1951; 92:419–431.
2. Choiniere L, Miller L, Ilves R, et al: A simplified method of esophageal pH monitoring for assessment of gastroesophageal reflux. *Ann Thorac Surg* 1983; 36:596–603.
3. Cooper JD, Jeejeebhoy KN: Gastroesophageal reflux: Medical and surgical management. *Ann Thorac Surg* 1981; 31:577–593.
4. Hill LD, Gelfand M, Bauermeister D: Simplified management of reflux esophagitis with stricture. *Ann Surg* 1970; 172:638–651.
5. Orringer MB, Sloan H: Collis-Belsey reconstruction of the esophagogastric junction. *J Thorac Cardiovasc Surg* 1976; 71:295–303.
6. Pearson FG, Langer B, Henderson RD: Gastroplasty and Belsey hiatus hernia repair. *J Thorac Cardiovasc Surg* 1971; 61:50–63.

2

Esophageal Stricture With Perforation Following Dilatation

A 63-year-old male smoker with chronic reflux esophagitis and a stricture has been intermittently dilated over a period of three years by his gastroenterologist. Following the most recent dilation, the patient was well for approximately two hours when he experienced mild epigastric pain and developed a sinus tachycardia. Both physical examination and result of chest x-ray film were normal. However, a barium swallow revealed a perforation just above the area of stricture.

Consultant: Alex G. Little, M.D.

DIAGNOSTIC APPROACH

There are two aspects to the diagnosis of this patient. First, is this a benign or malignant stricture? Although we are told that this is a chronic problem, it is possible for cancer to develop in a chronically inflamed site. If a recent endoscopy with biopsy has been performed proving the continuing benignancy of this lesion, one can accept that diagnosis; if not, re-endoscopy in the operating room is important. If a malignant etiology can be proved, the appropriate therapy is immediate esophagectomy with primary reconstruction. However, the remainder of this discussion will assume that the stricture is known to be benign.

Accordingly, the second aspect of diagnosis is that of diagnosing the perforation itself. It should be emphasized that, as in this case, the clinical manifestations can be minimal and the presentation therefore subtle. The diagnosis is obvious in a more florid situation in which the patient experiences immediate postdilation symptoms, physical examination reveals a mediastinal crunch and/or subcutaneous emphysema, and the chest x-ray film shows an air fluid level in the chest. Frequently, however, the patient has some, but mild, chest or epigastric pain and tachycardia, but no abnormal physical findings and a normal chest x-ray film. Regardless, if there is any real suspicion of a perforation, a barium swallow is mandatory. This is an examination with no important morbidity, and it is obviously preferable to obtain a few unremarkable studies than to miss the opportunity for an expeditious diagnosis of a perforation. In fact, a barium swallow is required even if there is overwhelming clinical evidence of a perforation, as it is quite important to localize the site of the leak so that the appropriate thoracotomy can be made. Barium is the appropriate contrast material to use, as it provides the maximum radiologic detail and is only severely injurious when it is mixed with fecal material, e.g., when a barium enema is performed in a patient with a colonic perforation. (*Editor's note:* One should add that water-soluble dyes are very hyperosmolar and may contribute to the edema of the mediastinitis by their irritant effect.)

The importance of a prompt diagnosis of an esophageal perforation relates to its impact on prognosis. When the diagnosis is made and the operation performed within 24 hours, primary healing can be expected and the mortality is approximately 10%. Conversely, when diagnosis is delayed and the operation performed after a longer interval than 24 hours, the mortality increases substantially and the chances of primary healing are greatly decreased. This emphasizes the benefits of a prompt diagnosis and, therefore, the need for a low clinical threshold of suspicion.

SURGICAL APPROACH

In the case presented here, diagnosis has been prompt, and it is clearly going to be possible to have the patient in the operating room within eight hours of perforation. There are several surgical options for treatment of this patient. That should not be viewed as a state of confusion but should allow the surgeon to recognize that there are multiple options and that treatment should be individualized for the patient and the disease. All operations, however, should be preceded by intravenous fluid resuscitation as required and administration of parenteral antibiotics.

I believe the critical issue to be the dilatability of the esophageal stricture. When the esophagus can be readily dilated, curtailment of the reflux with a successful antireflux operation will produce a good result after resolution of the perforation. Unfortunately, it is frequently the case in patients perforated during dilation that the stricture has been allowed to become a chronic, thickly scarred, noncompliant, and nondilatable stricture. In this setting, it is very unlikely that the distal esophagus will ever again be functionally or anatomically useful to the patients, and efforts at salvaging it, even if the perforation can be healed, are unlikely to result in a usable swallowing tube.

When the stricture is easily dilatable, my approach is the following. I approach the perforation through a left thoracotomy using an eighth interspace incision for perforations below the aortic arch (Fig 2–1). This is the situation

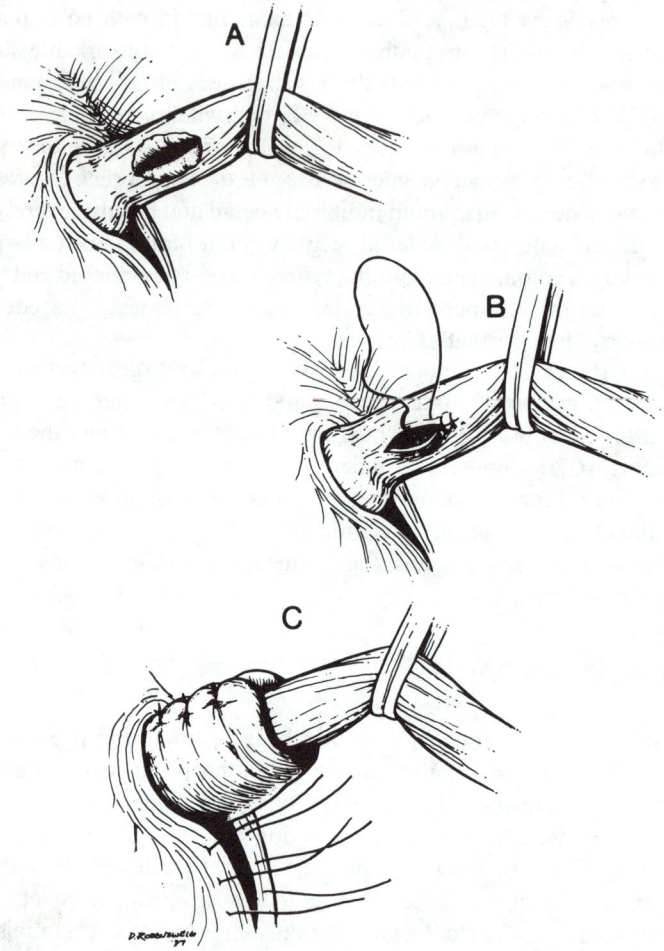

FIG 2–1.
A, the esophagus with a linear perforation near the gastroesophageal junction. The stomach has been mobilized; the hiatus dissected, and the esophagus mobilized up to the aortic arch. **B,** following debridement of the muscle, the mucosa has been closed with interrupted sutures, and the muscle is being closed in a separate layer over the mucosal suture line. **C,** Nissen fundoplication has been performed to treat the underlying problem of gastroesophageal reflux. The fundoplication also serves to bolster the suture line. The fundoplication suture line is actually along the right medial aspect of the esophagus that is temporarily turned to allow stitch placement.

for nearly all patients, as most strictures are in the distal esophagus. If the perforation is higher, a right thoracotomy or even neck approach is appropriate. Use of a double-lumen endotracheal tube allows the left lung to be collapsed, which gives ideal exposure and is well tolerated by most patients. The mediastinum is dissected and the esophagus mobilized from the aortic arch to the diaphragm. The area of perforation is then inspected. With early operation, local contamination is typically minimal. Following debridement of the edges of the perforation to healthy tissue, it is closed in two layers. It is crucial to close the entire mucosal defect, and the muscle layer should be opened sufficiently to guarantee this result. Following closure of the mucosa, the muscle is approximated separately to provide a two-layer closure. If the perforation is small, closure should be done transversely, but this is rarely the case. Choice of suture material is optional. I usually close the mucosa with either interrupted 4-0 Vicryl or Dexon or a running stitch of 4-0 Prolene. The muscle layer can be closed with any type of suture material; my preference is interrupted 4-0 Vicryl or Dexon sutures.

Once the perforation is closed, one must definitively address the underlying disorder. Otherwise either the perforation will releak in the face of a distal obstruction (i.e., the stricture) or the stricture problem will continue to be a long-term problem due to persistent reflux. Accordingly, if the patient's intraoperative condition remains satisfactory, an antireflux operation is performed. This requires opening the esophageal hiatus, but it should not result in peritoneal contamination as the perforation has been closed and the chest cleaned. The antireflux operation of choice depends upon the operating surgeon's experience and preference. A Nissen fundoplication serves to bolster the closed perforation partially or entirely, and therefore it has some additional appeal in addition to its antireflux properties. A flap of pleura can also be used to wrap and bolster the suture line, but the benefit of this maneuver is unproved. At the conclusion of the operation, I place a single but large (36-F) chest tube posterolaterally and remove it when the pleural fluid drainage has decreased below 200 cc/24 hours. The tube should not be placed near the suture line, as that encourages leakage. If the surgeon believes the suture line is unlikely to heal, primary closure is not the appropriate operation.

If it is not possible to carry out a standard antireflux surgery because the esophagus is shortened due to chronic esophagitis, a Collis gastroplasty with a Nissen wrap is a reasonable alternative. It is also legitimate to perform a Nissen fundoplication and leave the wrap in the chest. If this is elected, it is crucial that the esophageal hiatus be widely opened and sutured to the stomach. This avoids the risk of having a gastric pouch between a proximal obstruction, a competent Nissen, and a distal obstruction (the hiatus). When this caveat is adhered to, reflux is controlled and morbidity is not excessive.

When the stricture is not dilatable, the operation to be chosen is quite different. In this setting, I believe the diseased distal esophagus should be resected, reasoning that if the esophagus is not functional or anatomically useful to the patient, then a second operation will be required unless definitive surgery is carried out at this setting. Several options exist. The first option, performed through the left side of the chest, is to resect the distal esophagus and replace it by elevating the stomach into the chest. This option is not recommended because of the very high likelihood of iatrogenic reflux, even if attempts are made to create a competent esophagogastrostomy by adding a fundoplication. A second option is to replace the resected esophagus with a segment of colon, but this is not realistic, as without bowel preparation the risk of infection is too high. A third (and quite attractive) option, however, is replacement of the distal esophagus with a segment of jejunum. This functions very well and can be performed without preoperative bowel preparation. Through a left thoractomy through the eighth interspace, the esophagus is mobilized. The diaphragm is incised peripherally, near the chest wall, to gain exposure to the abdomen. A selected segment of jejunum is prepared by appropriate division of the vascular arcade, and the proximal end is advanced through the hiatus and sutured either end-to-end or side-to-end to the esophagus. The distal segment is anastomosed to the stomach. The jejunum works quite satisfactorily when used to replace the esophagus, and long-term results are good.

A fourth, and final, option is to perform a transhiatal resection of the entire thoracic esophagus and advance the stomach into the neck. This is a reasonable choice for certain patients, particularly those that are elderly, those whose physiologic status is not good, and those whose esophageal disease is so extensive that damaged esophagus would remain after a lesser resection. When the situation is appropriate, the operation is performed through a midline laparotomy, with the neck being opened through a cervical incision. The advantage to this approach is lower morbidity than for transthoracic operations. The stomach is advanced through the posterior mediastinum and into the neck for an end-to-side esophagogastrostomy. This is a well-tolerated operation and results are good, as the reflux problems are much less than when the esophagogastrostomy is in the chest.

In very carefully selected patients, nonoperative management is possible. The requirements are that the disruption be contained, i.e., not free into the pleural cavity; that the cavity be shown to drain back into the esophagus; that the patient have minimal symptoms; and that there be minimal evidence of sepsis. If all these criteria are met, the patient is then treated with parenteral nutrition and systemic antibiotics until healing occurs or one of the criteria can no longer be satisfied.

BIBLIOGRAPHY

1. Cameron JL, Kieffer RF, Hendrix TR, et al: Selective nonoperative management of contained intrathoracic esophageal disruptions. *Ann Thorac Surg* 1979; 27:404–408.

2. Little AG, Naunheim KS, Ferguson MK, et al: Surgical management of esophageal strictures. *Ann Thorac Surg* 1988; 45:144–147.
3. Maher JW, Hocking MP, Woodward ER: Supradiaphragmatic fundoplication: Long-term follow-up and analysis of complications. *Am J Surg* 1984; 147:181–186.
4. Nesbitt JC, Sawyers JL: Surgical management of esophageal perforation. *Am Surg* 1987; 53:183–191.
5. Polk HC: Jejunal interposition for reflux esophagitis in esophageal stricture unresponsive to valvuloplasty. *World J Surg* 1980; 4:731–736.
6. Skinner DB, Little AG, DeMeester TR: Management of esophageal perforation. *Am J Surg* 1980; 139:760–764.

Management:

1) Esoph. is dilatable.
   a) perforation closed in 2 layers (4-0 Vicryl).
   b) Antireflux op is performed — Nissen
   c) Drain c CT.

2) Stricture not dilatable
   Esophagectomy c jejunal interposition.

3

Pharyngoesophageal (Zenker's) Diverticulum

A 69-year-old woman in good general health presents with stable mild angina pectoris for which, after study, no coronary artery procedure is advised. In addition, she has noted daily cervical dysphagia and periodic episodes of oral regurgitation of fresh, bland, undigested food and saliva. On several occasions, she has awakened at night with paroxysms of coughing. During the past year, she has had two episodes of complete inability to swallow during meals, and on one of these occasions choking was so severe that the Heimlich maneuver was required to relieve her apparent airway obstruction. She has had one episode of pneumonia involving the superior segment of the right lower lobe of her lung, but this has cleared completely. On upper gastrointestinal (GI) series, she is found to have a 4-cm diverticulum, arising just cephalad to the indentation of the cricopharyngeus at C5 level. There is also a small sliding esophageal hiatal hernia. With further questioning, no heartburn or distal esophageal obstructive symptoms are uncovered.

Consultant: W. Spencer Payne, M.D.

MANAGEMENT

This patient is typical in age of most patients with Zenker's diverticulum. While both males and females appear to be equally affected, the incidence increases with age, reaching a peak in the eighth and ninth decades. Thus it is not unusual, as in this patient, to see concomitant but causally unrelated cardiovascular and other age-related conditions. It is generally held that Zenker's diverticulum develops as a consequence of cricopharyngeal dysfunction, which has been specifically defined as premature contraction of the upper esophageal sphincter. This appears to be entirely unrelated to any definable neurologic disease, and initiating factors remain unknown.

The chief indication for treatment is the presence of the diverticulum, irrespective of the severity of presenting symptoms or size. All such diverticula are associated with inevitable progression in size and severity of symptoms with time. We still see neglected diverticula of considerable size with advanced irreversible suppurative lung disease, with pulmonary insufficiency secondary to respiratory aspiration, and with severe nutritional failure. Less obvious but related problems include asthma, fever of presumed unknown origin, recurrent pneumonia, lung abscess, instrumental cervical esophageal perforation, and cancer arising in the diverticulum. One should keep in mind that medication by mouth in patients with Zenker's diverticulum may be greatly delayed in absorption or indeed may never pass beyond the cricopharyngeus, making medication blood levels difficult to maintain.

Of frequent concern are the patients with Zenker's diverticulum who are symptomatic of coronary artery disease. Such patients tolerate hypoxia related to hypopharyngeal food impaction or aspiration extremely poorly. However, they do tolerate surgical treatment of the Zenker's diverticulum well, with a mortality of 0.1%, identical to that of their disease-free cohorts. In some patients presenting with cardiovascular and respiratory distress, choking history is so severe that surgical treatment of the Zenker's diverticulum should be done at the time of coronary artery bypass to prevent postoperative hypoxic episodes.

It should be clear that Zenker's diverticulum is not a trivial condition, but with time can progress to significant disability, secondary disease, and death. It is important to deal with the condition in its trivial stage and not wait for serious complication before advising treatment. Thus, in the patient presented, the physician should urge prompt surgical intervention, especially since the patient has already demonstrated serious complication to her airway and lower respiratory tract.

A sliding esophageal hiatal hernia is nearly a universal finding in patients with Zenker's diverticulum. Its relationship causally is unclear. Its clinical importance is usually negligible, although on rare occasion gastroesophageal reflux symptoms and complications are dominant and require thorough assessment and treatment. One should not hesitate to perform antireflux surgery and Zenker's diverticula surgery with the patient under the same anesthesia, but the indication for such in our experience is extremely uncommon. Such combined surgery would not be indicated in the patient under discussion.

SURGICAL APPROACH

In the "usual" patient with Zenker's diverticulum and no other complications, a thorough history and an esophageal x-ray film demonstrating the diverticulum are all that are required preoperatively. Endoscopy is rarely indicated, and documentation of cricopharyngeal dysfunction by manometry adds little practical clinical information. Thus, in the patient under discussion, one should proceed with surgical treatment without further delay.

We generally provide a liquid diet the evening prior to operation and place the patient in a bed with the head elevated to minimize regurgitation.

The patient arrives in the operating room awake but premedicated parenterally. A rapid-induction–intubation anesthesia technique is employed, sealing the airway with a cuffed orotracheal tube to prevent intraoperative airway spillage.

After anesthesia is induced, the neck area is antiseptically prepared and draped. A primary oblique left cervical incision is made over the anterior length of the sternomastoid muscle, extending from the level of the hyoid bone to a point 3 to 4 cm above the left clavicle (Fig 3–1). This incision is carried deep through the skin, subcutaneous tissue, and platysma. The sternomastoid muscle is then gently retracted laterally, exposing the omohyoid as it crosses the anterior triangle of the neck. The omohyoid is an extremely important landmark, for the neck of the diverticulum and the cricopharyngeus lie just at the horizontal plane of the upper edges of this muscle. Thus, by blunt and sharp dissection just cephalad to the omohyoid, one can enter an avascular plane into the prevertebral, retropharyngeal space. Without dividing any muscles or vessels, but with gentle retraction of the larynx to the right and the carotid sheath to the left, the diverticulum can be seen and grasped with an Allis forceps and drawn cephalad into the incision. There are often rather flimsy fibrous connections between the anterior aspect of the sac and the posterior aspect of the upper esophagus that usually separate with traction on the fundus of the diverticulum.

When the entire sac is delivered into the wound, it is held at right angles to the long axis of the esophagus. At this point, the anesthesiologist can pass a 20- to 30 F catheter down the esophagus from the mouth without selectively intubating the diverticulum. This provides the surgeon a palpable endoesophageal landmark in the operative field. By sharp dissection, the connecting tissue around the neck of the Zenker's diverticulum is circumcised down to, but not through, the mucosa. This step brings into clear view the defect in the musculature of the posterior pharynx through which the mucosal sac protrudes. Immediately inferior to this round muscular defect lie the transverse fibers of the upper esophagus sphincter (cricopharyngeus muscle). Using a blunt-nose, right-angle forceps, a dissection plane is developed between the mucosa and muscularis immediately below the neck of the diverticulum. With muscle fibers in this area held on the stretch with the forceps and held away from the mucosa, a vertical extramucosal cricopharyngeal myotomy is performed for a distance of 3 cm inferiorly.

With the esophageal catheter still in a place, a TA* stapling device is applied across the neck of the previously dissected diverticulum. Depending on the actual size of the diverticular neck to be divided, we have employed TA-15 to TA-55, but most commonly the TA-30 is applicable. We believe it best to apply the clamp at right angles to the long axis of the esophagus, rather than parallel, and, of course, with the 20- to 30 F catheter in place as a mandril. These efforts are

---

*Auto suture Company, Division of United States Surgical Corp., Norwalk, Conn.

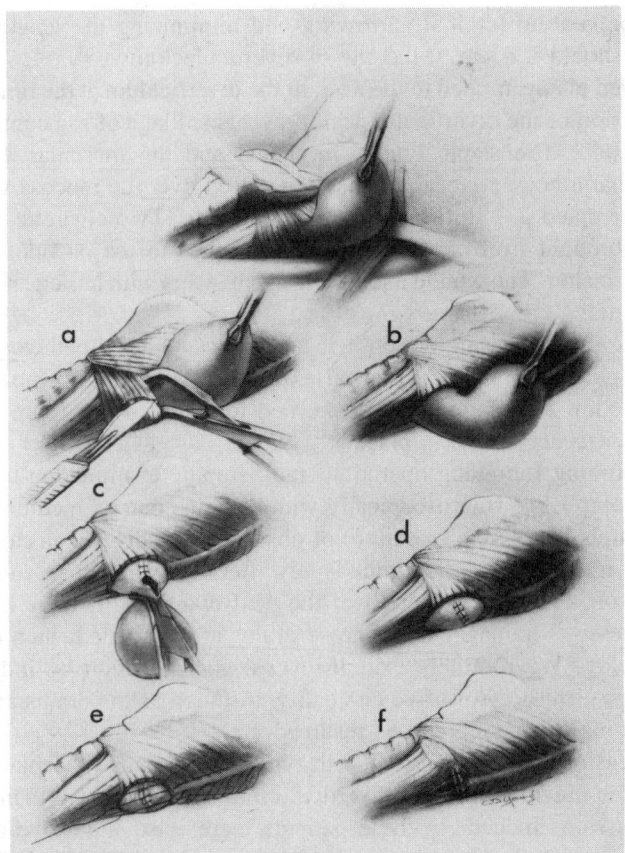

FIG 3–1.
One-stage pharyngoesophageal diverticulectomy with myotomy. This procedure is used to manage medium- and large-sized diverticula. *Top*, medium-sized diverticulum is exposed through left cervical incision. Note that omohyoid is retracted cephalad; diverticulum is dissected out to its neck, and apex of diverticulum is held cephalad. A right-angle forceps *(a)* is used to develop dissection plane between muscularis and mucosa just below neck of sac in preparation for extramucosal myotomy with scalpel. After 3-cm vertical myotomy is completed *(b)*, neck of mucosal sac appears to have widened. With 28 F catheter in esophagus *(c)*, curved clamp is placed across neck of diverticulum at right angle to long axis of esophagus at point of planned amputation. With cut-and-sew technique, sac is amputated stepwise and closed with fine vascular silk (5-0), placed so that tied knots are within esophageal lumen. Alternatively, a stapling device can be used. Diverticulectomy and closure are completed *(d)*. Vertical absorbable sutures are placed in edges of muscular defect after myotomy and diverticulectomy *(e)*. This completed transverse closure *(f)* provides muscular layer closure over mucosal suture line, which further minimizes leakage without restriction of cricopharyngeus. Drainage and closure are effected (see Fig 3–2). (From Payne WS: Esophageal diverticula, in Shields TW (ed): *Shield's General Thoracic Surgery*, ed 2. Philadelphia, Lea & Febiger, 1983, p 859. Used by permission.)

aimed at preventing luminal narrowing and minimizing the length of luminal narrowing should it occur at the site of diverticulectomy.

A curved clamp applied to the neck of the diverticulum at the time of stapling and transection of the diverticular neck prevents spillage of sac contents into the operative field. The staple line is inspected and the muscular defect in the posterior pharyngoesophageal area is then closed over the mucosa with a single row of interrupted 3-0 absorbable Lembert sutures. Two cigarette-size Penrose drains are brought from the retropharyngeal space to the outside at the lower end of the incision. The wound itself is closed in layers with buried and absorbable suture material.

An absorbent dressing is applied, and the esophageal catheter is removed before the patient awakens. Tracheal extubation is often accomplished in the operating room, and the patient is returned to the recovery room with only a peripheral intravenous line in place.

The morning following operation, radiographic examination of the esophagus is accomplished fluoroscopically with soluble contrast medium. If there is no demonstrable leak (extravasation) or obstruction at diverticulectomy site, the patient is permitted liquid diet immediately after the examination and progressed rapidly to soft and general diets over the next two days. If there is no clinical sign of excessive drainage, the Penrose drains are shortened, then removed by the fourth day. We routinely examine vocal cord function by indirect mirror laryngoscopy, irrespective of voice quality. As soon as the drains are removed, normal bathing or shaving can be resumed.

On occasion, patients present with typical symptoms of Zenker's diverticulum, but the magnitude of the diverticulum is less impressive than in the case under discussion. Indeed, in these patients there is so little diverticulum that only cricopharyngeal myotomy needs to be considered for relief of symptoms and the problem. Figure 3–2 outlines the technique we employ under these circumstances.

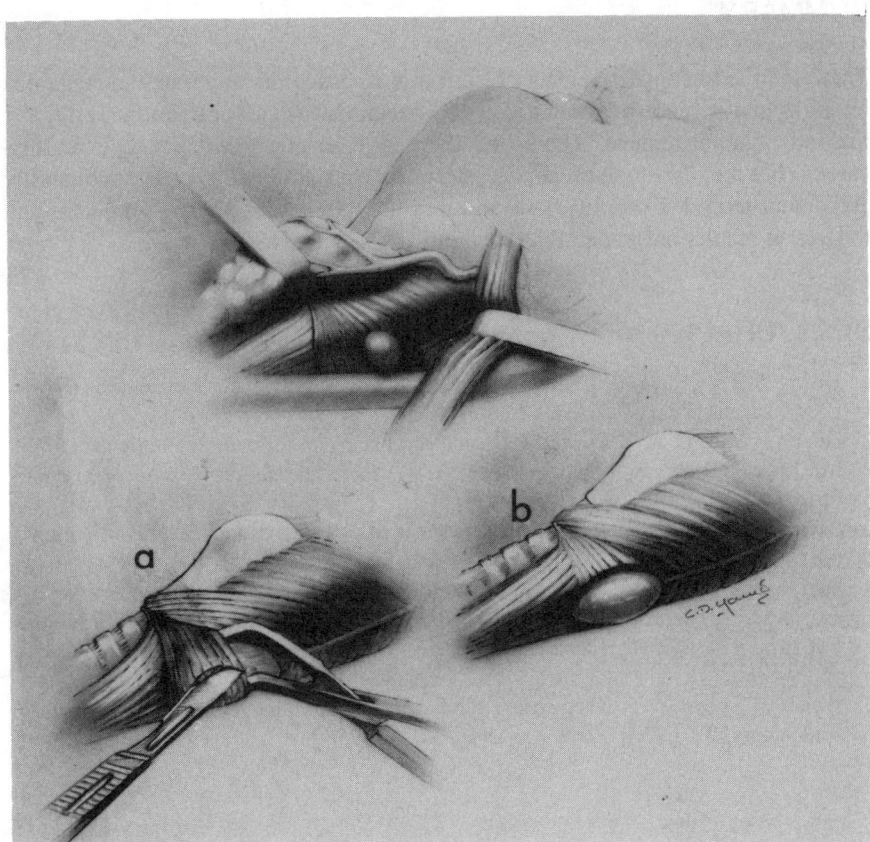

FIG 3-2.
Technique of cricopharyngeal myotomy. Myotomy alone is employed for treatment of small pharyngoesophageal diverticula. Surgical exposure of retropharyngeal space is gained through an oblique left cervical incision oriented along the anterior border of the sternomastoid muscle (not shown). Retraction of the sternomastoid and carotid sheath laterally and of thyroid, pharynx, and larynx medially provides necessary exposure of the diverticulum, which is located at a cervical level where the omohyoid crosses the surgical field. (Note that omohyoid in upper center of drawing has been retracted cephalad to show diverticulum.) After connective tissue is dissected from mucosal sac to identify defect in posterior pharyngeal wall *(a)*, a right-angle forceps is used to develop a dissection plane inferiorly between the muscularis and the mucosa. A posterior midline extramucosal myotomy is effected with a scalpel from the neck of the small sac and inferiorly for a distance of 3 cm. With retraction of the ends of the cut muscle *(b)*, an almond-shaped diffuse bulge of mucosa through the myotomy is seen. A small Penrose drain is brought from the region of the myotomy and retropharyngeal space through the lower end of the cervical wound to the outside, and platysma and skin are closed in layers around the drain. (From Payne WS: Esophageal diverticula, in Shields TW (ed): *Shield's General Thoracic Surgery*, ed 2. Philadelphia, Lea & Febiger, 1983, p 859. Used by permission.)

SUMMARY

There is little to support neglect of Zenker's diverticulum and much to be gained by early and prompt treatment. Surgical treatment is the only known effective method of management. There are alternative surgical methods to those discussed, but the one-stage procedures described have gained greatest applicability and safety record. Complications and mortality are exceedingly infrequent, and long-term results are generally excellent.

BIBLIOGRAPHY

1. Huang B-S, Payne WS, Cameron AJ: Surgical management for recurrent pharyngoesophageal (Zenker's) diverticulum. *Ann Thorac Surg* 1984; 37:189–191.
2. Huang B-S, Unni KK, Payne WS: Long-term survival following diverticulectomy for cancer in pharyngoesophageal (Zenker's) diverticulum. *Ann Thorac Surg* 1984; 38:207–210.
3. Payne WS, Reynolds RR: Surgical treatment of pharyngoesophageal diverticulum (Zenker's diverticulum). *Surg Rounds* 1982; 5:18–24.
4. Payne WS, Trastek VF: The role of stapling devices in the treatment of pharyngoesophageal (Zenker's) diverticulum, in Ravitch MM, Steichen FM (eds): *Principles and Practice of Surgical Stapling*. Chicago, Year Book Medical Publishers, 1987, pp 79–98.
5. Welsh GF, Payne WS: The present status of one-stage pharyngoesophageal diverticulectomy. *Surg Clin North Am* 1973; 53:953–958.

4

Dysplasia in a Barrett's Esophagus With Reflux

A 59-year-old man with long-standing heartburn previously relieved by antacids undergoes endoscopy. The esophagoscopic findings reveal columnar epithelium proved by biopsy at the level of 30 cm from the incisors. He begins to take histamine H_2-receptor blockers, metaclopamide, and antacids. Also elevation of the head of the bed and a weight reduction program are started. Six months later the endoscopy is repeated. Biopsies now show dysplasia in the columnar epithelium. Overnight esophageal pH monitoring documents free gastroesophageal reflux with decreased acid clearing and prolonged periods of low pH in the esophagus.

Consultant: David B. Skinner, M.D.

DISCUSSION

In 1950, Norman Barrett of London described the condition of a gastric type ulcer occurring in columnar epithelium lining the anatomical esophagus. The condition of the columnar-lined lower esophagus (CLLE) is now commonly referred to as Barrett's esophagus. However, at approximately the same time, Allison and Johnstone of Leeds, England, and Lortat-Jacob of Paris described similar findings. It is not clear which author should be credited with the first complete description of the condition as we know it today. From its earliest description as a clinical condition, Barrett's esophagus has been the subject of controversy.

As with most newly described conditions, this was initially thought to be rare, and sporadic cases of CLLE, some associated with adenocarcinoma of the esophagus, were reported during the 1950s and 1960s. By the 1970s, significant series of cases were being reported at both national and international meetings. By the 1980s, it was realized that the condition is not rare but is found in significant proportions of patients with abnormal gastroesophageal reflux or esophageal adenocarcinoma. A summary of my personal experience with the condition from 1974 to 1986 is presented in Table 4–1.

TABLE 4–1.
Barrett's Esophagus: The Chicago Experience

	1974–1982*	1983–July 1986	Total
Benign	23	46	69
Male	16	28	44 (63%)
White	21	45	66 (96%)
Malignant	20	15	35
Male	18	15	33 (94%)
White	20	15	35 (100%)
Total	**43**	**61**	**104**

*Adapted from Skinner DB, Walther BC, Riddell RH, et al: *Ann Surg* 1983; 198:554–565. Used by permission.

As more is known about Barrett's esophagus, the controversies about the condition intensify. There is no widely accepted definition. In the normal human esophagus, the most distal 1 to 2 cm of peristaltic tubular esophagus is normally lined with columnar (cardial-type) epithelium, so the mere presence of columnar epithelium in the lower esophagus is not abnormal. Arguments about the definition of Barrett's esophagus thus focus on how much esophagus must be lined with columnar epithelium or what cell type defines the abnormality. We have proposed that 3 cm or greater of the muscular tube of peristaltic esophagus lined with glandular epithelium is clearly abnormal and satisfies the definition for CLLE. However, there are patients in whom biopsy of the distal 3 cm of esophagus demonstrates intestinal metaplasia of the columnar lining, which is not a normal finding. Therefore, patients in whom the pathologist can identify the typical intestinal metaplasia cells associated with Barrett's esophagus may also be included within the definition of the abnormality. Disagreement about the precise definition leads to controversy about the incidence.

INCIDENCE

Since a CLLE can occasionally be identified in asymptomatic patients undergoing endoscopy for other conditions, the true incidence of Barrett's esophagus remains unknown. The symptoms that lead to endoscopic diagnosis are usually those of heartburn, regurgitation, or the dysphagia associated with esophageal malignancy. Not surprisingly, therefore, the proportion of patients with Barrett's esophagus having abnormal reflux or esophageal adenocarcinoma is high. In our practice, and that reported by others, approximately 10% to 15% of patients undergoing esophagoscopy for evaluation of reflux and its complications are found to have a Barrett's esophagus. In several series, the prevalence of Barrett's esophagus in patients treated for reflux-induced strictures is 50% or greater. In our series and in other series in which adenocarcinomas arising within the anatomical esophagus are classified as esophageal carcinoma, Barrett's esophagus is identified in the resected specimen in about 20% of patients undergoing surgery for esophageal carcinoma. It has only been in recent years that this condition has correctly been identified as among the common problems in digestive tract surgery.

ETIOLOGY

Controversy persists concerning the cause of Barrett's esophagus. Barrett initially classified the condition as congenital. Allison and Johnstone, noting the strong association with abnormal reflux, proposed that the condition was acquired in patients with long-standing reflux. Support for the congenital theory is derived from the embryological development of the esophagus, the finding of persistent islands of columnar epithelium in the cervical as well as distal esophagus, the identification of the condition in children, and the presence of the condition in asymptomatic patients and in patients in whom there is a well-healed, sharp line of demarcation between columnar and squamous epithelium in the mid-esophagus.

The acquired theory is supported by the high incidence (at least 90%) of documented abnormal gastroesophageal reflux in Barrett's esophagus patients undergoing pH studies, the repeated observations of proximal migration of the squamocolumnar junction over time, and experimental and clinical observations concerning the healing process in which columnar epithelium by proximal migration or by extension by submucosal glands is found to line the ulcerated esophageal mucosa in severe reflux esophagitis. However, the severity and high incidence of reflux in Barrett's patients may conceivably be part of a congenital syndrome rather than an acquired condition causing the columnar-lined esophagus. At present, there is no clear resolution to this controversy.

COMPLICATIONS

Since symptomatic acid peptic disorders are the most common reason for esophagoscopy, and Barrett's esophagus is an endoscopic diagnosis, it is not surprising that the incidence of severe esophagitis is high in the CLLE. In our series and that of others, acid peptic stenosis or stricture of the esophagus is present at the squamocolumnar junction in about one half of the patients with Barrett's esophagus. A penetrating ulcer in the columnar epithelium, as initially described by Barrett, is found in approximately 15% of our cases. Significant bleeding from the ulcer or esophagitis is found in approximately 10% of patients. At the time of presentation to our esophageal surgery clinic, approximately one third of the patients found to have Barrett's esophagus have an associated adenocarcinoma.

DIAGNOSIS

There are no typical symptoms that differentiate patients with Barrett's esophagus from those with uncomplicated gastroesophageal reflux or ulcerative esophagitis. The diagnosis of columnar-lined epithelium must be made by biopsy, and the site of the biopsy must be clearly identified relative to the upper and lower limits of the anatomical and peristaltic esophagus. Because the cell types in the columnar-lined esophagus are variable and include several distinct patterns, multiple biopsies should be taken.

Endoscopically, biopsies clearly taken from the mid-esophagus in patients with Barrett's epithelium may show typical cardial-type columnar cells, typical gastric fundic-type epithelium including parietal and chief cells, or an atypical metaplastic type of epithelium characterized by goblet cells. Other variations and combinations are seen and described. At endoscopy, the junction of the columnar epithelium with the squamous epithelium may be a sharp border without inflammation, proposed by some as evidence for a congenital origin, or the junction may show active ulcerative esophagitis, be highly irregular, and have typical flame-shaped projections upward into regions of squamous epithelium. The latter is proposed by some as evidence for the acquired variety of Barrett's esophagus.

MALIGNANCY

Of major concern today is the risk of malignancy arising in a Barrett's esophagus. From prospective follow-up studies of patients with initially benign Barrett's esophagus, the incidence of carcinoma developing is described between 1 in 72 to 1 in 400 patient years of follow-up. This makes the Barrett's esophagus condition the highest risk for carcinoma of any benign digestive tract abnormality. The condition occurs particularly in white male patients, in contrast with the demographics of squamous cell carcinoma. The carcinomata are always adenocarcinoma, classified as arising in Barrett's epithelium when regions of nonmalignant Barrett's esophagus are found adjacent to the tumor.

The most serious and significant harbinger of carcinoma is the presence of dysplasia, as reported in this patient. The pathologist's classification for dysplasia is still imprecise, but it attempts to distinguish among suspicious or indefinite for dysplasia, low-grade dysplasia, and high-grade dysplasia. In our experience, when high-grade dysplasia is found on a biopsy, there is a strong probability that carcinoma in situ, microinvasive carcinoma, or frank invasive carcinoma will be found within the Barrett's esophagus. High-grade dysplasia is regarded by us and others as an indication for esophagectomy of the type required for the treatment of esophageal carcinoma. In our practice, this is an attempted curative en bloc esophagectomy.

Management of low-grade dysplasia is more controversial. Two of our patients with low-grade dysplasia treated by fundoplication subsequently progressed to adenocarcinoma; they were fortunately diagnosed early by follow-up cytology studies, underwent a curative en bloc esophagectomy, and remain alive and well several years later. On the other hand, at least one of our patients with low-grade dysplasia treated by an antireflux repair did not demonstrate subsequent dysplasia on multiple repeat biopsies. Accordingly, it is not certain whether low-grade dysplasia inevitably progresses to carcinoma or whether it may be reversible. For this reason, we do not advocate resection for low-grade dysplasia, but close follow-up by repeated endoscopies or semiannual cytology studies is mandatory. When adenocarcinoma arising in Barrett's epithelium presents as a cause of dysphagia, the condition is often advanced and the prognosis is no better than that for patients with squamous cell carcinoma.

TREATMENT

Antireflux repair has proved to be as effective in patients with Barrett's esophagus as it is for patients with abnormal reflux or ulcerative esophagitis without the complication of CLLE. Initially, this was controversial because the Barrett's esophagus patients had more severe reflux and a lower-amplitude distal esophageal sphincter mechanism than did patients with other forms of reflux. However, long-term objective follow-up studies reported by us and others clearly documented the success of antireflux surgery in approximately 90% of patients with Barrett's esophagus.

What remains uncertain is whether the condition can be reversible and whether the potential progression to malignancy can be interrupted by a successful antireflux repair. Certainly, reversal back to a normal squamous epithelium is not common following successful antireflux surgery, and it is even doubtful whether true reversal occurs at all. Progression to adenocarcinoma in patients treated by successful antireflux surgery has been reported by several observers, but the success of the antireflux surgery has not always been demonstrated objectively, nor was it certain that such patients did not have low-grade or high-grade dysplasia prior to the antireflux repair. Other carefully controlled follow-up studies in patients with multiple biopsies of their Barrett's epithelium before and after antireflux surgery are necessary to resolve this controversy.

Resection for Barrett's esophagus today is indicated in those patients with a deep ulcer that penetrates outside the wall of the esophagus, patients with recurrence of esophageal stricture after an antireflux repair, and patients with recurrent esophagitis who are found to have an acid-secreting esophageal mucosa above the antireflux repair. The latter group prove resistant to medical and surgical treatment. Those patients demonstrated to have high-grade dysplasia should undergo resection as if they had carcinoma. Otherwise, an antireflux repair is recommended for all other patients with Barrett's esophagus who are symptomatic and have persistent esophagitis despite medical therapy.

In this case, management is dictated by the severity of dysplasia. A repeat endoscopy with more biopsies would be recommended. Since the diagnosis may differ among pathologists, we routinely have the slides reviewed by two or more pathologists regarded as experts in the classification of Barrett's esophagus. If the biopsies are seen to demonstrate high-grade dysplasia, a resection similar to that for esophageal carcinoma would be recommended. If low-grade dysplasia or indefinite findings for dysplasia are diagnosed, an antireflux repair would be carried out. If esophageal peristalsis is weak or ineffectual, as it often is in Barrett's esophagus, a partial fundoplication of the Belsey Mark IV or Hill type would be preferred to the total fundoplication of the Nissen type to avoid an incidence of postoperative dysphagia. In patients with Barrett's esophagus, a thoracotomy is generally preferred to increase mobilization of the esophagus and allow direct inspection of the region for signs of occult malignancy. If an antireflux repair is selected, careful follow-up with brush cytology examination at six-month intervals must be accomplished, as in this patient, in patients in whom dysplasia is suggested on the initial diagnosis.

BIBLIOGRAPHY

1. Iascone C, DeMeester TR, Little AG, et al: Barrett's esophagus. *Arch Surg* 1983; 118:543–549.
2. Skinner DB, Walther BC, Riddell RH, et al: Barrett's esophagus: Comparison of benign and malignant cases. *Ann Surg* 1983; 198:554–565.
3. Skinner DB, Little AG, Ferguson MK, et al: Selection of operation for esophageal cancer based on staging. *Ann Surg* 1986; 204:301–341.
4. Skinner DB, Belsey RHR: Barrett's esophagus, in *Management of Esophageal Diseases*. Philadelphia, WB Saunders, 1988.

[Handwritten notes:]

Indications of operation in pts c̄ Barretts

1) High grade dysplasia
2) Deep penetrating ulcers
3) Recurrent esoph stricture after antireflux op
4) Pts c̄ acid secreting mucosa above repair

5

Hiatus Hernia With Reflux Esophagitis

A 35-year-old, moderately obese woman is referred with a history of approximately three years of eructation and mild heartburn relieved by antacids. Endoscopy reveals grade 0 to 1 esophagitis, free reflux, and a small hiatus hernia. No evidence of stricture or ulceration is seen. On interviewing the patient, she admits to swallowing a great deal of gas when drinking liquid and significant eructation.

Consultants: Chris S. Ball, M.D.
Tom R. DeMeester, M.D.

In the management of this case, the following questions need to be answered:

1. Is this indeed gastroesophageal reflux disease?
2. What is its mechanism?
3. What complications have occurred?
4. How may the disease and its effects be corrected?

DIAGNOSIS OF GASTROESOPHAGEAL REFLUX

Symptoms of foregut disease are common in clinical practice and considerable overlap exists between symptom complexes arising from esophageal, gastric, duodenal, biliary tract, and lower intestinal disease. A careful, detailed inquiry about the symptoms, however, helps the clinician localize the problem and select the most appropriate line of investigation. Retrosternal heartburn and regurgitation of bitter-tasting fluid are the most common complaints in gastroesophageal reflux (GER). In the mild disease these symptoms may occur only postprandially or with strenuous exertion and postural changes, but symptoms occurring apart from such activities indicate more severe disease. Regurgitation of gastric fluid may cause a reflex-induced airway spasm with wheezing not unlike extrinsic asthma, while aspiration of the refluxate leads to choking and cough, often worse at night, and a tendency to recurrent chest infection. Other esophageal symptoms, dysphagia, odynophagia, and chest pain are indicative of motility disturbances in the absence of stricture or impaired hiatal flow. Epigastric burning, nausea, vomiting, and flatulence are less commonly found in simple GER and are more suggestive of other gastrointestinal disease.

The patient's complaints of heartburn would tend to focus our attention on esophageal investigation. Eructation of gas is more specifically a gastric or biliary symptom, but in this case the patient's eating habits and aerophagia may well be responsible. We are given the endoscopic finding of grade 0 to 1 esophagitis, which appears as mild erythema. This observation does not necessarily imply reflux disease. Drugs, infections (particularly *Monilia*), and trauma from repetitive vomiting can produce esophagitis in the absence of reflux disease. Conversely, acid reflux above the normal range will not always overcome mucosal resistance and produce inflammation. The basic pathophysiology of GER is abnormal esophageal exposure to gastric juice. Since both symptomatology and endoscopic findings fail to correlate with the abnormality, it is necessary to actually measure the exposure. The best way to accomplish this is prolonged pH monitoring of the distal esophagus.

Since its conception and development, ambulatory 24-hr pH monitoring has become the most widely accepted means of documenting acid GER. To do the test, we initially perform manometry using a five-channel water-perfused catheter passed transnasally and linked by transducers to a chest recorder. The lower esophageal sphincter is localized by the station pull-through technique; its pressure, overall length, abdominal length, and degree of relaxation with swallowing are measured. The esophageal body is assessed during a succession of wet and dry swallows. Finally, the upper sphincter pressure, length, and coordination with the pharyngeal contraction are measured. Digital recording of the data permits subsequent computer-assisted analysis of sphincter characteristics, wave form, and wave progression.

In performing pH monitoring, our preference is to use a glass pH probe with a combined reference electrode. This is positioned to lie 5 cm above the lower esophageal sphincter defined by manometry. The patient is instructed to remain ambulatory when upright and to follow dietary guidelines by consuming three meals at a pH between 5 and 7. Water only is permitted between meals. The pH is sampled every 4 to 6 seconds and values are stored digitally by a portable recording unit. The patient is encouraged to press an event button to indicate the timing of episodes of heartburn, belching, coughing, etc., and to keep a diary of events including the timing of meals and the time spent in the upright and supine positions. After 24 hours the probe is removed and the digital data transferred to a computer for analysis and display (Fig 5–1, A and B). Acid reflux is defined as a drop in esophageal pH to below 4, and values for percentage of total time, upright time, supine time, number of episodes, longest episode, and number of episodes lasting longer than five minutes are obtained. These six

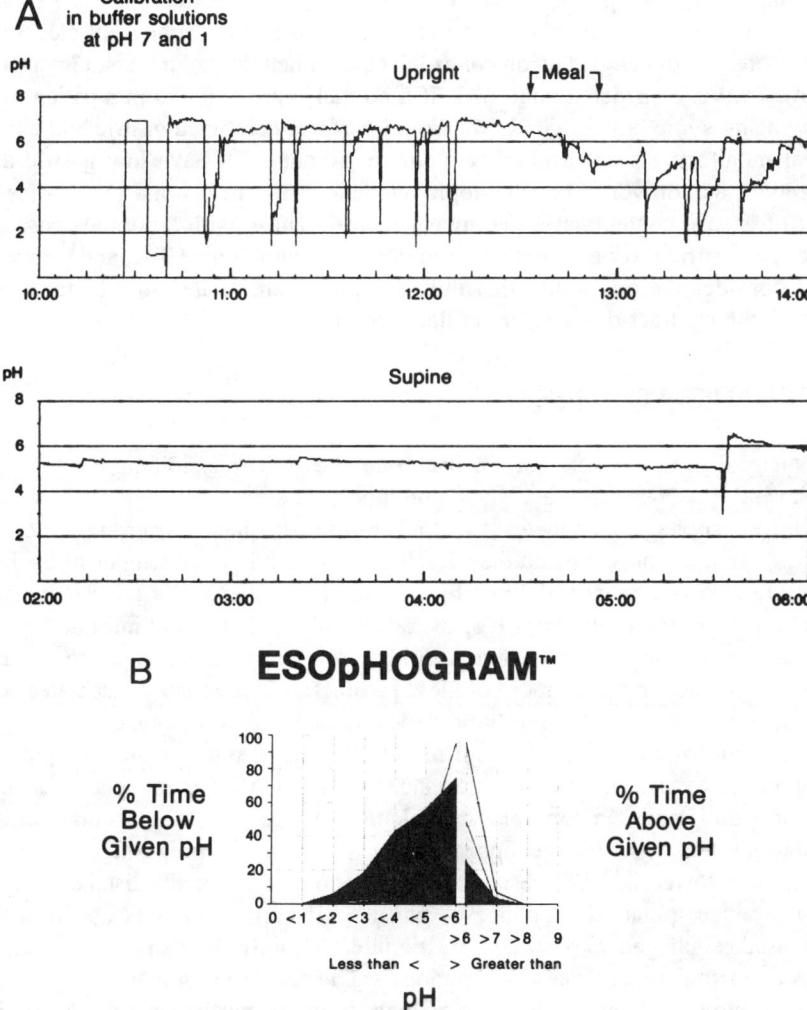

FIG 5–1.
A, graphic printout of a four-hour upright and supine segment of a 24-hour pH record. Multiple reflux episodes, signified by a drop in pH to below 4, are seen during the upright period, but rarely during the supine period. To determine if there is increased esophageal acid exposure requires computer analysis of the data base on the integration of six measurements, one of which is shown in Figure 5–1B. **B,** graphic display of ESOpHOGRAM showing the median and 90th percentile levels of the percent time of acid exposure in 50 normal individuals, using whole pH values above and below 6 as thresholds. The *black area* represents measurements made in a patient with acid reflux; it shows increased exposure over that seen in normal subjects below pH of 5, 4, 3, and 2.

parameters are incorporated into a composite score that reflects severity of acid reflux in terms of frequency, mucosal contact time, and esophageal clearance. The score was developed using control data from healthy volunteers, and a value above 14.0 is considered abnormal. If a normal score is found in a patient with convincing symptoms of GER, we would perform combined gastric and esophageal monitoring since a number of these patients will have low gastric acid secretion, achlorhydria, or pathologic duodenogastric reflux and may suffer reflux of gastric contents at a pH greater than 4. Those with a normal score and a normal gastric profile do not by definition have pathologic GER, and we would next consider the possibility that their symptoms are related to a hiatal hernia per se, biliary tract disease, or cardiac disease.

MECHANISM OF GER

Esophageal acid exposure may be increased above the physiologic level for any of several reasons. First, and most commonly, the high pressure zone we call the lower esophageal sphincter (LES) forms an inadequate barrier to reflux. The resting sphincter pressure and the overall and intra-abdominal lengths of the high pressure zone are readily defined by a manometric study. We have found that a sphincter pressure of 6 mm Hg, overall length of 2 cm, and intra-abdominal length of 1 cm are the minimum requirements for sphincter competence, and that a deficiency in one or more of these parameters is invariably associated with pathologic GER. The cause of these deficiencies are abnormalities in the length-tension ratio of esophageal smooth muscle. The LES pressure may be reduced temporarily by the ingestion of substances such as caffeine, chocolate, alcohol, nicotine, and drugs, in particular the calcium-channel–blocking agents, nitrites, and atropinic drugs. Endogenous substances, particularly progestogens in pregnancy, also lower the LES pressure. Second, poor motility in the distal esophagus may produce impaired clearance of physiologic reflux episodes and result in increased esophageal exposure to gastric juice. Usually, low-amplitude contractions and simultaneous mass contractions are detected during manometry, while a small number of reflux episodes of long duration, particularly during supine monitoring, produces the abnormal pH score. Third, gastric hypersecretion of acid is not uncommon in GER. Some studies have shown up to a 60% incidence, and it is our practice to carry out a gastric secretion analysis on all patients with positive pH scores. Physiologic reflux of intragastric fluid at a low pH may be responsible for the abnormal scores seen in individuals with normal motility and a competent cardia.

Fourth, a high intragastric fluid volume from delayed gastric emptying due to inflammation or ulceration of the pylorus and duodenum or a functional disorder of gastric, pyloric, and duodenal motility can augment physiologic reflux through a normal cardia. Some authors have found a significant incidence of

In symptomatic pts c̄ nl pH analysis a gastric analysis should be done.

unexplained delayed gastric emptying associated with GER. However, in our experience, such an association occurs also in symptomatic patients who do not reflux and, therefore, it appears to be independent of GER. Fifth, elevated intragastric pressure in excess of intra-abdominal pressure may overcome the LES pressure barrier to reflux. One cause of this is outlet obstruction of the stomach. Normally, this occurs during the physiologic act of vomiting, when the outlet of the stomach is obstructed by a strong antral contraction. Another cause is a previous vagotomy that interrupts the normal receptive relaxation of the stomach.

Finally, excessive gastric dilatation can shorten the normal overall length of the sphincter, resulting in incompetency and reflux of gastric contents into the esophagus. Excessive gastric dilatation can occur from aerophagia in patients who reflux and habitually swallow to clear the esophagus. Each pharyngeal swallow results in the propulsion of approximately 1 to 2 ml of air into the stomach. When the amount of air entering the stomach exceeds the capacity to evacuate it, gastric dilatation occurs, causing shortening of the sphincter and belching with further reflux. Gastric dilatation can also occur from a loss of secondary peristalsis, usually as a result of a collagen vascular disease or diabetes. In these patients, distention of the esophagus does not initiate a secondary peristalsis, and repetitive pharyngeal swallows are needed in order to propel food into the stomach. This again leads to aerophagia. Simple gluttony is another mechanism of gastric dilatation that results in shortening of the sphincter and significant postprandial reflux.

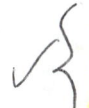
Any one of several of these factors might pertain to the case presented. Investigation with manometry, pH monitoring, gastric secretion analysis, and gastric emptying, together with a detailed history of drug therapy, dietary habits, and physical activity, will disclose which factors predominate in this patient.

COMPLICATIONS OF GER

In the case under discussion, endoscopic esophagitis in the absence of drug ingestion or infection must be considered a complication of the disease. It is a reversible condition, but, if left unchecked, chronic reflux can lead to ulceration, stricture formation, and columnarization of the distal esophagus. The importance of endoscopy in GER is not only to assess the extent and severity of complications, but also to facilitate the collection of histologic and cytologic specimens, particularly when the presence of Barrett's epithelium is suspected and dysplasia or frank malignancy must be excluded. Aspiration of refluxate causing vocal cord lesions, cough, and recurrent chest infections is another important complication of GER, especially when a coexisting motility disorder is present and can be suspected by visualizing erythema of the vocal cords during the endoscopic examination. Gamma camera imaging of the lung fields after oral ingestion of technetium isotope can confirm the event in suspected cases.

TREATMENT

In addressing the question of treatment, let us consider four possible results to the esophageal investigations outlined above.

1. Mild reflux only in the upright position on 24-hour pH monitoring and a mechanically normal cardia on manometry.—In these circumstances, initial management would involve an explanation to the patient of the possible mechanisms of reflux so that aggravating factors could be avoided. Dietary advice, particularly in regard to aerophagia, should be given. Those who are obese or smoke should be encouraged to lose weight or stop smoking. Antacids, alginates, and H_2-antagonists, particularly in the presence of confirmed gastric hypersecretion, would be used. Considerable improvement would be anticipated with this treatment, and surgical therapy should be resisted due to the inability to improve an already normal cardia. In some patients with this problem, biofeedback therapy has been effective.

2. Combined upright and supine reflux on 24-hour pH monitoring and a mechanically defective cardia on manometry.—These findings represent a more severe disease less likely to respond to conservative measures. In addition to the previous advice, the patient should be told to elevate the head of the bed, use extra pillows, and avoid food and drink later in the evening to minimize supine reflux. Treatment with combinations of alginates and H_2-antagonists would be given. If no improvement occurred in symptoms and/or endoscopic findings after eight weeks, an adequate response to further medical therapy would not be expected and the patient would be advised to have surgery. Our preference is for a transabdominal Nissen fundoplication. After mobilization, the right and left crura are approximated to narrow the hiatal opening, and a fundoplication performed over a 60-F bougie in the esophagus. A single "U"-stitch of polypropylene, with Teflon pledgets for support, maintains a wrap of 360 degrees over a length of 1 cm. By careful patient selection and consistent technique, pathologic GER is corrected in 93% of patients followed up over a ten-year period. Persistent dysphagia and gas bloat are rarely encountered.

Patients who respond to eight weeks of medical treatment and remain asymptomatic after cessation of the therapy are followed up. Those whose symptoms or esophagitis recur within one month are given maintenance therapy. Since they are likely to be drug dependent, surgical therapy should be discussed as an alternative.

3. **Esophageal acid exposure within the normal range on 24-hour pH monitoring and a mechanically defective cardia on manometry.**—This finding indicates the necessity to perform combined esophageal and gastric pH monitoring since a small percentage of refluxers have a relatively alkaline gastric environment due to hyposecretion, duodenogastric reflux, or previous surgery and hence alkaline gastroesophageal reflux. Failure of the symptoms or the esophagitis to respond to alginates or sucralfate would encourage us to recommend an antireflux operation. Those believed to have duodenogastric reflux and alkaline gastroesophageal reflux would undergo TcHIDA cholescintigraphy in hopes of confirming the diagnosis and would be treated with sucralfate or cholestyramine and alginates. Failure of medical therapy may necessitate a bile diversion procedure with Roux-en-Y duodenojejunostomy; when possible, this should be performed concomitant or subsequent to the antireflux operation.

4. **Esophageal acid exposure within the normal range on 24-hour pH monitoring and a mechanically normal cardia on manometry.**—In these patients, gastric pathology is suspected and they should undergo gastric pH monitoring. The gastric pH profile may show duodenogastric reflux or hypersecretion or suggest delayed gastric emptying by prolongation of meal effects. Gastric analysis, technetium sulfur colloid emptying scan, and TcHIDA scan would confirm these various possibilities.

If all tests of gastric function are normal, the heart and biliary tract should be investigated.

CONCLUSIONS

The patient described has mild reflux symptoms relieved by antacids and would be expected to be a mild refluxer during the upright period. It is likely that she has a mechanically normal cardia on manometry, and conservative therapy would suffice in these circumstances. She should be given dietary advice, particularly in regard to aerophagia. Surgical therapy should be resisted.

BIBLIOGRAPHY

1. DeMeester TR: Definition, detection, and pathophysiology of gastroesophageal reflux disease, in DeMeester TR, Matthews HR (eds): *International Trends in General Thoracic Surgery: Benign Esophageal Disease.* St Louis, CV Mosby Co, 1987, vol 3, pp 99–127.
2. DeMeester TR, Bonavina L, Albertucci M: Nissen fundoplication for gastroesophageal reflux disease: Evaluation of primary repair in 100 consecutive patients. *Ann Surg* 1986; 204:9–20.

3. DeMeester TR, Fuchs KH, Ball CS, et al: Experimental and clinical results with proximal end-to-end duodenojejunostomy for pathologic duodenogastric reflux. *Ann Surg* 1987; 206:28–38.
4. Johansson K-E, Ask P, Boeryd B, et al: Oesophagitis, signs of reflux, and gastric acid secretion in patients with symptoms of gastroesophageal reflux disease. *Scand J Gastroenterol* 1986; 21:837–847.

- Tc HIDA scan is useful in evaluating alkaline gastroduodenal reflux

- Tc sulfur colloid scan is useful in evaluating gastric emptying

- Gastric acid analysis is part of the w/u of pts c̄ GER.
- PH monitoring   "   "   "   "
- Manometry   "   "   "   "
- Endoscopy c̄ bx's

6

Symptomatic Paraesophageal Hernia

A 78-year-old woman in reasonable health is referred because of a retrocardiac shadow on her chest x-ray film. On further investigation with an upper GI series, it appears to be a paraesophageal hernia, with approximately 70% of her stomach within the chest. On further questioning, she reports occasional episodes when it is difficult to drink liquids and that solids do not pass. She has intermittent chest discomfort that is usually relieved by burping or antacids.

Consultant: Mark B. Orringer, M.D.

OVERVIEW

The case presented is quite typical of the clinical setting in which a paraesophageal hiatal hernia is encountered—an elderly, minimally symptomatic patient whose hernia is virtually an incidental finding on either a chest x-ray film or an upper gastrointestinal (GI) series. On standard chest x-ray the typical findings of a paraesophageal hiatal hernia are a double density behind the heart on the posteroanterior (PA) view and an air-fluid level in the posterior mediastinum on the lateral film (Figs 6–1 and 6–2). Such a posterior mediastinal air-fluid level can occur only with a huge paraesophageal diverticulum, a mediastinal abscess, or a paraesophageal hernia, which is by far the most common. Sliding hiatal hernias have no dependent intrathoracic portion to "trap" fluids, and the paraesophageal hernia or one of its variants (see below) is the *only* type of hiatal hernia in which an air-fluid level is seen. To determine the proper approach to the management of such a patient, it is appropriate to review the anatomical classification of hiatal hernias and to emphasize some of the important clinical features of this problem.

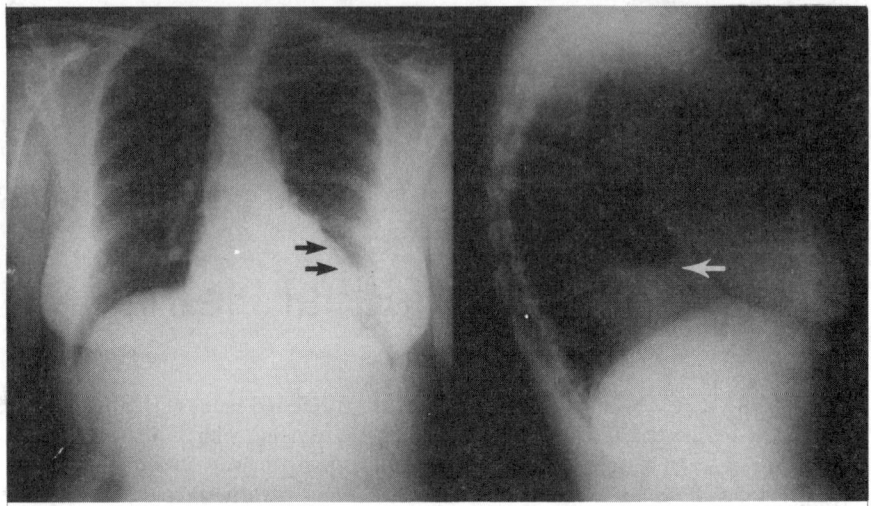

FIG 6–1.
The PA *(left)* and lateral *(right)* chest x-rays of 77-year-old woman with a retrocardiac density *(arrows)*. The lateral view shows an air-fluid level *(arrow)* in her paraesophageal hernia, known to be present for at least 15 years. She was minimally symptomatic and thought to be "too old for major surgery" by her internist.

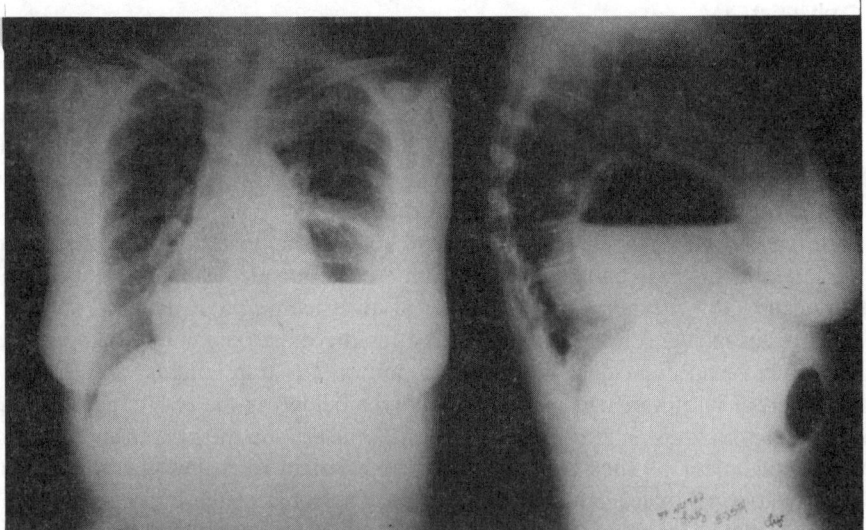

FIG 6–2.
The PA *(left)* and lateral *(right)* chest x-rays of same patient shown in Figure 6–1. Now 81 years old, this woman presented in extremis with chest pain, dyspnea, and hypotension from her distended strangulated intrathoracic stomach. She was operated on emergently and not only survived the operation but lived another eight years, dying of a myocardial infarction at age 89.

ANATOMICAL CLASSIFICATION

All hiatal hernias are not the same. While this statement seems self-evident, it is remarkable how common it is for physicians (including radiologists) to speak of the size of hiatal hernias as "moderate" or "moderate-to-large" without specifying the *type* of hernia to which they are referring. Anatomically, hiatal hernias are classified into four types. The type I, or sliding hiatal hernia, the most common, constitutes 95% of all diaphragmatic hiatal hernias and is recognized by the fact that the esophagogastric junction is the leading point of the hernia. The herniated stomach is not covered by a complete peritoneal sac but rather by peritoneum only on its anterolateral aspect. It is the type I hiatal hernia that is commonly, but not always, associated with gastroesophageal reflux.

In the type II (rolling) or pure paraesophageal hiatal hernia, the esophagogastric junction maintains its usual position fixed posteriorly within the hiatus; the gastric fundus, contained within a peritoneal sac, herniates through the anterolateral aspect of the hiatus. *It is extremely unusual to encounter a pure paraesophageal hiatal hernia.* With most paraesophageal hiatal hernias, there is both a sliding component, in which the esophagogastric junction is herniated into the chest, as well as a paraesophageal portion, with the anterior gastric wall or fundus herniated as described above. These combined, or type III, hernias are the most common variety of what is usually erroneously termed a "paraesophageal" hiatal hernia. The final variety of paraesophageal hiatal hernia, the type IV, is a paraesophageal hernia with other organs (colon, small intestine, or spleen) in addition to the stomach within the intrathoracic peritoneal sac.

CLINICAL FEATURES

The paraesophageal hiatal hernia (type II) and its variations (types III and IV) constitute 5% or less of all hiatal hernias and have a vastly different implication than the type I hernia. Unlike the latter, which may or may not be associated with gastroesophageal reflux and are most often satisfactorily treated medically, paraesophageal hiatal hernias may become quite large and are attendant with a variety of mechanical complications as are other abdominal wall hernias. They are notorious for being totally unpredictable regarding the likelihood of disastrous complications. Even with the knowledge that a paraesophageal hiatal hernia has been present and relatively asymptomatic for 15 to 20 years, one cannot predict with assurance that the patient will continue to have no difficulty from the hernia (see Figs 6–1 and 6–2). Paraesophageal hiatal hernias are almost certainly acquired, the average age of patients with this condition being older (about 67 years) than that of patients with sliding hiatal hernias. With time, as the herniated paraesophageal stomach is progressively "sucked" into the chest by negative intrathoracic pressure, the radiographic "upside-down stomach" is seen on contrast studies.

The complications of paraesophageal hiatal hernias include strangulation of the intrathoracic stomach, gastric volvulus with perforation, gastric outlet obstruction, bleeding, and bowel obstruction. Progressive distention of the incarcerated intrathoracic stomach may result in embarrassment of cardiorespiratory dynamics due to displacement of the heart and/or lungs. Gastric infarction may follow such extreme distention or occur with volvulus of the herniated stomach. Quite often the barium study in a patient with a paraesophageal hiatal hernia shows apposition of the esophagogastric and pyloroduodenal junctions. As the greater curvature of the stomach rotates to the patient's right, duodenal obstruction at the level of the diaphragm may occur and mimic ulcer disease.

Bleeding is a common complication of paraesophageal hiatal hernias, necessitating blood transfusion in as many as 20% to 50% of patients with this condition. The site of blood loss may be a gastric erosion at the point where the incarcerated stomach is "trapped" and partially compressed at the diaphragmatic hiatus (the so-called "rolling ulcer"), or an ulcer or gastritis in the herniated gastric fundus due to intermittent vascular insufficiency and obstruction. Paraesophageal hernias typically cause few if any symptoms until a catastrophic complication occurs. Patients may complain of vague indigestion, postprandial retrosternal fullness radiating around the left side to the back, or a gurgling sensation in the lower left part of the chest. Belching often relieves the "fullness" by decompressing the distended intrathoracic stomach. Extrinsic compression and displacement of the lower esophagus by the hernia may produce intermittent dysphagia that is unrelated to stricture formation. Shortness of breath or dyspnea on exertion may be caused by displacement of the lungs by a huge posterior mediastinal intrathoracic stomach projecting into both pleural cavities. Finally, in my experience, symptoms of gastroesophageal reflux are not at all uncommon in these patients; the reason for this will be discussed below.

TREATMENT

There is little debate that the patient with an obstructed or bleeding paraesophageal hiatal hernia requires surgical intervention. Controversy exists regarding: (1) the need for surgery in the relatively *asymptomatic* patient with a paraesophageal hiatal hernia; (2) the correct operative approach, i.e., transthoracic vs. transabdominal; and (3) the need for an antireflux procedure when repairing a paraesophageal hernia. The first issue is less controversial to surgeons who must treat the desperately ill, elderly patient with an incarcerated, strangulated, or perforated intrathoracic stomach. While the risk of operation in the typically elderly patient with a paraesophageal hiatal hernia may be high, it is clearly less than when an emergency procedure is required under dire circumstances. The incidence and magnitude of the serious complications that occur in patients with paraesophageal hiatal hernias are sufficiently great to justify elective repair whenever the patient's general condition permits, regardless of age or lack of symptoms from the hernia.

The described surgical approaches to paraesophageal hiatal hernias have been influenced by common misconceptions regarding the anatomy and physiology of this abnormality. In many standard textbooks, these hernias are designated "parahiatal," an allusion to the proposed anatomy in which the stomach is depicted as herniating into the chest, not through the diaphragmatic hiatus, but rather through a separate diaphragmatic defect adjacent to the normal hiatus. Thus, the hernia is termed parahiatal (adjacent to the hiatus), as there is supposedly a slip of diaphragmatic muscle between the hernia and the esophageal hiatus. This concept, however, is erroneous and simply ignores the usual anatomy found in these patients. Rarely, *if ever*, is the elusive slip of diaphragmatic muscle found, the paraesophageal hiatal hernia almost universally occurring through the true esophageal diaphragmatic hiatus.

One surgical school of thought emphasizes the normal posterior fixation of the esophagogastric junction in or near the diaphragmatic hiatus in these patients and approaches the problem purely anatomically and generally transabdominally by simply pulling the herniated stomach down out of the chest and narrowing the diaphragmatic hiatus. Occasionally the stomach is "tacked" to the anterior abdominal wall to prevent subsequent reherniation. Excision of the hernia sac is not regarded as necessary, and this relatively "simple" problem is managed in an equally simple fashion, ignoring any physiologic abnormality (i.e., gastroesophageal reflux) that might be present.

The other school, of which I am a part, approaches the paraesophageal hiatal hernia quite differently. Careful operative dissection in these patients, particularly through a transthoracic approach, indicates how uncommonly a pure paraesophageal hiatal hernia occurs. Much more often, in addition to the paraesophageal component, the esophagogastric junction is found above the diaphragmatic hiatus and the "paraesophageal" hiatal hernia is actually a *combined* (type III) sliding and paraesophageal hernia. It is a long-accepted principle in the repair of abdominal wall hernias in other locations that complete mobilization of the herniated viscus from the muscular defect is necessary to achieve complete reduction of the hernia with minimal chance of recurrence. Thus, unless the entire herniated cardia is mobilized away from its diaphragmatic hiatal attachments, the ideal tension-free reduction of the esophagogastric junction into the abdomen will not be possible. Complete mobilization of the esophagogastric junction translates into the need to reconstruct the cardia (i.e., to do an antireflux procedure) in every patient requiring repair of a paraesophageal hiatal hernia or one of its variants. Not only is better reduction of the hernia achieved with this approach, but also the commonly associated gastroesophageal reflux present in these pa-

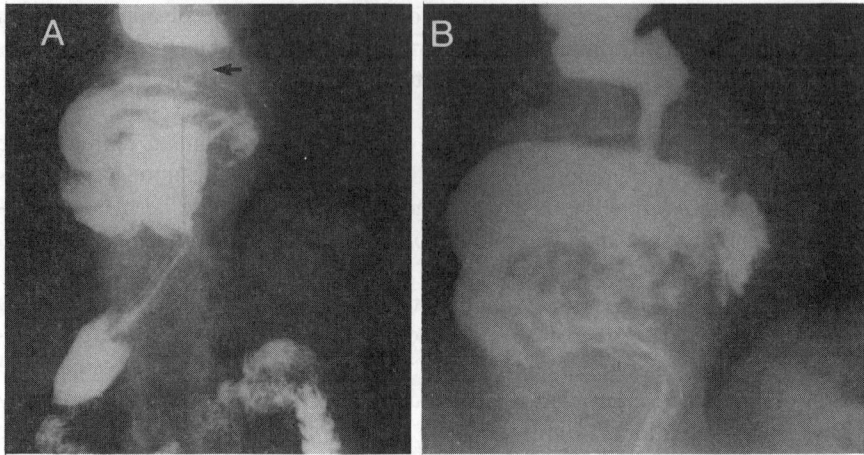

FIG 6–3.
A, barium study in an 85-year-old obese woman with an incarcerated "paraesophageal" hiatal hernia and a stricture *(arrow)* at the esophagogastric junction, which is clearly above the diaphragm in the chest. This is a *combined* (type III) hernia with both a sliding and paraesophageal component. **B,** detail of stricture in same patient shown in Figure 6–3. This "apple-core" lesion proved to be an adenocarcinoma arising in Barrett's epithelium, a testimony to the occurrence of significant gastroesophageal reflux in most patients with "paraesophageal" hernias. She was treated successfully with a transhiatal esophagectomy without thoracotomy and a cervical esophagogastric anastomosis.

tients is treated (Fig 6–3, A and B). DeMeester and associates have recently reported a 60% incidence of abnormal gastroesophageal reflux in patients with paraesophageal hiatal hernias studied preoperatively with 24-hour distal esophageal pH monitoring. To completely reduce a paraesophageal hernia and the esophagogastric junction well below the diaphragmatic hiatus, complete mobilization of the herniated stomach, esophagogastric junction, and adjacent lower esophagus is important. An antireflux procedure is indicated not only because many patients with paraesophageal hiatal hernias have associated gastroesophageal reflux to begin with, but also because once the cardia has been mobilized properly in the process of reducing the hernia, lower esophageal sphincter incompetence and gastroesophageal reflux may be induced.

My approach to the patient undergoing elective paraesophageal hernia repair is transthoracic, as I believe that this provides optimal exposure of the hernia, the esophagogastric junction, and the distal esophagus—all of which should be assessed in deciding the operation of choice. Esophagoscopy is performed after the patient has been anesthetized and intubated to evaluate the extent and degree of any esophagitis that may be present and, of course, to exclude the presence of neoplasm. While use of the flexible fiberoptic esophagoscope is currently in vogue, great care must be taken to avoid excessive air insufflation into the herniated stomach with resultant massive distention. A sixth or seventh interspace left posterolateral thoracotomy is utilized as for most transthoracic hiatal hernia repairs. Complete excision of the hernia sac is readily achieved through a transthoracic approach. The extent to which the hernia sac protrudes into the right chest is often dramatic. As the often thickened peritoneal sac is amputated at the hiatus, hemostasis either with electrocautery or a running chromic suture is appropriate, since intra-abdominal bleeding from the divided edge may occur.

It has been my observation, as well as that of others, that in many patients with type III hiatal hernias there is some degree of associated esophageal shortening. This may not necessarily be the result of reflux esophagitis. It appears that when the esophagogastric junction has been in the thorax for many years, as is often the case in these patients, relative shortening occurs; this is recognized as a subtle increased degree of tension on the lower esophagus seen after completion of a standard Belsey Mark IV or Nissen repair, both of which require a 3- to 5-cm intra-abdominal segment of distal esophagus. Therefore, in order to reduce the degree of tension on the lower esophagus and thereby minimize the chance of recurrent herniation and/or reflux, I have in recent years frequently utilized an esophageal-lengthening Collis gastroplasty in combination with a Nissen fundoplication in patients with paraesophageal hiatal hernias. This antireflux procedure has become an integral part of our operation. In patients in whom the esophagogastric junction, grasped with forceps, readily reduces several centimeters below the hiatus without producing undue tension on the lower esophagus, which is palpated above the hiatus, a standard antireflux operation (Nissen fundoplication or Belsey repair) is performed.

General surgeons who are accustomed to approaching these hernias transabdominally may view the transthoracic approach as unnecessary and fraught with increased morbidity. This is not the case, and it is only when one has had a repeated opportunity to evaluate the remaining tension on the lower esophagus after completion of an antireflux operation that an appreciation for these subtle findings can be gained. This assessment simply is not possible as readily through a transabdominal approach. Among 50 patients with paraesophageal hiatal hernias that we have operated upon during the past 12 years, 43 have undergone a combined Collis-Nissen reconstruction of the esophagogastric junction; 2, a Collis-Belsey repair; 3, a Nissen fundoplication; and 2, a Belsey repair. All of these operations have been transthoracic. There have been no operative deaths. One of the Collis-Nissen patients developed recurrent herniation four years postoperatively. Among the 24 Collis-Nissen patients in whom it was possible to perform preoperative standard acid reflux testing with the intraesophageal pH electrode, 19 (80%) were found to have abnormal gastroesophageal reflux. In postoperative follow-up (which averages 52 months), 95% have excellent subjective reflux control, and 87% have no reflux demonstrable with intraesophageal reflux testing (the standard acid reflux test).

Strangulation or perforation of an incarcerated paraesophageal hernia represents life-threatening emergencies. When a gangrenous stomach is found on transthoracic exploration, resection of nonviable tissue and control of infection are the primary considerations, and these patients are usually simply too sick to tolerate reestablishment of esophagogastric continuity. In most cases, a major portion of the stomach will be nonviable, but the esophagus is minimally involved. Necrotic stomach should be resected and viable stomach returned to the abdomen through the hiatus, which is then closed with heavy interrupted sutures. The distal esophagus should *not* be closed, oversewn, and left in this potentially infected field in the lower mediastinum. Rather, the entire thoracic esophagus is mobilized well into the neck through the thoracic incision. After irrigating the chest and mediastinum and inserting a large chest tube, the thoracotomy is closed. The patient is repositioned and turned supine. A feeding jejunostomy is inserted through a limited abdominal incision. Through an oblique left cervical incision paralleling the anterior border of the sternocleidomastoid muscle, the previously mobilized thoracic esophagus is delivered out of the wound and placed on the anterior thorax. Despite what has been written about the "tenuous" segmental blood supply of the esophagus, its submucosal collateral circulation is extensive. The totally mobilized thoracic esophagus, resting on the anterior chest wall, is attached to the patient only by its cervical end, which is nourished by collaterals of the thyroid arteries. If the distal tip is amputated, arterial bleeding is usually seen. Viable esophagus that can be used later for esophageal reconstruction should not be discarded as the cervical esophagus is amputated to "tailor" it for a traditional cervical esophagostomy, which is difficult to keep dry and to care for. Rather, a subcutaneous tunnel should be made on the anterior chest wall and as much viable esophagus preserved in construction of an anterior thoracic esophagostomy. This not only provides more esophagus for a later reconstructive operation, but it also creates a stoma that is much more easily cared for and covered by an appliance placed on the flatter anterior chest wall. Once the patient has recovered from the physiologic insult of the operation and any associated infection, restoration of alimentary continuity with a substernal intestinal conduit can be undertaken.

SUMMARY

Paraesophageal hiatal hernias are potentially lethal and should be repaired once diagnosed, whenever the patient's condition permits, regardless of the presence or absence of symptoms. Pure paraesophageal hiatal hernias are rare, and in most cases there is a sliding component in which the esophagogastric junction is above the diaphragm; gastroesophageal reflux is the rule, rather than the exception in these patients. An antireflux operation should be an integral part of the repair of a paraesophageal hiatal hernia. Many of these patients have relative esophageal shortening that is best assessed through a transthoracic approach, and an esophageal-lengthening Collis gastroplasty in combination with a fundoplication provides a tension-free reconstruction of the esophagogastric junction that should minimize the chance of later recurrence of the hernia and/ or reflux.

BIBLIOGRAPHY

1. Ellis FH Jr, Crozier RE, Shea JA: Paraesophageal hiatal hernia. *Arch Surg* 1986; 121:416–420.
2. Hill LD: Incarcerated paraesophageal hernia: A surgical emergency. *Am J Surg* 1973; 126:286–291.
3. Orringer MB, Sloan H: Combined Collis-Nissen reconstruction of the esophagogastric junction. *Ann Thorac Surg* 1978; 25:16–21.
4. Pearson, FG, Cooper JD, Ilves R, et al: Massive hiatal hernia with incarceration: A report of 53 cases. *Ann Thorac Surg* 1982; 35:45–51.
5. Walther B, DeMeester TR, LaFontaine E, et al: Effect of paraesophageal hernia on sphincter function and its implication on surgical therapy. *Am J Surg* 1984; 147: 111–116.

7

Myasthenia Gravis

A 51-year-old man initially experienced diplopia and some mild muscular weakness six months ago. His difficulty in vision persisted and an ophthalmologist referred him to a neurologist. A Tensilon test was positive, with increased strength. At the present time the patient complains of fatigue, some difficulty in swallowing, a weakened voice at the end of the day, and occasional diplopia. In addition to fatigue, the patient gets short of breath relatively easily, a change over the past three or four months.

Consultant: Josef E. Fischer, M.D.

OVERVIEW

The patient has myasthenia gravis, currently thought of as an autoimmune disease in which T-lymphocytes, produced by the thymus, produce an autoimmune antibody that reacts against acetylcholine receptors. There are other theories of myasthenia gravis, but the preceding theory has gained the most credence. The diagnosis, which often is disturbingly delayed, is frequently made by an ophthalmologist attending the patient because of difficulty in vision. Nonetheless, patients with protean symptoms such as weakness, fatigue, and dysphagia, in whom diplopia is not a prominent symptom, may elude diagnosis for one or two years. In this case, muscle weakness persisted for only six months, and the diagnosis was promptly made by a Tensilon test. Edrophonium chloride (Tensilon) is a short-acting cholinesterase inhibitor that prolongs the function of acetylcholine, and its administration usually results in sudden improvement in diplopia, dysphagia, and fatigue.

Whereas in the past, it was debatable as to whether patients should be treated with medication alone or undergo surgery, currently there seems to be little question that surgery is indicated. Although few randomized, prospective trials have been carried out, Buckingham and his colleagues, using computer-matched patients, showed that when patients were operated on for myasthenia gravis, 27 of 80 had drug-free remissions and an additional 26 patients were improved, whereas in the medically treated group only 6 of 80 had drug-free remissions and 13 of 80 were improved. In addition, survival was improved in the surgically treated group as opposed to the medically treated group.

The operation of choice is clearly a sternal split and extended thymectomy, currently employing radical dissection of the entire anterior mediastinum from phrenic nerve to phrenic nerve and from thyroid to diaphragm. This choice is based on several criteria, including (1) the embryology of the thymus, (2) the fact that the thymus does not have a true capsule, and (3) the fact that studies in patients who have undergone transcervical thymectomy frequently have residual thymus left in the mediastinum, and no one is certain as to how large a thymic remnant needs to be in order to precipitate myasthenia gravis.

The concept of the operation has gradually been extended because of the above mentioned facts. There are numerous thymic rests and thymic tissue frequently extends beyond the capsule, especially in the lower lobes. Thus, I believe that the operation should clear the mediastinum from diaphragm to thyroid and at least from phrenic nerve to phrenic nerve, and perhaps more widely when indicated (e.g., thymoma).

Since many studies have shown that one of the favorable factors in prognosis is a shorter duration of disease, operation should be undertaken as soon as the patient is stabilized. Different institutions use different modes of stabilization. In one large series reported by Olanow et al., steroids were not used, but the patients were repeatedly plasmapheresed until their respiratory status was stable, while in our institution the neurologist stabilizes the patient using steroids and pyridostigmine bromide (Mestinon) until respiratory status and general conditioning are reasonable, at which point operation is undertaken. Occasionally, patients may be plasmapheresed immediately preoperatively for stabilization, but in general this is not necessary. Pulmonary function tests are monitored carefully, both immediately preoperatively and perioperatively.

PREPARATION FOR OPERATION

The patient is admitted the day before the operation, and pulmonary function tests are obtained. The chest and shoulders are cleansed with Hibiclens. Intraoperative coverage is by hydrocortisone (300 mg/24 hours) if the patient is on steroids. In the few cases in which patients are not on steroids, ACTH is available in case the patient deteriorates immediately postoperatively; this has not been required in our series of 37 patients. The patient's hair is clipped the morning of surgery, since this has been shown by Alexander et al. to result in the lowest incidence of wound infection. Pyridostigmine therapy is stopped at midnight, since if it is given in the immediate preoperative period it may result in increased secretions. Antibiotics are used prophylactically for 48 hours, usually a second- or third-generation cephalosporin. Aminoglycosides are avoided, both in the irrigation solution as well as in perioperative antibiotics.

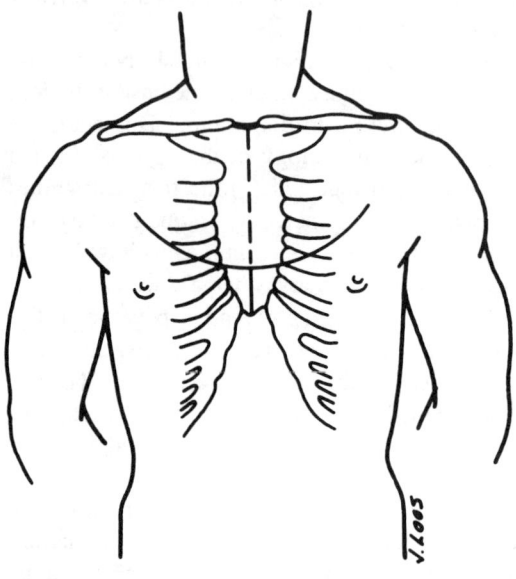

FIG 7–1.
The general outline for the incision that we have found to heal much more cosmetically than a vertical incision over the sternum. A large cephalad flap is developed from the curvilinear incision that generally hugs the contours of the breasts, depending on individual, and is extended caudad below the xyphoid. Approximately 8 inches of the cephalad flap can be developed, giving good exposure to the top of the sternum, the sternal notch, and to the upper portion of the dissection, especially the superior horns of the thymus as they approach the inferior border of the thyroid in the neck. The sternum is split (*dotted line*) in the usual fashion, as one would with a vertical incision directly over the sternum.

OPERATIVE PROCEDURE

Since many of these patients are young women, a cosmetic incision is important. While some have proposed a transverse incision, splitting the sternum transversely, I do not believe that it gives adequate exposure for an appropriate, complete dissection. Thus, we make a Y-type incision with a curvilinear flap, hugging the contours of the breasts (Fig 7–1). The incision is central, over the sternum, about 6 in. below the sternal notch, a distance that can be easily bridged by mobilizing the upper flap. The sternum is split vertically. The dissection begins at the diaphragm, taking the mediastinal fat off both pleura and the pericardium, leaving these structures bare (Fig 7–2). While much has been made of leaving the pleura intact, in my experience the pleura will be violated on both sides during an adequate mediastinal dissection. About midway across the pericardium or about the level of the atria, the thymus will gradually begin to blend imperceptibly with the mediastinal fat. The thymus is elevated off the pericardium and laterally. At about this level it derives some blood supply from the internal mammary; this branch should be tied with fine silk and divided.

The only delicate part of the dissection with respect to the thymus is the venous drainage, which enters the innominate vein posteriorly. It is easier to isolate by elevating the thymus from the innominate vein posteriorly and ligating these veins, which may number between one and five, in continuity. The dissection should also be completed from the area around both phrenic nerves, which can be easily identified as they course along the pleura. There is some nodal tissue in this area that must be excised. The thymus is then elevated from the innominate vein and the two cephalad horns of the thymus are dissected. This is the most difficult part of the dissection, since this is under the flap, and exposure is most difficult. The inferior parathyroids usually reside in this area and almost always can be identified and spared. After the cephalad horns of the thymus are dissected free, right-angle clamps are placed around the blood supply and tied, sparing the parathyroids. Hemostasis is then secured. Two No. 24 chest tubes are placed in the mediastinum, with their tips protruding into the respective right and left pleura. The sternum is wired with five large No. 4 wires placed through the sternum, as I believe it is extremely important to have a stable sternum. After being tightened, the tips of the wires are inserted in the crack of the sternum and the fascia and muscle are closed with a running 2-0 Dexon or 0 Dexon suture, and the subcutaneous tissue and skin closed with a subcuticular closure.

In the postoperative period, hydrocortisone is quickly tapered to the preoperative dose, with the remainder of the tapering left to be done by the neurologist over a prolonged period of time. The chest tubes are removed in 24 to 48 hours, and antibiotic therapy is discontinued. Patients are usually fed on the second postoperative day. Foley catheters or special monitoring are not required after the first 24 hours. In our series of 33 patients, only 2 have required reintubation. Our custom is to extubate the patients in the operating room but

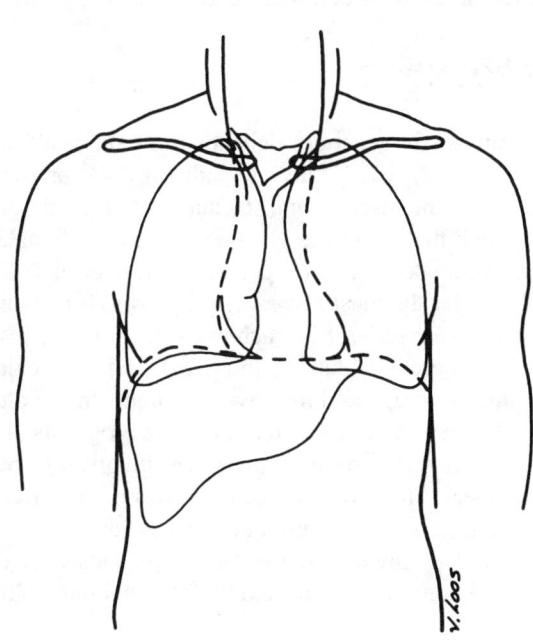

FIG 7–2.
Extent of dissection (*dotted lines*) includes the entire mediastinum from phrenic nerve to phrenic nerve and from the inferior border of the thyroid to the diaphragm. All fat is removed from the pericardium, the diaphragm, and the lateral parietal pleura.

to keep them overnight in their recovery room or in the intensive care unit to monitor blood gases as well as respiratory effort. Therapy with pyridostigmine is usually not restarted in the postoperative period. The patient is usually discharged on the fifth postoperative day. The most prominent postoperative pain is in the back due to spreading of the sternum, but this pain soon disappears. If the sternum is tightly wired, there should be no problem with sternal pain; indeed, most patients who have had both abdominal and transsternal procedures say that the abdominal procedures are by far the more painful.

If patients experience difficulty in the postoperative period weaning from the ventilator or develop a myasthenic crisis, a number of steps may be taken. If the patient is not receiving steroids, ACTH "rescue" (80 to 100 international units intravenously (IV) over six to eight hours daily for ten days) should be administered. If the patient is already receiving steroids:

1. Physostigmine or neostigmine 0.5 to 1.0 mg intravenously should be carefully titrated to maximum effect. Care should be exercised, as it is possible to overmedicate the patient; the patient may appreciate this as excessive salivation, sweating, increased weakness, etc.

2. Plasmapheresis daily for three days, then every other day.

3. Methylprednisolone 30 mg/kg IV daily for three days, then every other day.

Few patients should require these procedures alone or in combination, but they may be useful when required.

PROGNOSIS

Prognosis is generally dependent on six easily identifiable features, including: (1) age, (2) sex, (3) thymic pathology, (4) presence or absence of thymoma, (5) stage of the disease, and (6) duration of the disease. In general, sex and age are related; that is, in the younger age group, females tend to outnumber males by approximately 3:1 as reported by Mulder et al., Olanow et al., and Fischer et al. By far the most favorable prognosis is in young females without a thymoma, and in our series 82% achieved drug-free remission and all of the remainder were improved; that is, those that did not achieve drug-free remission had a reduced dosage and improved strength. In the older group (50 to 60 years old), males and females are equal, and the prognosis in this group is far less favorable. Whether this is because males are involved or because the patients are older is not clear. However, respectable rates of drug-free remission have been achieved even in this older group; in our series, drug-free remission was achieved in 46%. Overall, in my series, 89% of the patients were either in drug-free remission or were improved as indicated by less symptomatology and decreased drug dosage.

Another important factor is the duration of disease. Most authors believe that patients who have had the disease for less than two years tend to have a more favorable prognosis. In our series, however, mean duration of the disease prior to operation was three years, yet our results compare favorably with other previously published series. Therefore, the significance of this factor is unclear.

The pathology of the specimen is also a favorable factor if thymic hyperplasia is present. Again, in a patient receiving steroids, the thymus may involute. Although our series did not have an overwhelming majority of patients with thymic hyperplasia, our results are very favorable.

While current mythology has it that patients with thymoma have a distinctly less favorable prognosis, this is not the case in our series, as improvement was present in all of our five patients, including one patient with a malignant thymoma who has no disease evident 4 1/2 years after resection of a malignant thymoma and resection of an adjacent contiguous invaded left upper lobe; in the study by Olanow and associates, six of eight patients with thymoma were improved.

Finally, the stage of the disease, that is, the instability of a patient, does seem to be of some importance. The majority of our patients were stage II-B or III, and we did not have many patients in stage IV. Stage IV patients are rare at this point since steroids, plasmapheresis, and/or both tend to stabilize these patients prior to operation, but it is said that they have a poorer prognosis.

SUMMARY AND CONCLUSIONS

Myasthenia gravis is a surgical disease. Patients should be prepared for resection as soon as the diagnosis is made. The operation should be carried out through a sternal split and radical mediastinal dissection, with clearing of the mediastinum from diaphragm to thyroid and from phrenic nerve to phrenic nerve. Ninety percent of all patients can be expected to be improved, and in the most favorable group, the young female population without a thymoma, more than 80% should achieve drug-free remission. Medical therapy should be reserved for the rare patient in whom operation cannot be safely undertaken.

BIBLIOGRAPHY

1. Alexander JW, Fischer JE, Boyajian M, et al: The influence of hair-removal methods on wound infections. *Arch Surg* 1983; 118:347–352.
2. Buckingham JM, Howard FM, Bernatz PE, et al: The value of thymectomy in myasthenia gravis: A computer-assisted matched study. *Ann Surg* 1976; 184:453–458.
3. Fischer JE, Grinvalski HT, Nussbaum MS, et al: Aggressive surgical approach for drug-free remission from myasthenia gravis. *Ann Surg* 1987; 205:496–503.

4. Hankins JR, Mayer RF, Satterfield JR, et al: Thymectomy for myasthenia gravis: 14-year experience. *Ann Surg* 1985; 201:618–625.
5. Masaoka A, Nagaoka Y, Kotake Y: Distribution of thymic tissue at the anterior mediastinum. *J Thorac Cardiovasc Surg* 1975; 70:747–754.
6. Masaoka A, Monden Y, Seike Y, et al: Reoperation after transcervical thymectomy for myasthenia gravis. *Neurology* 1982; 32:83–85.
7. Mulder DG, Herrmann C, Buckberg GD: Effect of thymectomy in patients with myasthenia gravis: A sixteen-year experience. *Am J Surg* 1974; 128:202–206.
8. Mulder DG, Herrmann CH, Keesey J, et al: Thymectomy for myasthenia gravis. *Am J Surg* 1983; 146:61–66.
9. Olanow CW, Wechsler AS, Roses AD: A prospective study of thymectomy and serum acetylcholine receptor antibodies in myasthenia gravis. *Ann Surg* 1982; 196:113–121.

8

Solitary Pulmonary Nodule

A 63-year-old woman was noted to have a left upper lobe nodule 2.5 cm in its longest diameter on chest x-ray film (Fig 8–1). She was asymptomatic and had a 30 pack per year smoking history. The borders of the nodule were somewhat irregular. No previous chest x-ray films were available for comparison.

Consultant: Jack A. Roth, M.D.

The solitary pulmonary nodule is the most common presentation for asymptomatic lung cancers and benign lung tumors. This patient's presentation is typical and emphasizes several problems that continue to make management of this entity controversial. For this discussion, the solitary pulmonary nodule is defined as a nodular density appearing on the chest radiograph with the largest diameter less than or equal to 3 cm. For nodules larger than this, the likelihood of malignancy compared to a benign lesion exceeds 4:1.

The options for patient management include immediate surgery, attempt at biopsy, or observation. Disagreement over management reflects the fact that some patients in this group have potentially curable cancers that should be resected without delay, while other patients should not be exposed to the risks of surgery because they have benign lesions. Unfortunately, to date no test or procedure other than surgical excision can eliminate the possibility of cancer. Nevertheless, astute clinical judgment and knowledge of the probabilities for various outcomes can optimize patient management.

DIAGNOSIS

The patient described above presents with a typical history. She has no symptoms as would be expected from a small lesion not contiguous with major bronchi or invading extrapulmonary structures. There is no clinical evidence for metastases or another primary tumor. The patient has a long cigarette-smoking history that doubles the probability of the nodule being cancer. The borders of the nodule are indistinct, which suggests but is not conclusive for cancer. The single most

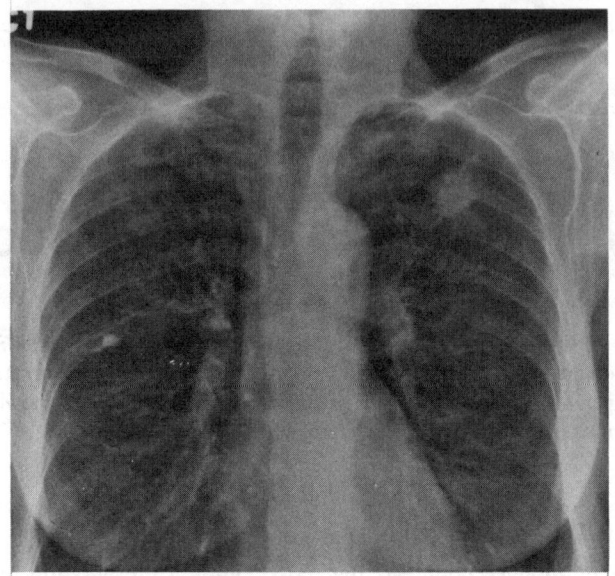

FIG 8–1.
Chest x-ray film of 63-year-old patient under consideration. A solitary nodule with an irregular border is noted in the left upper lobe. No hilar or mediastinal adenopathy was present.

important point in the evaluation is the availability of a previous chest x-ray film. Comparison with a previous study may show the nodule was present and unchanged for several years. Because most benign nodules either do not change in size or have doubling times greater than 450 days, no change on a two-year or more follow-up film indicates the lesion is benign. If the follow-up time is less than two years, the interpretation must be qualified because some malignancies have slow doubling times. Unfortunately, as occurred with this case, previous films are frequently not available.

Differential Diagnosis

The most common benign lesion presenting as a solitary pulmonary nodule is a granuloma, perhaps due to fungal disease or tuberculosis. Other common benign lesions include a slowly resolving circumscribed pneumonia, lung abscess, lipoid pneumonia, or hamartoma. A number of uncommon lesions have been described including pulmonary sequestration, inflammatory pseudotumor, bronchogenic cyst, pulmonary infarct, rheumatoid nodule, infected, fluid-filled bulla, bronchial adenoma, or arteriovenous malformation.

Most malignant nodules are primary lung carcinomas. Solitary metastases are infrequent, and a solitary metastasis from an asymptomatic primary cancer is very rare. Therefore, an extensive radiographic evaluation for an occult primary cancer is not necessary. It is also unproductive to perform a metastatic evaluation if it is believed the nodule is a primary cancer. In the absence of symptoms, metastases are rarely detected by radiographic studies.

Historical Factors

Although the patient's history cannot (with the exception of a previous chest x-ray film) give definitive diagnostic information, it can contribute to an overall assessment of the probability of malignancy. Cummings and co-workers have correlated the likelihood of malignancy in a solitary nodule with several historical factors. The probability of a nodule being cancer increases with age. A direct correlation was also noted for smoking and the number of cigarettes smoked per day; those patients who had ceased smoking had a lower probability of malignancy directly correlated with length of time the patient had not smoked. For a patient with the lowest risk of malignancy (a 35-year-old nonsmoker with a 1-cm nodule), the risk was 1%. This exceeds the operative mortality by at least a factor of 2; therefore, even in this low-risk group, I believe surgery is indicated. In comparison, the probability of malignancy for a 50-year-old, one pack per day smoker with a 2-cm nodule was 34%.

Radiologic Studies

The radiographic appearance of the nodule may provide information related to the probability of malignancy. The appearance is classified by "edge characteristics" (i.e., the margin of the lesion as seen on computed tomography (CT) scans on a scale of 1 to 4, where type 1 indicates sharp and smooth, type 2 indicates moderately smooth, type 3 indicates some irregular undulation or slight spiculation, and type 4 indicates grossly irregular with spiculations). This classification is not completely reliable. In the study by Siegelman and co-workers, some primary cancers and many metastases were classified as type 1 or 2, and a significant percentage of nodules were indeterminate.

The detection of occult calcification in nodules by CT scans has been used by Zerhouni and co-workers to determine malignancy. Direct comparison between scanners is difficult, and therefore reference phantoms have been developed to simulate the anatomy on the thorax and facilitate calibration. Unsuspected calcification was demonstrated in 55% of histologically benign nodules by this technique. However, almost 60% of the nodules studied were classified as indeterminate. In addition, one nodule with central calcification proved to be malignant for a false negative rate of 1.5%. Thus, this technique does not appear to be useful for the majority of cases, and false negative results can occur. This emphasizes the need for definitive histologic diagnosis. Certain patterns of calcification are characteristic of benign lesions. These include central, concentric, diffuse, or punctate (popcorn) calcification. If one of these patterns is identified, the lesion may be followed with serial chest roentgenograms.

Other Diagnostic Techniques

In the past, recommendations for preoperative evaluation have included delayed cutaneous hypersensitivity testing and collection of sputum cytologies. Both of these tests are uninformative. Skin test reactions usually do not give useful diagnostic information, as many patients with lung cancer have been exposed to fungal or mycobacterial pathogens. Peripheral lesions rarely communicate with large bronchi, and therefore sputum samples will not contain malignant cells.

Flexible fiberoptic bronchoscopy should be performed routinely. The purpose of this is not to obtain a diagnosis, but to ascertain the existence of any other coexisting lesions such as second primary cancers or other pathologic conditions of the tracheobronchial tree.

Percutaneous needle aspiration has been recommended to obtain a diagnosis for solitary nodules; the accuracy for this procedure in diagnosing malignancy is over 90%. The procedure can be performed on an outpatient basis with the patient under local anesthesia. Fluoroscopy or CT scans are useful for localization. The most frequent complications are pneumothorax and hemoptysis. Pneumothorax occurs in 30% of procedures in most series, but it requires a chest tube in less than 10% of cases. The problem with the technique is the significant incidence of nondiagnostic biopsies that cannot be interpreted to mean a cancer risk is not present. If the patient is a surgical candidate, then needle biopsy is superfluous. A negative biopsy is not adequate assurance that cancer is not present, and thus surgery is required. If cancer is diagnosed, surgery will also be performed. The one exception is obtaining the diagnosis of small-cell cancer. If clinical suspicion for this is high, then needle biopsy is indicated. Very few small-cell cancers present as peripheral solitary nodules, and even if the nodule is a small-cell carcinoma, resection is not an unreasonable initial treatment. This technique is very useful for the patient who is a poor surgical risk or for the patient for whom documentation of metastatic disease is important before therapy is initiated.

The diagnostic techniques discussed above are not sufficiently accurate to exclude malignancy in this group of patients. Therefore, exploratory thoracotomy is indicated. The preoperative evaluation should be minimized, using routine blood studies, bronchoscopy, and pulmonary function tests, if indicated.

TREATMENT

During the evaluation, a decision must be made as to whether the patient can tolerate surgical resection. If the patient does not have a history of pulmonary disease, is not symptomatic, and can walk up two flights of stairs without dyspnea, a lobectomy should be well tolerated. If the patient has a smoking history, if the chest x-ray film shows evidence of emphysema, or if the patient gives any indication of impaired pulmonary function, spirometry should be obtained. If the FEV1 is less than 1.8 L, a quantitative-ventilation-perfusion xenon scan is extremely useful for determining the FEV1 for the residual lung following resection. If the residual FEV1 is less than 1 L, the operative risks for lobectomy become unacceptably high. Some retrospective studies have suggested that nonanatomical resection of the nodule may yield survival rates equivalent to lobectomy. I consider wedge or segmental resection an acceptable alternative to lobectomy in the patient with lung cancer in a peripheral nodule.

PROGNOSIS

The operative mortality should be less than 3% for lobectomy and less than 1.5% for lesser resections overall; this will vary with the patient's age and medical condition. If the patient has lung cancer without metastases to regional lymph nodes, the prognosis is very favorable. Over 60% of these patients will be alive five years later without evidence of cancer.

SUMMARY

The patient described above underwent bronchoscopy, which was normal. Pulmonary function studies showed an FEV1 of 1.5 L, but the quantitative-ventilation-perfusion xenon scan indicated the patient would have adequate reserve following lobectomy. At thoracotomy, a needle biopsy revealed squamous cell carcinoma on frozen section, and a left upper lobectomy was performed with mediastinal node dissection. All mediastinal and hilar lymph nodes were negative for tumor, and the patient was discharged after an uncomplicated recovery.

BIBLIOGRAPHY

1. Bennett WF, Smith RA: Segmental resection for bronchogenic carcinoma: A surgical alternative for the compromised patient. *Ann Thorac Surg* 1979; 27:169–172.
2. Cummings SR, Lillington GA, Richard RJ: Estimating the probability of malignancy in solitary pulmonary nodules. *Am Rev Respir Dis* 1986; 134:449–452.
3. Cummings SR, Lillington GA, Richard RJ: Managing solitary pulmonary nodules: The choice of strategy is a "close call." *Am Rev Respir Dis* 1986; 134:453–460.
4. Ginsberg RJ, Hill LD, Eagan RT, et al: Modern thirty-day operative mortality for surgical resections in lung cancer. *J Thorac Cardiovasc Surg* 1983; 86:654–658.

5. Hoffman TH, Ransdell HT: Comparison of lobectomy and wedge resection for carcinoma of the lung. *J. Thorac Cardiovasc Surg* 1980; 79:211–217.
6. Siegelman SS, Khouri NF, Leo FP, et al: Solitary pulmonary nodules: CT assessment. *Radiology* 1986; 160:307–312.
7. Zerhouni EA, Stitik FP, Siegelman SS, et al: CT of the pulmonary nodule: A cooperative study. *Radiology* 1986; 160:319–327.

9

Breast Mass

A 43-year-old woman presents with a 2-cm mass on the right breast at approximately the 11 o'clock position. There is no peau d'orange or dimpling and no axillary adenopathy. Family history is negative for breast cancer. She has not been examined recently by a physician. The mass is nontender but firm.

Consultants: D. Lawrence Wickerham, M.D.
Bernard Fisher, M.D.

The obvious concern is that the mass could be a breast cancer. How should the diagnosis be established? What is the preferred surgical intervention? Should radiation therapy be employed? Is systemic adjuvant therapy indicated? The following outline provides answers to those and other questions describing our management of such a patient.

ESTABLISHING THE DIAGNOSIS

Pertinent History

Obtaining a complete medical history from the patient, with special emphasis directed toward her breasts, is appropriate in that it may provide insight into the nature of her mass. It is highly unlikely, however, that such information will provide us with a definite diagnosis or alter our approach to her management. Since the patient being considered is most likely premenopausal, the mass, particularly if it is of brief duration, may represent a cyst despite the fact that it is nontender. Cysts may be nontender and cancers tender, or vice-versa. Such a symptom in itself is meaningless relative to establishing a diagnosis. Historic information concerning the duration of the presence of a mass is likewise deceptive. The description by a reputable historian of a palpable mass occurring "overnight" may suggest the presence of a cyst, particularly if it is tender.

The patient's menstrual history is pertinent. Is she having regular menses? Does the mass change in relation to her menstrual cycle? Is she taking medication? Hormonal replacement therapy is increasingly common. While there is good epidemiologic evidence that estrogens do not significantly increase the risk of developing a breast cancer, there remains concern that should a breast cancer be present, estrogens may stimulate its growth. Thus we do not recommend continuing estrogen/progesterone replacement therapy in patients with known or suspected breast cancer.

While this particular patient has no family history of breast cancer, there may be other risk factors that make it more likely the mass is cancer. Is she nulliparous? Was her first child born when she was over the age of 30? Did she have a previous breast cancer or a previous biopsy showing hyperplastic changes? These factors are known to result in an increased risk of developing a breast cancer. While it is uncommon to examine a patient exposed to high-dose radiation such as that experienced in Nagasaki, Hiroshima, or Chernobyl, patients who have received radiation for benign conditions such as postpartum mastitis, acne, and birth marks may not be infrequently encountered, and such exposure cannot be ignored. Diagnostic x-ray film taken over prolonged periods of time for conditions such as scoliosis or pneumothorax for tuberculosis have been reported to increase the risk of developing breast cancer. Consequently, the patient should be interrogated concerning such exposure. It is strongly emphasized that information regarding the presence or absence of any of these risk factors in a patient is of little or no consequence relative to definitively establishing her diagnosis or determining her management. Such knowledge is important for establishing an appropriate follow-up program of women without a mass or with benign disease.

Our patient should be interrogated as to whether she has had a previous mammogram that revealed a finding of concern or whether it was reported as "normal." Hopefully, the films will be available for comparison with a more current study. The American Cancer Society recommends a baseline mammogram for women between the age of 35 and 40. During her 40s a woman is advised to have mammograms yearly or every other year depending on her degree of risk, findings from physical examination, and previous mammograms. It is recommended that in those over the age of 50, mammograms be performed once a year. The National Cancer Institute is more conservative in their recommendations. They recommend yearly mammograms for women over the age of 50 because randomized clinical trials have shown a mortality benefit for that age group. Only if women in their 40s are at increased risk do they advise that mammograms be carried out. Since mammography is the single most effective method for detecting small, often nonpalpable breast masses that can be treated by breast-conserving surgery, it is our view that they be judiciously employed in women under 50, particularly if they are symptomatic or at higher than usual risk for breast cancer, as well as in women 50 years or older.

Physical Examination

A careful physical examination of both breasts, axillae, supraclavicular, and cervical nodal areas is in order after completion of the history. The 2-cm lesion in the upper outer quadrant of the right breast in the patient being discussed is not fixed, and there are no overlying skin changes. There is unlikely to be nipple discharge, crusting or eczema-like change of the nipple or areola, and erythema of the breast. The opposite breast and regional nodes are also likely to be normal. Thus, this particular cancer is classified as T_1 (tumors less than or equal to 2.0 cm), N_0 (clinically negative axillary nodes), and M_0 (no overt evidence of distant disease). Clinical staging is a notoriously poor predictor of histologic staging and is being rapidly displaced or augmented by "biologic" staging.

The estimation of clinical tumor size is difficult, especially in premenopausal women. We have observed that 40% of patients thought to be clinically node-negative had, upon histologic examination, one or more positive nodes. Of those thought on physical examination to be clinically node-positive, 25% were found on histologic examination to have no tumor in their axillary nodes. The mass in the patient under discussion is described as firm, but this does not preclude the possibility of a cyst or even a fibroadenoma. Fibroadenomas in a woman of this age are not rare but are routinely excised to preclude the remote possibility of an associated cancer and to eliminate patient anxiety engendered by their presence.

Fine-Needle Aspiration

The next step in establishing the diagnosis of a mass is to perform a fine-needle aspiration. This procedure should be carried out at the time of the initial office visit subsequent to the physical examination. Local anesthesia is rarely employed for such a procedure. We prefer to use a 21-gauge, 1 1/2-in. needle attached to a 20-cc leur-lock syringe. The syringe is fastened to a holder that helps create negative pressure in the syringe while carrying out the aspiration. When cyst fluid is obtained, if the fluid is grossly bloody, if the mass itself does not completely disappear following aspiration, or if the fluid is guaiac positive, it is submitted to a pathologist for cytologic examination. While all fluid aspirated may be submitted for examination, the yield of positive findings is extremely low when the preceding characteristics are absent. Patients who have had cysts aspirated should be reexamined in four to six weeks or sooner should the mass reappear. Repeat aspirations of recurrent cysts are not infrequent, but biopsy must be considered after one or two such procedures.

Should the mass prove to be solid, several passes are made through different planes of the tumor to obtain sufficient and representative material for examination. The contents of the needle and syringe are expelled on a glass slide, smeared, and fixed according to the preference of the cytologist. This technique allows for a rapid and highly accurate diagnosis by an experienced pathologist. Tru-cut or core-needle biopsies are less popular because they are more painful to the patient and often produce a hematoma. They may also fail to obtain samples representative of the tumor mass. Multiple samples from the same mass in small tumors are difficult to obtain by such a technique. Nonetheless, some pathologists prefer to examine and make their diagnosis from material obtained by such biopsies rather than by aspiration cytology.

Let us assume that the patient being discussed has had a fine-needle aspiration and that the smears have been diagnosed as cancer by a pathologist with expertise in cytology. If the material obtained is adequate and properly prepared, the false-negative rate should be low. False-positive results can be encountered, but this too should decrease with the experience of the pathologist. Just as with mammography, a negative cytology in our patient would not preclude proceeding with open biopsy if clinical and/or mammographic findings warrant the effort. Such would seem to be the case in our patient.

Mammography

Subsequent to needle aspiration cytology, all patients should have a bilateral mammogram even if the clinical diagnosis of cancer is obvious. This is done to detect multiple lesions in the same breast or abnormalities in the opposite breast. If a core-needle rather than a fine-needle biopsy is to be done, it is better that the mammogram be carried out before the procedure, since such a biopsy may perturb the breast sufficiently to distort the mammographic findings. Our preference is for xeroradiograms, especially in young women. This technique provides better edge enhancement, allowing for differentiation between normal but dense breast tissue and either benign or malignant tumor masses; also, the chest wall is better visualized. In general, xeroradiography is more comfortable to the patient because less compression is required. Xeroradiograms do deliver a slightly higher radiation dose to the patient, but this is not apt to be clinically significant. Newer developments in xerograms, not yet widely available, reduce the dose to that delivered by film screen studies that, in general, are satisfactory. There are, however, a distressing number of poor-quality film studies being done in this country.

Consequently, a mammogram is obtained in the patient under discussion. It cannot be too strongly emphasized that a negative mammogram in the presence of a palpable mass does not preclude the removal of tissue for making a histologic diagnosis of the lesion. Positive clinical findings often override a negative mammogram relative to patient management. This would be the case in our patient should she have a negative mammogram.

DECISION-MAKING RELATIVE TO THE SURGICAL PROCEDURE

Recently, one of us (BF) has described our recommended strategy for the management of a primary breast cancer. The need for such an algorithm arose following our publication of findings from two clinical trials conducted by the

National Surgical Adjuvant Breast and Bowel Project (NSABP). Results of one of the studies (Protocol B-04) clearly demonstrated that alternative therapies are as efficacious as radical mastectomy. In that study, between 1971 and 1974, 1,600 patients were randomly assigned to radical mastectomy or a total (simple) mastectomy without axillary dissection if they were clinically node-negative. One half of those having a total mastectomy received irradiation to the chest wall and regional lymph nodes. Patients judged clinically node-positive were randomized to be treated by either a radical mastectomy or a total mastectomy and regional radiation. After 12 years of follow-up, there was no significant difference in disease-free survival, distant disease-free survival, or survival among the three node-negative patient groups and the two node-positive patient groups. Aside from indicating no advantage for radical mastectomy, the findings of that study confirm previous findings indicating that postoperative regional radiation following mastectomy, while slightly decreasing the incidence of local and regional recurrence, does not affect survival. Irradiation of internal mammary nodes has not been demonstrated to improve survival in this or any other study. Moreover, there is no justification for axillary radiation if an axillary dissection has been carried out. Another important finding from that trial indicates that through ten years of follow-up, only 4% of patients developed a cancer in the opposite breast, an incidence considerably less than the 1% per year risk often quoted by others but one that is in keeping with our own findings from a previous trial. We do not biopsy (random or mirror-image) the opposite breast unless there is clinical or mammographic justification.

The early results of Protocol B-04 provided justification for beginning another study in 1976 (Protocol B-06) to determine the worth of lumpectomy (segmental mastectomy). In that trial, 2,200 women having breast cancers less than or equal to 4 cm with no skin fixation or evidence of skin involvement were randomly assigned to receive a modified mastectomy or a lumpectomy and axillary dissection with or without breast radiation. Both clinically axillary node-negative or positive-node patients were eligible. A lumpectomy was defined as removal of the tumor together with an adequate amount of fat or normal breast tissue so that the resected specimen margins were histologically free of tumor. The precise extent of this "free margin" was not mandated. Axillary dissections removing at least the lower two levels of nodes were carried out through separate incisions to improve the cosmetic outcome. We emphasize that axillary *dissection*, rather than axillary *sampling*, is the procedure carried out with resection of the two lowest levels of nodes. In our trial, it was required that a mastectomy be performed if specimen margins free of tumors could not be obtained or if there was a recurrence of tumor in the ipsilateral breast subsequent to lumpectomy.

The published five-year results and the unreported seven-year findings continue to indicate that there is no difference in survival among any of the three treatment groups. Recurrence of tumor in the operated breast has been observed in approximately 30% of those treated by lumpectomy without radiation, in comparison to 8% in those receiving breast radiation. Radiation administered only to the breast and not to regional nodes seems to be of benefit; we have not defined a group that should not receive local irradiation following lumpectomy. No interstitial radiation or external beam boost was employed. Radiation therapy was begun within a few weeks of lumpectomy when wound healing had occurred. The time of radiation administration may vary relative to the type of systemic adjuvant therapy employed. Axillary node-positive patients received adjuvant chemotherapy.

The results of our study, as well as those reported by Veronesi et al. from a trial conducted by the National Cancer Institute of Milan in a subset of patients ($T_1N_0M_0$) treated by quadrantectomy, have led us to conclude that lumpectomy and axillary dissection followed by breast radiation is the optimal choice for the local-regional treatment of almost all tumors less than or equal to 4 cm. Consequently, it would seem that the patient under discussion is an ideal candidate for such treatment should she have a cancer.

Referring to our previously mentioned algorithm, if the result of this patient's needle biopsy was positive and she was judged suitable for breast conservation, we would proceed with a lumpectomy and axillary dissection using general anesthesia. If her cytology was nondiagnostic or negative, but her clinical and/or mammographic findings were suspicious for cancer, we would perform her biopsy as if it were a lumpectomy, i.e., with the patient under general anesthesia so that an adequate amount of tissue could be excised to ensure free margins. Should frozen section confirm the diagnosis of cancer, then the axillary dissection could be carried out, avoiding a second procedure.

We cannot too strongly emphasize that in all patients with tumors that can be treated by breast conservation, if needle biopsy cannot be done and an open biopsy is performed, it must be carried out as if a lumpectomy were being performed. If it is performed without paying attention to specimen margins, it is an inappropriate biopsy. Thus, the operation carried out to establish the diagnosis becomes the definitive treatment of the breast. (*Editor's note:* This is an important point that has not received sufficient emphasis. Inadequate excisional biopsies carried out under less than ideal conditions probably contribute to a relatively high incidence of local recurrence seen in certain series.)

A FEW TECHNICAL CONSIDERATIONS

In all lumpectomies, which include diagnostic excisional biopsies, make the incision directly over the mass regardless of its location. Avoid circumareolar incisions and "tunneling" to distant masses. Curvilinear incisions in the upper or lower half of the breast produce satisfactory cosmesis. Do not undermine skin flaps, and removal of skin is undesirable. Employ meticulous hemostasis and make no attempt to obliterate "dead space" by approximating breast tissue or fat. No drain is placed in the operative site. Subcutaneous fat is approximated and the skin is closed by use of a fine continuous subcutaneous suture.

The presence of a pathologist at the time of biopsy is desirable. In addition to establishing the diagnosis and obtaining a tumor aliquot for hormonal receptor analysis, the pathologist can aid in deciding whether specimen margins are free of tumor. If gross tumor is seen to be close to the resected specimen margin, additional tissue is immediately removed from the area in question. Multiple frozen sections of margins are not routinely done, as specimen margins grossly tumor-free rarely will be found to contain microscopic tumor.

SYSTEMIC ADJUVANT THERAPY

Should our patient receive systemic therapy? While breast conservation procedures have been shown to be equivalent to breast removal, they have not improved prognosis. Only with systemic therapy is that apt to be accomplished.

Chemotherapy or chemo-hormonal therapies have repeatedly demonstrated an alteration in the natural history of this disease, with an improvement in disease-free survival and survival. A recent NIH Consensus Panel reviewed the use of adjuvant therapy for breast cancer. They recommended the routine use of combination chemotherapy for node-positive premenopausal women. In postmenopausal node-positive women who have positive hormone receptors, tamoxifen, an oral anti-estrogen, was the recommended treatment. For node-negative patients and node-positive postmenopausal women with negative receptors, adjuvant treatment was not recommended but could be considered in women at increased risk of recurrence. The panel emphasized the need for entering all eligible patients into ongoing clinical trials. We strongly agree with this recommendation. Although improvements in breast cancer treatment have occurred largely as a result of clinical trials, optimal therapy is yet to be achieved.

BIBLIOGRAPHY

1. Fisher B: Reappraisal of breast biopsy prompted by the use of lumpectomy: A position paper on surgical strategy. *JAMA* 1985; 253:3585–3588.
2. Fisher B, Bauer M, Margolese R, et al: Five-year results of a randomized clinical trial comparing total mastectomy and segmental mastectomy with or without radiation in the treatment of breast cancer. *N Engl J Med* 1985; 312:665–673.
3. Fisher B, Redmond C, Fisher ER, et al: Ten-year results of a randomized clinical trial comparing radical mastectomy and total mastectomy with or without radiation. *N Engl J Med* 1985; 312:674–681.
4. Fisher B, Wolmark N, Fisher E, et al: Lumpectomy and axillary dissection for breast cancer: Surgical, pathologic and radiation consideration. *World J Surg* 1985; 9:692–698.

5. National Institutes of Health: Consensus Development Conference on Adjuvant Chemotherapy for Breast Cancer, Sept 9–11, 1985. Bethesda, Md, US Department of Health and Human Services, Public Health Service, National Institutes of Health, Vol 5, No. 12, 1986.
6. Veronesi U, Saccozzi R, Del Vecchio M, et al: Comparing radical mastectomy with quadrantectomy, axillary dissection and radiotherapy in patients with small cancers of the breast. *N Engl J Med* 1981; 305:6.

10

Bilateral Carcinomas In Situ

A 46-year-old woman undergoes routine mammography because of a strong family history of breast carcinoma in a mother and sister. Although there is no lesion palpable, there are suspicious microcalcifications in identical areas in both breasts.

Consultant: Donna L. Stahl, M.D.

This case represents a very difficult management problem for breast surgeons today because there is no common agreement among surgeons on how to treat preinvasive cancer of the breast, with a wide disparity of surgical options ranging from radical mastectomy to follow-up alone. This report will examine both lobular carcinoma in situ and intraductal carcinoma, describe in detail their natural history, and present treatment options. A conclusion will be reached on how to treat this patient that most likely will not meet with universal agreement. Please note that the term "minimal breast cancer" has been purposely avoided to exclude any type of primary invasive disease in this discussion.

TERMINOLOGY

Lobular carcinoma in situ (LCIS) and intraductal cancer (IDC) are both considered noninvasive diseases. Other descriptive terms include "intraepithelial cancer" and "preinvasive cancer." Although there may be gray areas, the basic criteria for the histologic diagnosis of these preinvasive cancers have been accepted (Figs 10–1 and 10–2). The established histopathologic diagnosis is based on the fact that there is no evidence of tumor involvement beyond the basement membrane as seen in the light microscope. Yet, Fisher et al. did find that the integrity of the basement membrane in intraductal carcinoma may not be a reliable indicator of invasive disease, since a defect in that membrane may be found upon electron microscopy. In spite of this problem, it is indeed important that we strive to obtain an accurate diagnosis since there are differences in the biologic behavior between these two cancers—both in the propensity to invasion and in ultimate prognosis. Both of these factors will be discussed.

With the increased use of mammograms and with the expansion of screening programs, earlier and smaller cancers are being detected. The patient under

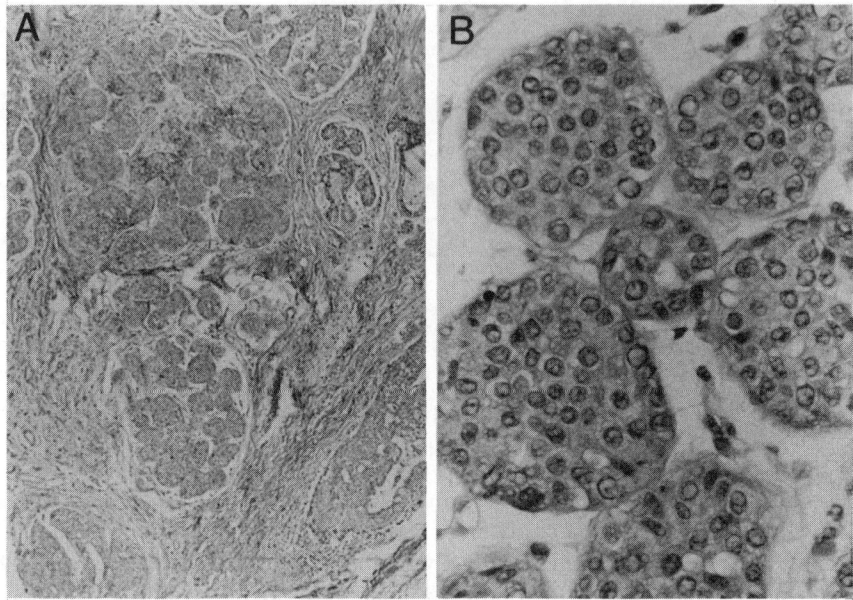

FIG 10-1.
Lobular carcinoma in situ. **A,** note swollen acini of varying size in lobule filled with neoplastic cells. **B,** higher magnification of acini shows contrast between small, uniform, hyperchromatic nuclei in center and more pleomorphic cells with larger nuclei.

discussion illustrates the benefits of mammogram when lesions are found that are nonpalpable. In the NCI-ACS Breast Cancer Detection Demonstration Project reported in 1982, 38% of the cancers found on screening mammography were less than 1 cm, and 68% of these cancers were noninvasive (81% intraductal, 19% lobular carcinoma in situ). The National Breast Cancer Survey of the American College of Surgeons collected data from 498 hospitals in 1978 and found that the incidence of noninvasive carcinomas in resected specimens in the lobular and ductal group was 3.2%. Thus, screening mammography, which has come into widespread use since that report, has certainly increased the percentage of earlier cancers being found.

In regard to this case presentation, there are two principal areas that must be addressed: (1) establishing the diagnosis; and (2) selecting the proper treatment.

DIAGNOSIS

Since the lesions found on mammogram in this patient were nonpalpable, bilateral needle localizations should be performed to ensure excision of the suspicious area. This is usually done on an outpatient basis with the patient under local anesthesia (with or without sedation) or under general anesthesia. I prefer general anesthesia when both breasts are to be biopsied. After the lesion has been removed, the specimen must be radiographed to ensure that the suspicious calcifications have been removed (Fig 10–3). Because the tissue is generally soft and the involved area may be small in caliber, the pathologist will usually defer a firm diagnosis for 24 hours. In fact, at the Institut Gustave Roussy, the histologic diagnosis of noninfiltrating cancer by frozen section has been shown by Jotti and associates to be unreliable: it is sensitive in only 30% for IDC and 0% for LCIS. Even when the removal of the calcifications have been confirmed, the remaining breast tissue must be carefully examined and palpated, as Hutter stated that the calcifications in LCIS may not be the true cancer. The malignant lesion may be situated close to the calcifications but not included in the suspicious area found on mammogram.

TREATMENT

Next, one must select the best treatment once the diagnosis of preinvasive cancer has been made. The proper therapy of preinvasive breast cancer is based upon a working, accurate knowledge of the natural history of this disease. Four principal features will be discussed in relationship to this natural history: (1) multicentricity, (2) bilaterality, (3) evolution of preinvasion to invasion, and (4) the risks of invasive cancer.

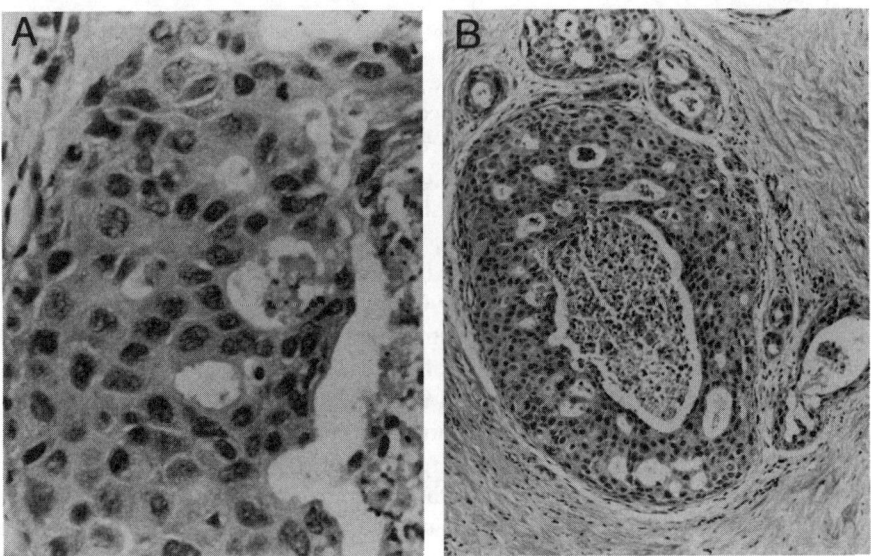

FIG 10–2.
Intraductal carcinoma. Note the frequent abnormal miotic figures and variation in cell size and shape.

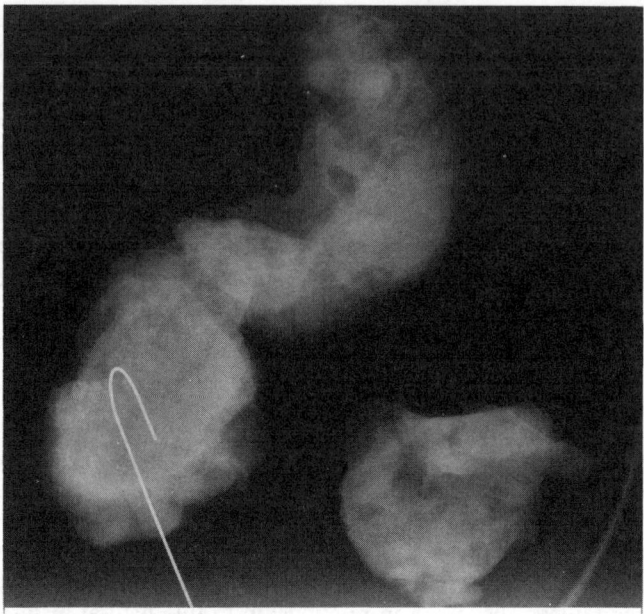

FIG 10–3.
Example of a radiographed needle localization specimen. Calcifications near the curve of the wire represent lobular carcinoma in situ.

Multicentricity

Preinvasive breast cancer should not be considered only a focal problem. It is a diffuse disease. Multicentricity may occur in both IDC and LCIS. (Please note that there is a difference between the terms multicentricity and multifocal; multicentricity describes the disease in other quadrants of the breast, while multifocal disease relates only to the local biopsy site itself.) During the 1970s and 1980s, various studies described extensive sectioning of mastectomy specimens following a biopsy for preinvasive cancer. A frequently cited report is that by Rosen from Memorial Sloan-Kettering Cancer Center in 1981. In a consecutive series of 53 patients having biopsy-proved intraductal carcinoma, multicentric preinvasive cancer was found in 34 (64%) of the cases. Six percent of patients had foci of invasion in other quadrants, and 94% was of the infiltrating ductal type.

In 1982, Lagios and associates quoted an incidence of about 32% multicentricity with IDC and a 21% overall frequency of occult invasion. They made a significant contribution to the understanding of multicentricity when they described the importance of size differentiation. Twenty-four cases had tumors 2.5 cm or larger in diameter; of these, 13 (54%) had multicentric foci. In contrast, of 29 cases in which lesions were less than 2.5 cm in size, 4 (14%) were multicentric. Therefore, the larger lesions showed a greater likelihood of multicentricity. This feature of preinvasive breast cancer is very perplexing to surgeons. How can they rationally abandon a total mastectomy in favor of breast salvage while realizing that multicentricity is present?

In regard to LCIS patients, Rosen reported on a consecutive series of 122 biopsies with preinvasive cancer. Mastectomies were performed in 103 of these cases. Residual preinvasive cancer involved quadrants other than the biopsy site in 60% of patients with LCIS; the lesions consisted of LCIS in 88% of these cases. Invasive cancer was found in 4%. In 1984, Hutter reported similar results when he described a 60% to 90% rate of multicentricity in mastectomy specimens for LCIS, with a 4% to 6% invasive cancer elsewhere in the breast.

Bilaterality

Since multicentricity can exist in one breast, then what of the other side? Having recently summarized four case series, Jotti and associates reported a bilateral percentage of LCIS at 42.4% and IDC at 13.4% (simultaneous or subsequent). They also stated that if contralateral biopsies were negative, subsequent contralateral carcinomas were rare. Other reports, including a recent study by Frykberg et al., have cited a bilateral percentage in LCIS as high as 69%. The mirror-image nature of bilaterality in lobular carcinoma is well appreciated. In fact, if there is no localizing sign in the contralateral breast, a blind biopsy may be taken of the upper outer quadrant since 60% of the breast tissue is located there. On the other hand, a mirror-image biopsy is recommended if the original biopsy site is other than the upper outer quadrant, since 40% of contralateral malignant disease will be found upon biopsy.

Route of Preinvasion to Invasion

Once the diagnosis of in situ cancer has been made, can this progress to a more invasive type? It does seem logical in IDC, since intraductal components may be appreciated in at least three fourths of all invasive cancers of the breast. In 1969, Gallager and Martin described a hypothetical progression of intraductal carcinoma in which epithelial hyperplasia led to atypical hyperplasia to a latent or static stage and finally to frank invasion. This progression may be nonobligate or discontinuous. In contrast, lobular carcinoma in situ is a risk marker for the formation of cancer in that breast rather than a precursor lesion per se, and, interestingly, when a patient with LCIS develops an invasive cancer, it is usually of the ductal type. It is proposed that IDC and LCIS may coexist in the same breast. Since it is estimated that it takes LCIS up to 20 years to become clinically detectable, the ductal form may appear over a shorter period of time. Hence, an infiltrating ductal cancer may emerge in this breast earlier than infiltrating lobular cancer.

Risks of Invasion

What is the risk of invasive breast cancer developing in a patient who has had preinvasive cancer of the breast upon biopsy? Rosen demonstrated a progression of ipsilateral invasive cancer occurring in about 40% of patients who had prior breast biopsies positive for IDC, a progression that occurred over an average of ten years of follow-up. In addition, in 1982, Page and associates stated that 28% of patients treated with biopsy alone (without wide excision) developed invasive cancer in the ipsilateral breast in a 15-year follow-up period.

The transition in lobular carcinoma in situ was longer. In 1967, McDivitt and associates described the total risk of developing a homolateral lobular invasive cancer as 15% at 10 years and 35% at 20 years. In 1981, Rosen estimated that it would take up to 20 years for lobular carcinoma in situ to change into an invasive cancer. He studied 77 patients at risk to develop subsequent breast cancer for a total of 1,789 patient years. In that group of 77 cases, 28 were ultimately found to have cancer. This is a ninefold increase in the frequency risk associated with LCIS over that of an age-matched control population from the Connecticut Tumor Registry, and death from breast cancer was 10.7 times more frequent than expected. In 1982, Tulusan and associates quoted a surprisingly high 16% rate of subsequent invasive cancer within 24 months of a diagnosis of LCIS, although some of these were very small occult cancers.

RECURRENCE

Appreciating the problems of multicentric foci, local recurrences following biopsies, cancer transformation, and the presence of occult invasive cancers, surgeons have frequently included mastectomies in their treatment strategies for preinvasive breast cancer. Various nonrandomized studies have examined cure rates after mastectomies. In 1978, Betsill and associates found a 98% cure rate in their mastectomy patients for IDC. In the Brigham experience reported by von Rueden and Wilson, there were no failures following mastectomy in a group of 45 patients. Yet, when the American College of Surgeons compared their five-year cure rates for radical and conservative surgery, the results were similar. For LCIS, the cure rates were as follows: wedge resection, 80.6%; total mastectomy, 77.3%; and radical surgery, 92.2%. For IDC, similar results were obtained: wedge resection, 66.7%; total mastectomy, 62.2%; and radical surgery, 71.5%. In addition, the recurrence rate at five years in noninvasive cancer was similar, with conservative surgery at 7.0% and radical surgery at 7.7%. It should be noted that the recurrence rate was 5% higher in IDC (10.4%) than in LCIS (2.5%). I must emphasize that these are five-year results only; this is not considered long-term follow-up.

Today, with the trend toward more conservative surgery for small invasive breast cancers, it is inevitable that the question of breast salvage and radiation for preinvasive disease is raised, i.e., whether radiation treatment can ultimately control this local disease. Danoff conducted a prospective, nonrandomized study of 40 patients with intraductal carcinoma from 1976 to 1983. Patients were treated with breast salvage and radiation treatments in which 5,000 rads was given to the breast and 1,000 rads was given as a boost to the primary. After five years, the recurrence rate was about 10%. It should be noted that three recurrences of central primaries in this study occurred only among those four patients who presented with a nipple discharge. In addition, there is an ongoing prospective, randomized clinical trial underway by the National Surgical Adjuvant Breast Project (NSABP) comparing women who have had segmental mastectomy with or without radiation treatment.

SURGICAL APPROACH

The patient described is essentially perimenopausal and has a strong family history of breast cancer. Let us first propose that the breast biopsy demonstrated bilateral lobular carcinoma in situ, since there is a mirror-image finding. In regards to LCIS, a family history of malignant disease of the breast is found in 15% to 20% of the patients, which is the same as women who have had invasive cancer of the breast. This patient may be offered the following treatment options on her ipsilateral breast:

1. No further surgery, if the needle localization margins are clear.
2. Conservative surgical procedures: Wide reexcision or quadrantectomy with or without axillary node dissection, with or without radiation treatment or breast reduction.
3. Aggressive surgical approach: Radical mastectomy, modified radical mastectomy, simple mastectomy with or without low axillary node dissection, or subcutaneous mastectomy with or without reconstruction.

What of the contralateral breast? The options would appear to be the same for LCIS in the second breast. In view of this patient's age and family risk, I would recommend a bilateral simple mastectomy with low axillary node dissection (Level I) with or without immediate breast reconstruction. If the breasts are small or moderate in size, the nipple may be removed, preserving a considerable amount of skin, which makes immediate breast reconstruction more feasible.

Why low axillary node dissection? Axillary metastasis can occur in about 1% of patients with preinvasive cancer when invasion has not been demonstrated. Specifically, Jotti and associates reported a 1.7% axillary node involvement in IDC and a 2.8% node involvement in LCIS.

Certainly, the other options may be offered to this patient as listed. Yet, she must be fully informed of the risks that accompany her decision, particularly if follow-up alone is chosen. Even our best attempts at follow-up may not be enough. Remember that in 50% of all instances of LCIS, there may be no x-ray film findings whatsoever. Therefore, much of the follow-up may depend on clinical grounds alone. Also remember, however, that metastasis may occur within the first 10 to 20 doubling times at which the stage of cancer is not even detectable.

What if the biopsies returned intraductal carcinoma? From the data presented, there would seem to be a high risk for invasive cancer at a future date. Lagios and associates have attempted to list characteristics of patients who are at higher risk to evolve into an invasive form of ductal carcinoma: (1) tumors greater than 2.5 cm in diameter; (2) nodular breasts that are difficult to evaluate by palpation; (3) multiple microcalcifications present on the mammogram; and (4) significant family history and/or contralateral breast cancer. I might add that nipple discharge and a central tumor may indicate a high recurrence problem, as noted in the Danoff study. While Lagios and associates would offer this patient a mastectomy, they would offer limited breast surgery to patients who meet the following criteria: (1) tumors 2.5 cm or less in extent, with evidence that the surgical resection encompasses the tumor; (2) the breasts are very easy to palpate; (3) there is low radiographic density; and (4) there are no risk factors present.

Applying the criteria used by Lagios and associates to the described patient, I would recommend bilateral simple mastectomy with low axillary node dissection (Level I) with or without immediate breast reconstruction. In this situation, I believe it is imperative to remove the nipple, due to the risk of possible cancer involvement of the nipple in the future.

As one can see from the list of surgical options available to patients, there is not just one "best" treatment modality. The patient must be evaluated on an individual basis. The final decision must take into consideration the patient's psychological makeup. If she has a great fear of ultimately developing an invasive breast cancer and finds it difficult to save her breasts, then mastectomy would be the best procedure to perform. On the other hand, if she is stoic, has focal noninvasive cancers, and wishes breast salvage, then conservative surgery would seem to be the better choice. Regardless of the decision, a final plea is made that both the patient and the family be informed of any risks that are involved in whatever decision is made.

For the future, more scientific work remains to be done in preinvasive breast cancer. More randomized, prospective studies will help to further define the optimal treatment for patients with preinvasive breast cancer.

Acknowledgment

I want to thank Dr. John A. Wirman, Associate Professor of Pathology, for his help with the pathology photographs.

BIBLIOGRAPHY

1. Baker LH: Breast Cancer Detection Demonstration Project: Five-year summary report. *Cancer J for Clinicians* 1982; 32:194–225.
2. Betsill WL Jr, Rosen PP, Lieberman PH, et al: Intraductal carcinoma: Long-term follow-up after treatment by biopsy alone. *JAMA* 1978; 239:1863–1867.
3. Fisher ER, Sass R, Fisher B, et al: Pathologic findings from the National Surgical Adjuvant Breast Project (Protocol 6): I. Intraductal carcinoma (DCIS). *Cancer* 1986; 57:197–208.
4. Frykberg ER, Santiago F, Betsill WL Jr, et al: Lobular carcinoma in situ of the breast. *Surg Gynecol Obstet* 1987; 164:285–301.
5. Gallager HS, Martin JE: Early phases in the development of breast cancer. *Cancer* 1969; 24:1170–1178.
6. Hutter RVP: The management of patients with lobular carcinoma in situ of the breast. *Cancer* 1984; 53:798–802.
7. Jotti GS, Petit JY, Contesso G: Minimal breast cancer: A clinically meaningful term? *Semin Oncol* 1986; 13:384–392.
8. Lagios MD, Westdahl PR, Margolin FR, et al: Duct carcinoma in situ: Relationship of extent of noninvasive disease to the frequency of occult invasion, multicentricity, lymph node metastases, and short-term treatment failures. *Cancer* 1982; 50:1309–1314.
9. McDivitt RW, Hutter RVP, Foote FW Jr, et al: In situ lobular carcinoma: A prospective follow-up study indicating cumulative patient risks. *JAMA* 1967; 201:96–100.
10. Page DL, Dupont WD, Rogers LW, et al: Intraductal carcinoma of the breast: Follow-up after biopsy only. *Cancer* 1982; 49:751–758.
11. Recht A, Danoff BS, Solin LJ, et al: Intraductal carcinoma of the breast: Results of treatment with excisional biopsy and irradiation. *J Clin Oncol* 1985; 3:1339–1343.
12. Rosen PP, Braun DW Jr, Kinne DE: The clinical significance of preinvasive breast carcinoma. *Cancer* 1980; 46:919–925.
13. Rosen PP: Clinical implications of preinvasive and small invasive breast carcinomas. *Pathol Annu* 1981; 16:337–356.
14. Rosner D, Bedwani RN, Vana J, et al: Noninvasive breast carcinoma: Results of a national survey by the American College of Surgeons. *Ann Surg* 1980; 192:139–147.
15. Tulusan AH, Egger H, Schneider ML, et al: A contribution to the natural history of breast cancer: IV. Lobular carcinoma in situ and its relationship to breast cancer. *Arch Gynecol* 1982; 231:219–226.
16. von Rueden DG, Wilson RE: Intraductal carcinoma of the breast. *Surg Gynecol Obstet* 1984; 158:105–111.

PART II

Gastric

11

Perforated Duodenal Ulcer

A 60-year-old man develops sudden, severe epigastric pain three hours prior to admission. His physical examination reveals board-like rigidity of the abdomen and absent bowel sounds. For the past 12 years, he had intermittent epigastric pain relieved by antacids and food. He had a history of 40-pack-years of cigarette smoking and was known to use alcohol, even though his pain was aggravated by both. His stool is guaiac negative and his temperature is 101° F.

Consultant: Paul H. Jordan, Jr., M.D.

DISCUSSION

The severe epigastric pain and board-like rigidity of the abdomen certainly suggest the presence of peritoneal irritation, and the suddenness of the onset indeed points to peritonitis resulting from a ruptured viscus. On this basis, one might make the diagnosis of an "acute" abdomen and recommend operation. Although this course of action would be correct in most instances, I believe that the surgeon must commit to a specific diagnosis preoperatively. To do less results in the surgeon's thought processes becoming dull. The thoughtful evaluation required to make a precise diagnosis in a patient with an acute abdomen is necessary to avoid overlooking aspects of a case that have important bearing on its management. (*Editor's note:* I agree wholeheartedly with Dr. Jordan; the essence of making the correct preoperative diagnosis is in the best interest of the patient, both from the standpoint of allowing the surgeon to review alternative surgical procedures and operative tactics prior to operation, as well as allowing emotional and material preparation for complex and/or prolonged procedures. Nonetheless, the essence of surgical decision-making, especially with respect to the acute abdomen, I believe to be as follows: (1) Does this patient require operation? (2) If so, when? (3) What incision should I use? (4) What am I likely to find?)

Attempting to solve the mysteries of the acute abdomen provides the surgeon with one of the most exhilarating exercises to hone his diagnostic acumen. Bacon, in his essay on Delay, had this to say: "A correct diagnosis is the basis of firm counsel. To obtain this there is surely no greater wisdom than when to time the beginning and onset of things. The dextrous hand must not be allowed to reach before the imperfect judgment.''

The most common presentation of a perforated peptic ulcer is heralded by an abrupt onset of severe epigastric pain that rapidly involves the abdomen; the pain causes most patients to seek medical attention within 6 to 12 hours. Evidence of peritonitis is manifested by the appearance of an acutely ill patient who complains bitterly of pain and who avoids movement and resists examination because to do so exacerbates the pain. In the elderly, a more benign pain pattern and a paucity of findings can deceive the patient and the physician, causing delayed treatment of the abdominal catastrophe.

The abdomen is rigid and diffusely tender to gentle examination, but perhaps maximally tender in the epigastrium. The findings are modified by the degree of contamination and resulting inflammation within the abdomen. This in turn is dependent on the size of the perforation, the amount of gastric contents at the time of perforation, the elapsed time after perforation, and whether the perforation sealed spontaneously.

The extent to which the peritoneal surfaces are exposed to gastrointestinal contents will determine the severity of the peritonitis (the "chemical burn") and the loss of fluid from the intravascular space. When patients are first seen, they may have a deceptively normal pulse rate and blood pressure, and the severity of their illness may be underestimated. With longer intervals of time after perforation, the patient may develop hypovolemia, shock, and anuria. Leukocytosis develops rapidly. The serum amylase level may increase two to three times the normal value due to peritoneal absorption of salivary and pancreatic amylase after spillage of gastrointestinal contents into the peritoneal cavity.

In this case, the diagnosis of a perforated peptic ulcer suggested by the history and physical examination would have been supported had we been told that intra-abdominal air was present. This can be suspected by the loss of liver dullness on percussion and confirmed by the demonstration of a pneumoperitoneum on an upright chest or left lateral decubitus x-ray film. Pneumoperitoneum can be demonstrated in 60% to 85% of patients with a perforated peptic ulcer. Support for the diagnosis of a perforated ulcer can also be obtained if orally administered diatrizoate meglumine (Gastrografin) is seen in the abdominal cavity on radiographic study.

In view of the history and physical findings, this case seems to represent a straightforward perforated viscus, most likely a perforated ulcer. The diagnosis is not always so obvious and one must consider other diagnoses such as pancreatitis, perforated cholecystitis, diverticulitis, or appendicitis. An ulcer that seals spontaneously soon after perforation or one that perforates and is contained in the lesser sac may defy accurate diagnosis. Peritoneal aspiration of a cloudy, bile-stained fluid, positive for amylase, will be helpful in establishing a diagnosis of peritonitis, but it is not specific for perforated ulcer. Even intraperitoneal air is not specific for perforated ulcer, but usually the amount of air is smaller when it results from perforations of the gastrointestinal tract other than the stomach and duodenum.

TREATMENT OPTIONS

Treatment options are initially whether to operate or not to operate. Since the initial recognition of perforated ulcers, nonoperative treatment has been one method for their management. As Fronmuller, who first described the Heineke-Mikulicz pyloroplasty, pointed out, nonoperative treatment was a method of euthanasia since in his day everyone treated in this way died. This remains the situation today because of the seriously ill patients who are usually relegated to this therapy. In the opinion of most authors, nonoperative treatment is not the method of choice for healthy individuals, nor can it be expected to save the lives of patients who are literally dead when first seen. Nonoperative treatment may benefit an occasional patient too ill for operation even though the ulcer is not sealed, but it is difficult to identify this potentially small number of patients.

Most patients with perforated duodenal ulcer are treated by simple closure of the perforation or by a primary definitive operation. A definitive operation not only takes care of the immediate problem of perforation, but also provides protection against the occurrence of further ulcer disease. The major controversy concerning treatment of perforated ulcer is which of these two methods is best.

Surgeons who prefer definitive therapy usually reserve this form of therapy for patients with "chronic" ulcers and simple closure for those with "acute" ulcers. The patient under discussion clearly conforms to one with a chronic ulcer. Unfortunately, the differentiation between acute and chronic ulcers cannot always be so easily made. This is partly due to a lack of consensus by different authors as to what constitutes a chronic ulcer history. Our ability at the time of perforation to differentiate between acute or chronic ulcers based on the duration of ulcer symptoms is further compromised because the patient's past history of pain fades into insignificance when compared with the pain caused by perforation. At the operating table, the surgeon can attempt to distinguish between an acute and chronic ulcer on the basis of duodenal deformity and induration surrounding the perforation. The inflammation caused by peritoneal contamination frequently makes this distinction imprecise. We remain unconvinced of the reliability of our differentiation into acute and chronic perforated duodenal ulcers or of the utility of selecting the method of operative treatment based on such a differentiation.

In some series of acute ulcers, as many as 75% of patients have no further ulcer symptoms after simple closure of a perforation. In these studies, 25% of patients continue to have symptoms that may require subsequent definitive treatment. In the case of chronic ulcers, it is the reverse; 75% of patients have subsequent ulcer symptoms following simple closure, and 35% to 60% require reoperation. These results suggest that the surgeon's chance of identifying the patient with an acute ulcer who will benefit or the chronic ulcer patient who will not benefit from primary definitive treatment is poor.

SIMPLE CLOSURE VS. DEFINITIVE TREATMENT

Simple closure is preferred by most surgeons for all patients who represent an increased operative risk. Many surgeons consider it safer than a definitive operation even for a good-risk chronic ulcer patient, such as the patient under discussion, even though many of these patients will require reoperation.

In a prospective study, Boey et al. evaluated major medical illnesses, preoperative shock and long-standing perforation (more than 24 hours) as risk factors affecting mortality following surgery for perforated ulcers. The mortality rate increased progressively with increasing numbers of risk factors: 0%, 10%, 45.5%, and 100% in patients with 0, 1, 2, and 3 risk factors, respectively. Simple closure is therefore more prudent than definitive surgery if any risk factor is present. The available evidence suggests that in the absence of risk factors, the mortality rates following simple closure and definitive surgery are the same and should be less than 2%.

As indicated previously, we lack the criteria for precise selection of patients likely to benefit from definitive operation. To illustrate this point, one author believes that if one excludes men between 40 to 60 years of age, only 18% of patients with perforated chronic duodenal ulcers will ever require definitive surgical treatment. On the other hand, others believe that patients who perforate before the age of 30 are most likely to have recurrent ulcer symptoms.

In my opinion, there is no satisfactory way to select precisely at the time of perforation those patients who will eventually require or benefit from definitive therapy. Previous ulcer symptoms and the presence or absence of a chronic ulcer are not accurate predictors of the need for definitive ulcer operation. For this reason and because of the fact that operative mortality for definitive surgery and simple closure is equal in patients without risk factors, we recommend definitive operation for all perforated ulcer patients who are without risk factors. We estimate that 25% of our patients with perforated duodenal ulcer are best treated by simple closure because of the presence of significant risk factors. Age is a contraindication to definitive surgery only in the sense that coexisting severe disease that contraindicates such treatment occurs with increasing frequency with advancing age.

Simple Closure

The traditional treatment of perforated duodenal ulcer is surgical closure of the perforation, copious irrigation of the peritoneal cavity, and use of an antibiotic with broad coverage. The techniques used to effect closure include plication, abutment, or the use of a free or vascularized omental patch. Our choice is to fashion carefully a vascularized tongue of omentum that will reach to the perforation without tension that might cause rotation and obstruction of the duodenum. To avoid any encroachment on the pyloric lumen, the patch is held in place by a ring of interrupted sutures, rather than by imbricating sutures tied over the omental patch. The latter technique may constrict the pyloric lumen. (*Editor's note:* Agreed! For some reason, the message that "plication" (imbrication of the ulcer) often results in duodenal obstruction is difficult to convey, and many patients suffer prolonged duodenal obstruction.)

Definitive Surgery

DeBakey's initial report gave impetus to definitive surgery, and his subsequent reports demonstrated that resection in properly selected patients can be performed with a mortality of 1%. Most authors agree that antrectomy or hemigastrectomy and vagotomy are the best operations to prevent recurrent ulcer and, from this point of view, might be the best operation for the patient under discussion. Unfortunately, these operations are associated with a number of undesirable postoperative gastric sequelae, including dumping, diarrhea, early satiety, reflux gastritis, and weight loss, to name a few. These symptoms are deterrents to our use of the conventional definitive operations because they might occur in some patients operated on for perforated ulcer who might never have developed ulcer symptoms or required definitive operation. Postgastrectomy sequelae can be of greater concern to patients than their ulcer complaints and loom especially large if ulcer symptoms before operation were minimal or nonexistent.

At one time, truncal vagotomy and a pyloroplasty that incorporated the perforation were considered a more acceptable operation than vagotomy and hemigastrectomy for perforated duodenal ulcer. This operation was considered technically easier and therefore safer than vagotomy and hemigastrectomy. It was also expected that gastric sequelae would be less frequent and less severe than those following vagotomy and hemigastrectomy. Two randomized, prospective studies compared simple closure with vagotomy and pyloroplasty for treatment of perforated duodenal ulcer. After simple closure, subsequent operation was necessary in 17% and 33% of patients in the two studies. By contrast, after vagotomy and pyloroplasty the reoperation rate was 6% in both studies. In a prospective, randomized study to compare truncal vagotomy and drainage with vagotomy and hemigastrectomy in the treatment of perforated duodenal ulcer, the operative mortality was 0% and 2% and the reoperation rate was 6% and 2%, respectively. Unfortunately, the frequency of dumping, diarrhea, and weight loss was essentially the same after both operations.

Clearly, recurrent ulcers were less frequent after truncal vagotomy and pyloroplasty than after simple closure. However, the postoperative gastric sequelae were no less after truncal vagotomy and pyloroplasty than after truncal vagotomy and hemigastrectomy, and the recurrent ulcer rate was greater. Truncal vagotomy and pyloroplasty as well as truncal vagotomy and hemigastrectomy are acceptable definitive operations for perforated duodenal ulcer. The choice should depend on existing technical factors that govern the relative safety of the two operations. However, both operations are associated with an unacceptable rate of gastric sequelae for those patients who would not have required a definitive operation to prevent return of ulcer symptoms.

The ideal operation for definitive treatment of perforated duodenal ulcers should have a negligible mortality, provide protection against recurrent ulcer, and not inflict undesirable gastric sequelae if it is performed on patients who would not have required definitive treatment to prevent recurrent ulcers. Based on excellent results obtained with parietal cell vagotomy in the elective treatment of duodenal ulcers, it was logical to evaluate this operation for the treatment of perforated duodenal ulcers.

In a prospective, randomized study by Boey et al. in 1982, recurrent symptoms occurred in 9% and reoperation was required in 6% of patients after truncal vagotomy and pyloroplasty, compared with 3% recurrence of symptoms and no reoperations after parietal cell vagotomy. In a prospective study by Ceneviva et al. in 1986, there was a 5% recurrence rate after parietal cell vagotomy compared with a 58% recurrence rate after simple closure.

We treated 88 patients with perforated ulcers by parietal cell vagotomy and closure of the perforation with an omental patch (Fig 11–1), without consideration as to whether the ulcers were acute or chronic. There was one operative death and a recurrent ulcer rate of 6%. Numerous other studies, including our own, support the low recurrence rate and the virtual absence of undesirable gastric sequelae and mortality after parietal cell vagotomy. For these reasons, I would have considered the patient under discussion an ideal candidate for partietal cell vagotomy and omental patch closure.

SUMMARY

Perforated duodenal ulcer was first successfully treated in 1894. It occurs predominantly in young men. Use of tobacco and alcohol seem to be exacerbating factors. Although the frequency of ulcer disease has declined in the United States, the number of perforated ulcers has changed only slightly except in older patients, in whom the frequency has increased, particularly in women. Circumstantial evidence suggests that this is due to increased use of nonsteroidal anti-inflammatory drugs.

The diagnosis of perforated duodenal ulcer was not difficult to make in the patient presented, but it can be much more difficult in elderly patients, particularly

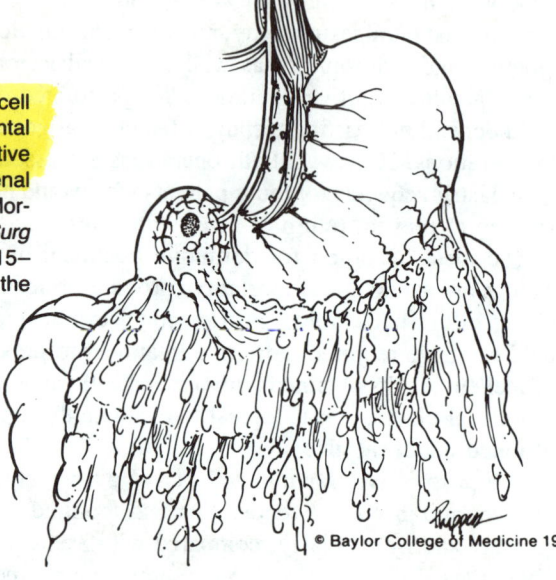

FIG 11–1.
The author considers parietal cell vagotomy, combined with omental patch closure, the ideal definitive treatment of perforated duodenal ulcers. (From Jordan PH Jr, Morrow C: Perforated peptic ulcer. *Surg Clin North Am* 1988; 68(2):315–329. Used by permission of the author.)

when they are in the hospital for other conditions. One must be vigilant, as such patients left undiagnosed and untreated will die.

Nonoperative treatment has limited application in the management of perforated duodenal ulcer. Simple closure of the ulcer is still the most widely used procedure. Being unable to predict accurately the individuals at risk to develop recurrent ulcer after simple closure, and since the mortality in patients without risk factors is equal for simple closure and definitive surgery, definitive treatment is appropriate for patients such as the one under discussion. Truncal vagotomy and pyloroplasty or hemigastrectomy are commonly used for treatment of perforated duodenal ulcers. My concern about the use of these operations is the occurrence of gastric sequelae in patients that might not have needed a definitive operation. For this reason, parietal cell vagotomy and patch of the ulcer is my treatment of choice when definitive management is indicated and the operation is technically possible.

BIBLIOGRAPHY

1. Boey J, Lee NW, Koo J, et al: Immediate definitive surgery for perforated duodenal ulcers: A prospective controlled trial. *Ann Surg* 1982; 196:338–344.
2. Boey J, Choi SKY, Alagaratnam TT, et al: Risk stratification in perforated duodenal ulcers: A prospective validation of predictive factors. *Ann Surg* 1987; 205:22–26.

3. Ceneviva R, de Castro e Silva O, Castelfranchi PL, et al: Simple suture with or without proximal gastric vagotomy for perforated duodenal ulcer. *Br. J Surg* 1986; 73:427–430.
4. Frommüller F: Operation der Pylorusstenose Erlarying der Diktorurde der Median Fakultät der Universität. Erlangen, 1886.
5. Jordan GL Jr, DeBakey ME, Duncan JM: Surgical management of perforated peptic ulcer. *Ann Surg* 1974; 179:628–633.
6. Jordan PH Jr, Korompai FL: Evolvement of a new treatment for perforated duodenal ulcer. *Surg Gynecol Obstet* 1976; 142:391–395.

12

Adenocarcinoma of the Stomach

A 69-year-old woman in rather ill health because of chronic rheumatoid arthritis presents with anemia and on examination is found to have a guaiac-positive stool. Radiographic and endoscopic examinations reveal a flat lesion high in the fundus of the stomach measuring 2 cm. Biopsy is positive for adenocarcinoma of the stomach.

Consultant: Robb H. Rutledge, M.D.

OVERVIEW

The patient, a chronically ill 69-year-old woman with rheumatoid arthritis, enters the hospital because of a carcinoma of the stomach. Her diagnosis was made by endoscopy, the only way to diagnose an early cancer since findings of x-ray films are frequently inconclusive. With the vigorous use of endoscopy, the percentage of resected gastric tumors that are Stage I (limited to the mucosa and submucosa) and Stage II (extension into but not through the serosa with negative nodes) has increased from 4% to 16%.

The Japanese have described early gastric cancer as that limited to the mucosa and submucosa with or without lymph node metastases. Survival for these patients approaches 80% to 90%, in contrast to 10% to 15% for advanced gastric cancer. Early endoscopy discovers more of these patients. One third of early gastric cancers are in the fundus. The patient's 2-cm flat lesion suggests that she may have a Type 2 early gastric cancer (Japanese endoscopic classification: Type 1, protruded; Type 2, superficial; Type 3, excavated). However, there is no way to know preoperatively if she is in this fortunate group. She needs careful preoperative, operative, and postoperative management to give her the best chance of cure and the least chance of complications or distressing gastrointestinal side effects.

PREOPERATIVE MANAGEMENT

The patient's history, physical examination, and routine laboratory tests evaluate her general medical condition, nutritional status, transfusion needs, and any obvious metastatic disease. Administration of medicine for arthritis that might contribute to intraoperative bleeding is stopped. The remaining gastrointestinal tract and gallbladder are investigated to eliminate a second malignancy, bleeding source, or gallstones that might require a concomitant cholecystectomy. A computerized tomography (CT) examination is not done routinely since hepatic metastases can be evaluated intraoperatively. However, a positive CT scan occasionally will allow a percutaneous biopsy diagnosis and avoid a fruitless laparotomy in a relatively asymptomatic patient.

Total parenteral nutrition is given for seven to ten days preoperatively if the patient is malnourished (albumin value less than 3.0 gm/dl, weight loss greater than 10% of body weight, or total lymphocyte count less than 1,500/cu mm). Otherwise, it is started when convenient and continued for seven to ten days postoperatively to decrease the chance of septic complications. (*Editor's note:* The need for and efficacy of perioperative parenteral nutrition in *malnourished* patients with malignancy is still controversial. It is likely that ultimately decreased complications will result, but one must balance this against stimulation of tumor growth, especially when excessive nutritional support i.e., calories and protein in excess of need, is utilized.)

Perioperative antibiotics are used because a stomach with carcinoma usually is hypochlorhydric and contains many bacterial pathogens. Cultures taken at the preoperative endoscopy allow specific antibiotic therapy. Otherwise, therapy with a cephalosporin (currently cefoxitin) is begun with anesthesia and continued for two or three postoperative days. (*Editor's note:* Some, including the editor, use oral antibiotics (aminoglycosides) as well, although improved efficacy of combined oral and parenteral antibiotics remains unproved, but there is much suggestive evidence of efficacy.)

OPERATIVE MANAGEMENT

Although some prefer a thoracoabdominal approach for a fundic lesion, I use an upper midline incision because of simplicity and safety. A Thompson or similar retractor elevates the ribs and sternum to give excellent exposure of the hiatus. If necessary, the xiphoid can be excised, the sternum split, or the incision extended into the left side of the chest.

A thorough exploration assesses the liver, peritoneal surfaces, regional lymph nodes, and resectability of the tumor. If unresectable metastases are present, good palliation may still be achieved by a wedge resection or proximal partial gastrectomy, providing there is no gross tumor at the anastomosis. A resection is preferred to a bypass for palliation. At times, no procedure is worthwhile. If the tumor is localized and resectable, a curative operation is performed.

The best choice is a total gastrectomy, including 3 cm of duodenum with the subpyloric nodes, the lesser and greater omentum with the right gastric and gastroepiploic nodes, the spleen with its hilar nodes, and the distal 2 cm of esophagus with the cardiac and left gastric nodes. An extended lymph node dissection, including the hepatic and coeliac nodes along with the body and tail of the pancreas, is not done routinely since any increase in operative survival is offset by increased morbidity and mortality.

A total gastrectomy is not recommended for every gastric carcinoma, but is used for resectable tumors of the cardia, fundus, and body of the stomach. A subtotal resection is usually used for antral tumors.

A proximal partial gastrectomy is not the preferred curative operation in this patient. The resection margins may be inadequate because of skip areas and multicentricity. The regional node dissection is not as complete. The remaining distal stomach may be a poor reservoir and have stasis unless a pyloroplasty is added. The esophagogastric anastomosis is more likely to have both early and late problems. Early, a leak is more difficult to treat than a leak after a Roux esophagojejunostomy because of associated gastric, biliary, and pancreatic leakage. Later, the esophagogastrostomy is more likely to have alkaline reflux and subsequent stricture.

Microscopically clear resection margins are important in improving survival rates. Palpation and gross inspection are not reliable for evaluation. Submucosal infiltration is more extensive proximally than distally, and it increases with the depth of tumor penetration. Frozen section examinations of the resection edges are done to rule out proximal and distal submucosal spread. Further excision is performed if needed to obtain clear margins. An in situ gross margin of 9 cm proximally and 6 cm distally will usually, but not always, be free of microscopic tumor invasion at the resection edges.

The most difficult part of the operation is the retrocolic esophagojejunostomy. Recently, many surgeons have used an EEA stapler for this. Stapled anastomoses are safe, but late strictures have been a problem. I have preferred the two-layer, end-to-side anastomosis (Fig 12–1). The inner layer may be either interrupted or continuous, depending on the size of the esophagus. A careful inner continuous catgut suture is just as reliable as the more traditional inner interrupted silk layer. The esophageal stay sutures illustrated help line up the anastomosis and keep the muscularis and mucosa together so that full-thickness bites are easily achieved in the inner layer. An end-to-end esophagojejunostomy is also satisfactory, but the end-to-side technique has better jejunal blood supply and allows anastomotic support by suturing the jejunum to the diaphragm posteriorly and anteriorly.

The most important principle in reconstruction after total gastrectomy is diversion of bile and pancreatic juice from the esophagus. This alkaline reflux

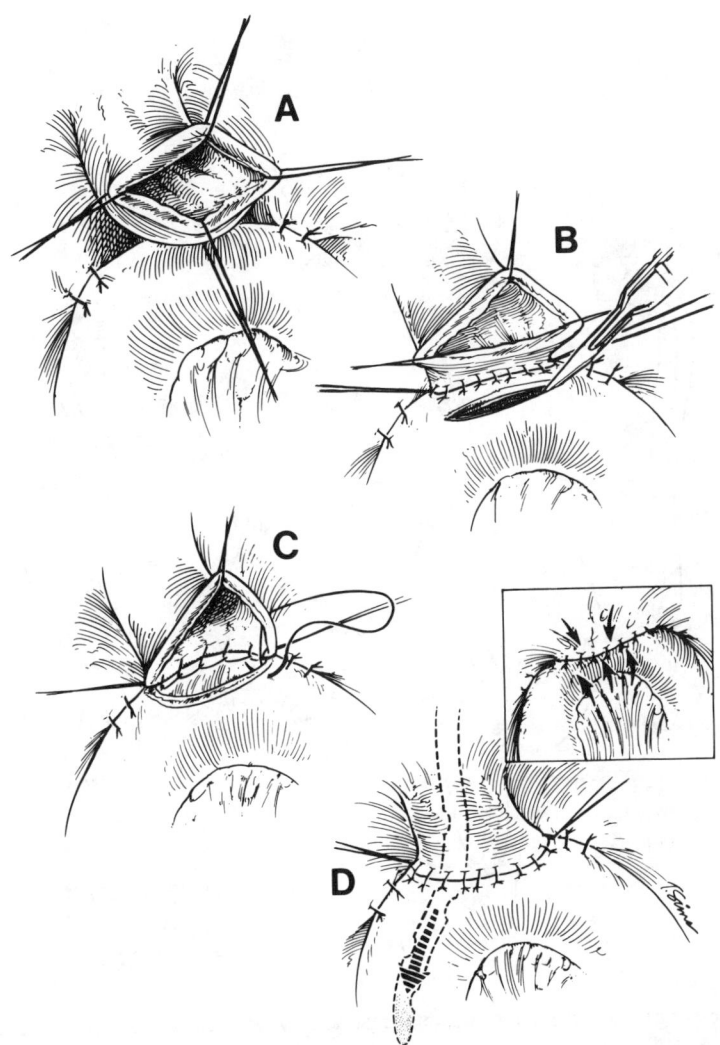

FIG 12–1.
Technical steps in end-to-side esophagojejunostomy. **A,** jejunum sutured to diaphragm posteriorly to support anastomosis. Esophageal stay sutures line up anastomosis and keep esophageal mucosa and muscularis together. **B,** posterior seromuscular layer of interrupted 3-0 silk sutures have been tied and the jejunum opened. **C,** full-thickness inner posterior layer of continuous locking chromic catgut continued anteriorly as a baseball stitch. **D,** completed anterior outer layer with Levin tube passed into either limb of Roux-19. (*Inset*, diaphragmatic peritoneum sutured over anterior layer of anastomosis.)

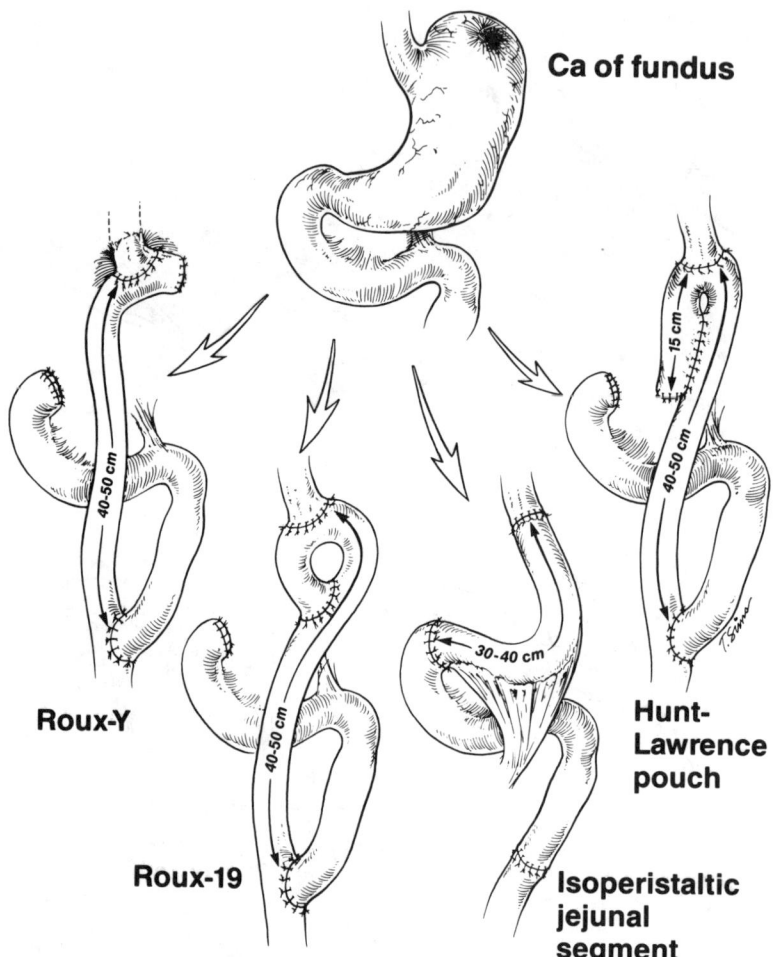

FIG 12–2.
Several methods of reconstruction after total gastrectomy for carcinoma of fundus of stomach.

is prevented by a long 40- to 50-cm Roux jejunal loop. The prevention of reflux is more important than the construction of a reservoir for a good nutritional result. The jejunum between the esophagus and the Roux jejunojejunostomy hypertrophies and takes on some reservoir function.

After the esophagojejunostomy, I usually complete the reconstruction as a Roux-19. This gives some reservoir effect, avoids a blind pouch, and has two jejunal limbs for outflow from the esophagojejunostomy.

Other reconstructions are shown in Figure 12–2. The Roux-Y is simple and works well. An isoperistaltic jejunal segment between the esophagus and duodenum takes longer, but it has the advantage of retaining duodenal function. It must be at least 30 to 40 cm long to prevent alkaline reflux. A Hunt-Lawrence pouch is more complex. If the pouch is made too close to the esophagojejunostomy, the intervening jejunal circulation is precarious. Other double and triple limb jejunal reservoirs have also been used, but none of the pouches are clearly superior to the simpler Roux-Y or Roux-19.

A stuffed Penrose drain is left near the esophagojejunostomy and brought out the left upper quadrant. (*Editor's note:* Most authors, including the Editor, use closed suction drainage systems to minimize contamination present with "two-way" drains.) The Levin tube is passed through the esophageal anastomosis into either jejunal limb of the Roux-19 and left on gravity drainage. Some surgeons use a catheter duodenostomy for early decompression and later postoperative enteral feeding. Others prefer a catheter jejunostomy. (*Editor's note:* Count me among these.) I have not used either method routinely, but have relied on total parenteral nutrition.

POSTOPERATIVE MANAGEMENT

Antibiotic therapy is stopped on the second or third day. About the fifth postoperative day, a water-soluble contrast study is done to confirm the integrity of the anastomosis and demonstrate good jejunal transport. Liquids are then begun, and the drain is removed from the left upper quadrant. Total parenteral nutrition is continued until oral intake is adequate. The diet is increased to six small feedings of a high-protein, high-fat, low-carbohydrate diet (anti-dumping diet) during the second postoperative week. Before hospital discharge, the patient receives a pneumococcal vaccine injection (Pneumovax) and prescriptions for cyanocobalamin (vitamin B_{12}) and iron.

If the postoperative x-ray film shows an esophageal leak, the drain is left in place, total parenteral nutrition is continued, and oral feeding is withheld until the leak has healed. Further drainage of infection is sometimes required to attain healing, but a major revision is rarely needed.

Occasionally the final pathology report will show microscopic submucosal invasion at the resection edges despite a clear-margins intraoperative frozen-section report. I have not reoperated in this situation. This report does not preclude a long-term survival. As many as 15% of five-year survivors have positive margins. This type of report is more likely to occur in a patient with full-thickness gastric wall involvement and positive nodes who may benefit from adjuvant therapy, but not from further surgery.

The ultimate prognosis depends on the extent of tumor penetration of the gastric wall and lymph node involvement. Early gastric cancer limited to the mucosa and submucosa has an excellent prognosis even with regional node involvement (approximately 70% five-year cure). More advanced resectable cancer has only a 15% five-year cure. The presence of positive lymph nodes more than 3 cm from the tumor markedly decreases the chance of cure.

The possibility of increasing five-year survival rates in patients with positive nodes or full-thickness penetration by using adjuvant chemotherapy or irradiation has not been proved. Both methods are currently being tested. The best drugs presently available are a combination of 5-fluorouracil, doxorubicin (Adriamycin), and mitomycin C (FAM), and therapy should be begun within the first postoperative month. Since many early recurrences are local or regional, adjuvant postoperative x-ray therapy is also being evaluated.

If the above patient has positive lymph nodes or full-thickness tumor penetration, she should be made aware of the current status of these methods of adjuvant therapy. Although I would be more aggressive in a younger patient, I probably would not urge her to take them because of the present lack of evidence that they would be of benefit to her.

CONCLUSIONS

The liberal use of endoscopy has brought encouraging news in the treatment of patients with carcinoma of the stomach. Carcinomas in more patients with Stage I and Stage II disease are being discovered, explored, and resected. More early gastric cancer is being found. Better cure rates and nutritional results are being obtained. More effective adjuvant therapy is still needed, but the overall outlook is much improved.

BIBLIOGRAPHY

1. Bozzetti F, Bonfanti G, Bufalino R, et al: Adequacy of margins of resection in gastrectomy for cancer. *Ann Surg* 1982; 196:685–690.
2. Carter KJ, Schaffer HA, Ritchie WP: Early gastric cancer. *Ann Surg* 1984; 199:604–609.
3. Fielding JWL, Fagg SL, Jones BG, et al: An interim report of a prospective, randomized, controlled study of adjuvant chemotherapy in operable gastric cancer: British Stomach Cancer Group. *World J Surg* 1983; 7:390–399.
4. Re Mine WH, Priestley JT: Trends in prognosis and surgical treatment of cancer of the stomach. *Ann Surg* 1966; 163:736–745.
5. Sekons DH, McSherry CK, Calhoun WF, et al: Contribution of endoscopy to diagnosis and treatment of gastric cancer. *Am J Surg* 1984; 147:662–665.

13

Benign Gastric Ulcer

A 45-year-old man with a history of 40-pack-years of cigarette smoking is investigated for anemia and a guaiac-positive stool. On review of his history, he complains of intermittent epigastric pain, aggravated by food and sometimes, but not always, relieved by antacid. On upper gastrointestinal studies and subsequent endoscopy, a 1.5-cm, sharply punched out, apparently benign gastric ulcer high in the lesser curvature approximately 1 cm from the gastroesophageal junction is detected. Endoscopic biopsies are repeatedly returned benign. The ulcer heals with therapy with histamine H_2 antagonists; however, when the therapy is stopped, the ulcer promptly recurs, with recurrence of symptoms.

Consultants: Raymond Pollak, M. B., FRCS
Lloyd M. Nyhus, M.D.

The history presented is the common stereotype of a 45-year-old man with symptoms of ulcer dyspepsia and findings on physical examination of a guaiac-positive stool. Risk factors for the occurrence of peptic ulcer disease include a history of cigarette smoking (40 packs per year) and being male. Appropriate investigations revealed the presence of a high-lying gastric ulcer on the lesser curvature, close to the gastroesophageal (GE) junction. While the position of this benign gastric ulcer was somewhat unusual (5% of gastric ulcers occur close to the GE junction), the ulcer healed predictably on appropriate medical management. The prompt recurrence of the ulcer after cessation of medical therapy was not entirely unexpected, because the natural history of gastric ulcers is for 50% to recur within six months of completion of a successful course of medical therapy. This is especially true when preexisting risk factors, such as excessive cigarette smoking, are still present. Thus, the problem at hand is the management of the high-lying, benign ulcer of the lesser curve of the stomach.

INCIDENCE

A peptic ulcer will develop during a lifetime in 5% to 10% of the population of the United States. In 1975 the annual costs for the management of and the economic losses caused by peptic ulcer disease were approximately 1.3 to 2.6

billion dollars. The annual incidence is about 1.6%, i.e., 4 million ulcers per year. Important risk factors include cigarette smoking, which is especially implicated in ulcer recurrences and in a retardation in the rate of healing, and the use of salicylates, steroids, and nonsteroidal anti-inflammatory agents. Diet, alcohol, and coffee-drinking have no clear association with ulcers.

In general, unlike that of duodenal ulcers, the incidence of gastric ulcers has not changed during the 20th century. There has been, however, a marked reversal in sex ratios, gastric ulcers becoming more common in men (male:female ratio 1:27:1). Also unlike the situation in the 19th century, gastric ulcers rarely occur in persons younger than 40 years of age; thereafter, the incidence rises with age.

ETIOLOGY

Modern thought on the pathophysiology of the causation of gastric ulcers has concentrated on the ability of gastric acid to cause mucosal injury. As a rule, the presence of gastric acid is required for ulceration of the mucosa to occur. What initiates the initial injury, however, has been the subject of intense investigation. Currently, the role of duodenogastric reflux caused by a possible defect in the pyloric sphincter mechanism has been implicated as a prime factor in gastric mucosal injury. This injury then exposes the mucosal cells to a back diffusion of hydrogen ions, which results in cellular dysfunction and death, and leads to mucosal slough and ultimate ulceration. Together with the incompetent pylorus and increased bile reflux, other features of note in patients with gastric ulcers are fasting and postprandial hypergastrinemia, hyposecretion of gastric hydrochloric acid and pepsin, decreased basal acid output and decreased 12-hour overnight acid secretion, decreased gastric mucosal blood flow, and delayed gastric emptying. (*Editor's note:* The apparent paradox between hyposecretion of acid compared with that of the normal population can be best resolved by viewing the etiology of peptic ulcer disease as the result of a balance between aggressive and defensive factors; in the case of a peptic ulcer, the aggressive factors "win.")

Gastric ulcers are a heterogeneous group of disorders that appear to have a variety of pathophysiologic associations. Because of this fact, they have been divided into three types. Type I ulcers occur in the middle third of the stomach and are the classic gastric ulcers that have as their probable causation the reflux of duodenal contents with gastric mucosal injury (57% of patients). Type II gastric ulcers are associated with concomitant duodenal ulcers, which occur in about 40% of patients, especially when the gastric ulcer is distal to the incisura. The associated duodenal ulcer usually points to the benign nature of the gastric ulcer and does not appear to affect the rate of healing of the gastric ulcer (21% of patients). Type III ulcers are the so-called prepyloric ulcers. Like duodenal ulcers, they may be associated with extremely high levels of gastric acid output as a primary etiologic factor (22% of patients). (*Editor's note:* Because duodenal mucosa usually extends proximally beyond the pylorus into the stomach, these ulcers are in fact ulcers in duodenal mucosa, and are, as the authors state, high-acid peptic ulcers. Patients with pyloric channel ulcers usually do poorly while receiving medical therapy; most come to surgery.)

Of recent intense interest has been the discovery of *Campylobacter pyloridis* as a factor in the causation of peptic ulcer disease. The organisms are found commonly in patients with nonautoimmune chronic gastritis and have been seen in up to 80% of patients with gastric ulcers. *C. pyloridis* is a spiral gram-negative organism and has a specific ability to hydrolize urea. It can be demonstrated in histologic specimens by special silver stains, and its pathogenicity has been suggested in volunteers who have ingested it. The role of *C. pyloridis* in causing or potentiating ulcer formation may result from the initial disruption of mucus production by other factors such as duodenogastric reflux. The organism is susceptible to bismuth, but less so to cimetidine, carbenoxolone, and sucralfate. It is also sensitive to a number of antibiotics including tetracycline, erythromycin, penicillin, cephalothin, and metronidazole.

DIAGNOSIS

The accuracy of the clinical diagnosis of gastric ulcers approximates 50%, gastric ulcer being difficult to distinguish from nonulcer causes of dyspepsia. Pain is the most common presenting symptom (90% of patients). The pain is epigastric in 46% of patients, and it usually does not radiate. In 24% of the patients, the pain is aggravated by food and usually occurs approximately one hour after a meal. More than 43% of patients may have nocturnal pain. Despite the often dramatic visceral pain syndrome presented by these patients, 25% of gastric ulcers may be asymptomatic. There may also be associated anorexia, nausea, vomiting, or weight loss. There is often no correlation between ulcer symptoms and the actual presence of an ulcer; this association is even worse in older patients.

Because of the potential for a misdiagnosis, a number of specialized investigations have been used to confirm the clinical suspicions. Traditionally, roentgenographic procedures have been used for the initial diagnosis of gastric ulcers. However, upper gastrointestinal roentgenograms are difficult to compare because observations are very observer-dependent. Experienced roentgenographers using double-contrast techniques can achieve an accuracy of more than 80%. Nevertheless, x-ray studies still prove incorrect in almost 30% of cases. In addition, 3% to 7% of ulcers that appear to be benign on roentgenograms are found to be malignant during a surgical procedure. Despite these facts, roentgenography may be preferred initially by some patients and for the definition of associated abnormalities or other disease processes.

Because roentgenographic findings are often incorrect, endoscopy has become the mainstay of the diagnosis of gastric ulcers. In a series of 153,000 endoscopies, only 37 (0.024%) revealed carcinoma within the ulcer when the study was performed for duodenal ulcer disease. However, 5% to 10% of gastric ulcers are malignant and, as such, every gastric ulcer should be subjected to endoscopic biopsy. Ulcers larger than 2 cm in diameter also have a greater chance of being malignant. In addition, Japanese surgeons have reported that 70% of gastric ulcers that harbor a malignant lesion may heal, thus emphasizing the point that even after gastric ulcers heal, they should be subjected to follow-up routine endoscopy and biopsy.

TREATMENT

The selection of patients for therapy is based on three factors: (1) the natural history, (2) the effectiveness of therapy, and (3) costs. The goals of therapy are control of symptoms, healing of the ulcer, and prevention of recurrence and complications. Spontaneous healing may occur in 50% of patients with gastric ulcers, the ulcers recurring in the other 50% within the first year; 80% may recur on a long-term basis. Ten percent of patients with gastric ulcers have complications largely consisting of bleeding, perforation, or stenosis. While it is widely accepted that medical therapy is effective, especially in terms of relieving symptoms, the natural history may not be affected at all. Recurrences seem to be prevented by continuous prophylaxis, but no reduction in complication rate has been achieved by medical therapy.

MEDICAL THERAPY

Hydrochloric acid production is central to all ulcers, so production of acid has to be decreased or the acid neutralized if it is present. Another approach is to enhance mucosal defenses. Dietary therapy has proved to be of little value. Caffeine does increase acid output, but so do some caffeine-free beverages. Thus, whether it is prudent to restrict caffeine intake is not a settled issue.

Anticholinergic agents are also known to decrease acid production, but are less potent than H_2-receptor blockers. Their effectiveness, however, as assessed endoscopically, is unproved. (*Editor's note:* This seems more a function of funding sources than design. When endoscopy was generally available for evaluation, the H_2 blockers were being evaluated; funding was available for the H_2 blockers, but not for anticholinergics, which were "old therapy.") Anticholinergics are sometimes used to complement H_2-receptor blockers, especially in situations of hypersecretory states such as the Zollinger-Ellison (Z-E) syndrome.

The use of antacids is limited by the rate of stomach emptying and acid production, as well as by the potency of the antacid used. The presence of magnesium in some preparations may lead to diarrhea, and aluminum in others may lead to constipation. Calcium-containing solutions may cause acid rebound with calcium-stimulated acid secretion. The pain relief seems to be independent of healing when a potent antacid combination of aluminum hydroxide gel (dried), magnesium hydroxide, and simethicone (Mylanta II), 30 ml, is used one and three hours after meals and at night. The rate of healing of gastric ulcers with antacids (50%) rises with the use of H_2-receptor blockers to approximately 80%. Antacids in tablet form tend to be less potent and should not be used because they are expensive if used properly and cost twice as much as an H_2-receptor blocker used for six weeks.

The H_2 receptor antagonists such as cimetidine and ranitidine are currently the agents of choice for the management of gastric ulcers of all types. Ranitidine is thought to be four to ten times as potent as cimetidine. A new agent, famotidine, appears to be five to eight times as potent as ranitidine (50 to 80 times better than cimetidine). Eighty percent of gastric ulcers heal when H_2-receptor blockers are used, compared with 35% to 40% for matched placebo groups. A 300-mg dose of cimetidine decreases acid secretion by 70% for four to five hours. Ranitidine, 150 mg orally twice a day for approximately eight weeks, heals 90% of gastric ulcers. Recurrences (50% to 80%) can be prevented with 150 mg of ranitidine given at bedtime. Side effects are few at these doses. Cimetidine has anti-androgen side effects in the high doses used for the Z-E syndrome. Also, drug interactions occur with cimetidine (P-450 system) and treatment may be switched to ranitidine.

Other agents used include sucralfate, a sulphated sucrose complex with aluminum hydroxide. It binds free protein in the ulcer base. Side effects are few and ulcers heal at the same rate as when treated with H_2-receptor blockers. Combination with an H_2-receptor blocker is no more effective than sucralfate alone. Patient compliance is poor, however, because of a metallic taste and constipation, as well as a cumbersome dosage schedule (i.e., 30 to 60 minutes before meals). Omeprazole, an inhibitor of the proton pump mechanism, has been used at a single bedtime dosage to decrease acid production for 24 hours; 80% to 90% of ulcers treated with this agent heal in two weeks, in contrast to a healing rate of 50% with ranitidine. Prostaglandins have also been shown to decrease acid and gastrin secretion, and they may stimulate gastric bicarbonate secretion. They may also increase mucus production and mucosal blood flow. A number of these agents, such as misoprostol, have been tested and are awaiting approval. Tricyclic antidepressant drugs are in the evaluation phase and have good healing potential for ulcer disease. They have anticholinergic effects and also block H_2 receptors. Trimipramine, 250 mg/day, and cimetidine, 300 mg three times a day and at night, heal ulcers at rates of 86% and 100%, respectively.

Thus, as for the patient under discussion, the initial management of a gastric ulcer, once a malignant lesion is definitively excluded, is medical. Treatment should consist of an appropriate H_2-receptor antagonist such as ranitidine for at least six to eight weeks of therapy. Antacids and sucralfate should not be combined, because such therapy is more expensive and is not more efficacious than either agent used alone if taken properly. Although therapy is likely to be more successful with hospitalization, hospital treatment is largely impractical. The patient should be encouraged to stop smoking and to omit salicylates and nonsteroidal inflammatory drugs. Once the ulcer has healed, and repeat endoscopy has confirmed this finding in the absence of malignant change, H_2-receptor blockers may be used prophylactically to prevent ulcer recurrence.

Ulcers recur almost 50% of the time, usually within the first six months of treatment. They recur in older patients with chronic medical illnesses or because of the continuing use of anti-inflammatory agents. Thus, for maintenance therapy to be an alternative to surgical treatment of recurrent ulcers, the drug must be effective, safe, and inexpensive, and patient compliance must be good. Age, in particular, appears to affect recurrence; the patient's sex and the size or position of the ulcer do not. Gastric acid output or hemorrhage similarly does not appear to affect the rate of ulcer recurrence. Furthermore, recurrences tend to be smaller than at sites different from the original ulcer. When carefully managed, recurrent ulcers heal at the same rate as the initial ulcer on appropriate medical therapy. Coexisting duodenal ulcers may occur in up to 40% of patients, especially when the ulcer is distal to the incisura. An associated duodenal ulcer usually points to the benign nature of the gastric ulcer, but it appears not to affect healing when managed appropriately. Recurrences in the latter group are common.

SURGICAL THERAPY

Surgical therapy for gastric ulcers is indicated when: (1) the ulcer fails to heal after three months of effective H_2-receptor antagonist therapy; (2) there is no long-term control, especially of recurrent ulcers, many of which may be asymptomatic; (3) there is poor compliance with medical therapy or its side effects; (4) complications such as perforation, hemorrhage, or fibrosis occur; and/or (5) dysplasia or carcinoma is present within the ulcer. The Billroth I operation is curative in more than 95% of gastric ulcers, with minimal major morbidity. This is especially applicable to Type I ulcers. For Type II ulcers, a vagotomy may be required to decrease acid production satisfactorily. Type III, prepyloric ulcers are often treated like duodenal ulcers, largely because of the extremely high acid production occurring in such instances, and because (as noted above) these are ulcers in duodenal mucosa.

It is apparent that our patient has suffered a recurrence of the high lesser curve ulcer following what appeared to be adequate medical management. He has an important risk factor for recurrence, namely the excessive smoking of cigarettes. The position of the ulcer 1.5 cm from the GE junction presents a particular challenge, since the goal of surgical therapy is to achieve reduction of acid secretion, resection of the ulcer, improvement in delayed gastric emptying, and removal of the area of chronic gastritis. The largest experience in the management of these juxtaesophageal gastric ulcers comes from Chile, where a collected series of 246 such ulcers has been reported by Csendes et al. Although the generally quoted incidence of these ulcers in the Western world is approximately 5%, these high-lying juxtaesophageal ulcers constituted 27% of a total collected series of 1,000 gastric ulcers. The male:female ratio was 176:70, and the mean age of the patients was 53 years (range, 25 to 82 years). To the great credit of Csendes and his colleagues, endoscopy was performed in almost all patients, especially in the late follow-up period (more than 90% of patients).

For the management of these high-lying gastric ulcers, the authors divided the procedures into those that leave the ulcer in situ and those that resect the ulcer. Procedures that left the ulcer in situ included gastrojejunostomy, pyloroplasty alone, vagotomy and pyloroplasty, and a wedge resection of the ulcer. These four procedures were associated with a recurrence rate that varied from 12% for the vagotomy and pyloroplasty to a high of 50% for gastrojejunostomy. However, when they used the Kelling-Madlener procedure (a distal gastrectomy leaving the ulcer in situ), the long-term recurrence rate was only 5% to 10%.

The second category of procedure was resection of the ulcer. These procedures included total gastrectomy, proximal gastrectomy, and esophagogastrostomy, or "mesogastrectomy." These three procedures resulted in a high mortality and were not recommended. A subtotal gastrectomy using the Shoemaker procedure or a Pauchet procedure provided excellent results with no recurrences and a 2% mortality. A Csendes gastrectomy, which uses a subtotal gastrectomy with esophagogastrojejunostomy, also was reported to give satisfactory results.

We favor resection of the ulcer, together with a distal gastrectomy. This has been achieved as a modification of the Pauchet maneuver, in which a generous distal gastrectomy is performed and a freehand excision of the ulcer is made along the lesser curvature to incorporate the ulcer at the juxtaesophageal position. (*Editor's note:* Because of hypochlorhydria and the use of H_2 blockers, these patients should receive an aminoglycoside orally preoperatively, as the stomach is unlikely to be sterile.) The closure is then performed as a standard Billroth I operation (Figs 13–1 to 13–4).

Thus, when assessing operations for high gastric ulcers close to the GE junction, the morbidity and mortality, recurrence rate, and side effects of the operation need to be considered. The Pauchet or Shoemaker operation, which in essence is an antrectomy with excision of the proximal tongue of mucosa containing the ulcer can be employed or a rotation gastrectomy using the Tanner method can be used when the ulcer is situated on the posterior wall of the

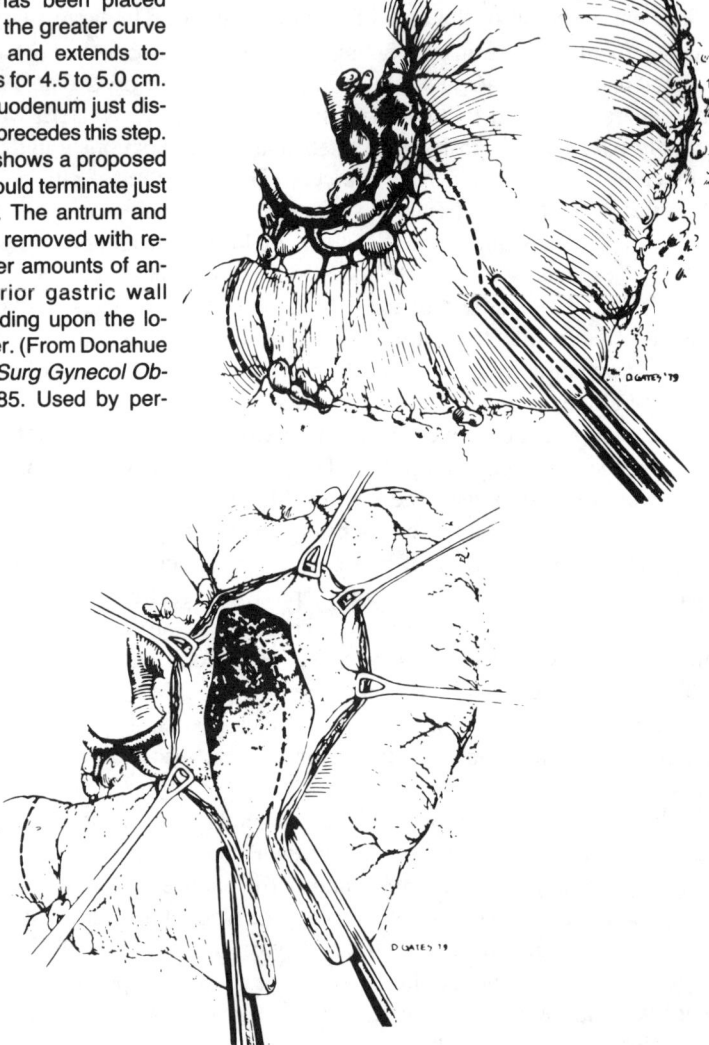

FIG 13–1.
A Payr clamp has been placed perpendicular to the greater curve of the stomach and extends toward the angulus for 4.5 to 5.0 cm. Division of the duodenum just distal to the pylorus precedes this step. The *dotted line* shows a proposed resection that would terminate just above the ulcer. The antrum and the ulcer will be removed with respectively greater amounts of anterior or posterior gastric wall included, depending upon the location of the ulcer. (From Donahue PE, Nyhus LM: *Surg Gynecol Obstet* 1982; 155:85. Used by permission.)

FIG 13–2.
A freehand completion of the excision proceeds rapidly, and bleeding is temporarily stopped with Babcock clamps. The posterior location of the ulcer accounts for the narrow amount of anterior resection and the generous amount of the posterior wall in the planned resection. A suture should be placed just after the apex of the incision has been created to take advantage of the remaining stomach as a traction device and to avoid retraction of the proximal part of the stomach. (From Donahue PE, Nyhus LM: *Surg Gynecol Obstet* 1982; 155:85. Used by permission.)

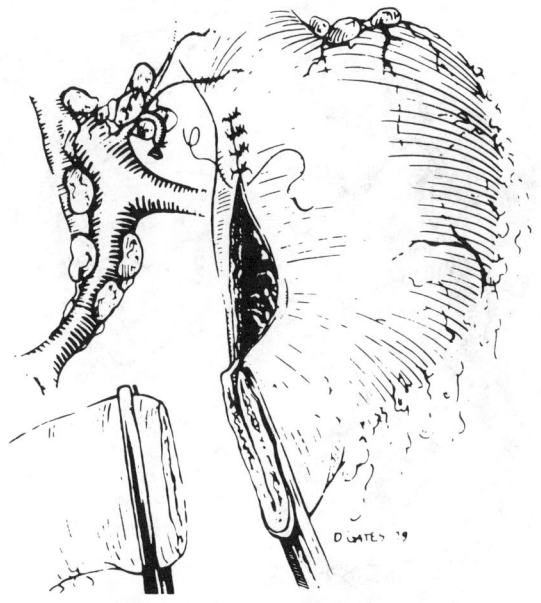

FIG 13–3.
A two-layer anastomosis is always advisable. We prefer an inner layer of running lock sutures of 00 chromic catgut. A larger needle will facilitate rapid placement of this hemostatic stitch, and interrupted nonabsorbable sutures complete the tubularization of the remaining part of the stomach. (From Donahue PE, Nyhus LM: *Surg Gynecol Obstet* 1982; 155:85. Used by permission.)

stomach. The modern modification of this procedure as performed by Donahue and Nyhus has, in our experience, proved most successful with minimal postoperative morbidity and mortality and no recurrences to date. (*Editor's note:* I agree! A Billroth I reconstruction has late metabolic advantages (better fat, iron, and calcium absorption) and should, in my opinion, be utilized, preferably following gastric resection if duodenum is suitable, which it usually is in Type I gastric ulcers.)

CONCLUSION

A 45-year-old patient with an ulcer high on the lesser curve close to the GE junction was initially examined and treated appropriately. Risk factors for recurrence, however, existed in this patient because he was a heavy smoker and did not receive prophylactic H_2-receptor antagonist therapy to maintain the healed state. Our plan of management was to perform a second endoscopy to exclude the presence of a malignant lesion within the ulcer. Having satisfied ourselves

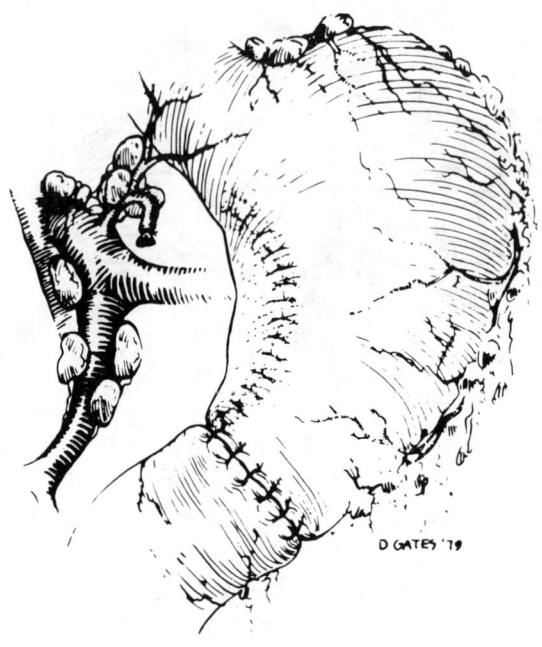

FIG 13–4.
The suture line has seemingly rotated posteriorly, a fact explained by the posterior location of the ulcer and the consequent resection of more of the posterior than the anterior lesser curvature. If the ulcer had been situated more anteriorly, the suture line would appear to have rotated anteriorly. (From Donahue PE, Nyhus LM: *Surg Gynecol Obstet* 1982; 155:85. Used by permission.)

that, in fact, the ulcer was not malignant in nature, we attempted treatment with medical therapy such as an H_2-receptor blocker. Furthermore, the patient was counseled and encouraged to give up cigarette smoking and to avoid factors thought to promote ulcer recurrence, perhaps by restricting caffeine intake and adjusting his diet. If the medical therapy and other measures are unsuccessful, operative therapy is recommended. Our operation of choice would be a modified Pauchet operation as described by Donahue and Nyhus, that is, a distal gastric resection with a freehand excision of the ulcer. This procedure has been associated with minimal postoperative morbidity and mortality, and there have been no long-term recurrences. These results would be expected for our patient.

BIBLIOGRAPHY

1. Brooks FP: The pathophysiology of peptic ulcer disease. *Dig Dis Sci* 1985; 30(suppl):15S–29S.

2. Csendes A, Braghetto I, Calvo F, et al: Surgical treatment of high gastric ulcer. *Am J Surg* 1985; 149:765–770.
3. Donahue PE, Nyhus LM: Surgical excision of gastric ulcers near the gastroesophageal junction. *Surg Gynecol Obstet* 1982; 155:85–88.
4. Gugler R: Current diagnosis and selection of patients for treatment of peptic ulcer disease. *Dig Dis Sci* 1985; 30(suppl):30S–35S.
5. Rathbone BJ, Wyatt JI, Heatley RV: *Campylobacter pyloridis:* A new factor in peptic ulcer disease. *Gut* 1986; 27:635–641.
6. Rudick J: Gastric ulcer, in Nyhus LM, Wastell C (eds): *Surgery of the Stomach and Duodenum*, ed 4. Boston, Little Brown & Co, 1986, pp 243–261.
7. Siepler JK, Mahakian K, Trudeau WT: Current concepts in clinical therapeutics: Peptic ulcer disease. *Clin Pharm* 1986; 5:128–141.

14

Bleeding Duodenal Ulcer

A 75-year-old man with no previous upper gastrointestinal history presents with a sudden onset of hematemesis, melena, and syncope. On admission to the emergency ward, a nasogastric aspirate is grossly positive for blood. Iced saline lavage does not clear the stomach. Emergency endoscopy reveals a 0.5-cm, sharply punched out, duodenal ulcer with a bleeding vessel that does not respond to bicap coagulation. After eight hours in the hospital, he remains tachycardic and orthostatically hypotensive despite the transfusion of 4 units of packed cells and appropriate crystalloid and colloid.

Consultant: Ashby C. Moncure, M.D.

INITIAL APPROACH

Prior to the consideration of the operative approaches in the management of hemorrhage complicating duodenal ulcer, it is appropriate to focus on the initial management of this patient. Each patient presenting with a major clinical problem must have a formally designated managing physician or surgeon who is to be the primary "decision-maker." This principle is of great importance, particularly in those patients with major gastrointestinal hemorrhage. (*Editor's note:* An important point! Medicine by committee is always difficult, but in emergency situations the patients almost always suffer from lack of clear-cut decision-making.)

The initial management of the patient with active gastrointestinal hemorrhage involves both diagnostic and therapeutic maneuvers, each giving way to the other as circumstances dictate. Identification of the location of the bleeding site and the nature of the disease state, as well as the extent and activity of the hemorrhage, are the diagnostic mission of the managing physician or surgeon. As this diagnostic mission is being accomplished, the patient must undergo volume resuscitation, and the major effort in managing the patient will, upon occasion, shift back and forth to and from diagnostic and therapeutic maneuvers. In the extreme example of major life-threatening hemorrhage, the diagnostic maneuver may indeed be prompt operative intervention. If the hemorrhage is of a less pressing extent, one may have the opportunity to employ endoscopic investigation of the esophagus, stomach, and duodenum if the patient is believed to have upper gastrointestinal bleeding suggested by a history of hematemesis, previous history or physical findings suggesting diseases predisposing to upper gastrointestinal hemorrhage, or blood or guaiac-positive material within the nasogastric aspirate.

The prompt establishment of a large-bore intravenous portal for blood and fluid replacement is of the highest priority in the management of such patients, assuming adequacy of airway and gas exchange. A baseline hematocrit reading is promptly obtained; blood for type and crossmatch is obtained, and a Foley catheter placed to monitor urinary output. If the nasogastric aspirate suggests massive bleeding, an Ewald tube will facilitate gastric evacuation and ice-water lavage can be initiated.

If massive upper gastrointestinal hemorrhage continues, the patient should be transported promptly to the operating suite in anticipation of esophagoscopy to be followed by laparotomy unless an esophageal source for hemorrhage is seen. Placement of a Linton or Sengstaken-Blakemore tube in those patients suspected of variceal hemorrhage secondary to portal hypertension may be tried as an initial quick trial, and, if hemorrhage abates, preparation for elective endoscopy and possibly variceal sclerotherapy may be undertaken.

If the upper gastrointestinal hemorrhage ceases or is of such extent that volume resuscitation is readily accomplished, early upper gastrointestinal endoscopy should be undertaken to localize the bleeding point and, if possible, to determine the disease process. Specifically, barium contrast examination should not be the initial diagnostic maneuver. Flexible fiberoptic endoscopy has enabled prompt diagnosis of the source of upper gastrointestinal hemorrhage to be achieved in greater than 90% of cases, and hence has become the major diagnostic tool utilized in the early evaluation of this clinical problem. In recent years, endoscopic control of the bleeding point in certain circumstances (variceal sclerotherapy and coagulation of ulcer base or bleeding vessel within the ulcer) has frequently been achieved as well. Cauterizing with laser light delivered by flexible fiberoptic systems, currently in its infancy, may prove to enhance further control of bleeding within an ulcer.

Angiographic assessment of the upper gastrointestinal tract is reserved for those cases in which the source of hemorrhage remains obscure after endoscopy or in which endoscopy suggests the source of hemorrhage to be secondary to diffuse gastric mucosal lesions ("stress gastritis"). Angiographic demonstration of bleeding can be anticipated to be successful if the rate of bleeding exceeds the level of 0.5 to 2.0 ml/minute. In the event of failure to demonstrate hemorrhage, one can leave the catheter in place in anticipation of restudy if hemorrhage again ensues.

If hyperemic gastric mucosa is seen angiographically, in the absence of evidence of bleeding from other sources, intra-arterial vasopressin may successfully control the hemorrhage. An alternative technique to control bleeding from a specific site, such as an ulcer, is selective embolization of the bleeding vessel with angiographic techniques. Inherent in this approach is the risk of both peripheral emboli to major organs, such as the liver, and ischemic necrosis of the neighborhood tissue that may lead to hollow viscus perforation.

Finally, it should be mentioned that technetium-labeled red blood cells have been utilized in an effort to document the site of bleeding in patients with gastrointestinal hemorrhage. This technique is quite sensitive in indicating active bleeding, but it has generally offered little assistance to the clinician in localizing the site of hemorrhage. (*Editor's note:* Labeled red blood cell scans are useful if bleeding rate exceeds 0.1 cc/minute, but (as stated) they often only indicate the approximate area of extravasation.)

Fortunately, the majority of patients presenting with upper gastrointestinal hemorrhage cease bleeding and, while undergoing observation for the resumption of hemorrhage by careful monitoring of vital signs and serial hematocrit readings, specific therapy can be directed at the underlying condition causative of the hemorrhage, if known. Operative management is employed in those patients with persistent or repetitive hemorrhage at the level of approximately 4 to 5 units of blood transfused. The elderly, those patients with gastric ulcers or chronic duodenal ulcers, and those patients seen to have a visible vessel in the ulcer base when endoscopically evaluated are more likely to suffer continuing or repetitive hemorrhage.

OPERATIVE APPROACH

The operative approach in the management of hemorrhage complicating duodenal ulcer is designed to control the active arterial hemorrhage initially and thereafter to control the further formation of gastric acid. Ligation of the bleeding point alone has been proved to be an unreliable method of management and is associated with a high incidence of recurrent hemorrhage. When ligation has been performed with distal gastric resection and vagotomy, control of active and recurrent hemorrhage has been the rule. Others have reported a favorable experience with ligation combined with pyloroplasty and vagotomy, stating that although early recurrent hemorrhage has been a problem following this procedure, the overall mortality has improved because it is a "lesser" procedure in a critically ill population of patients.

It is the view of the author that in this modern era of skilled administration of general anesthesia and accurate monitoring of hemodynamic status, the operative procedure utilized should be the optimal procedure to ensure long-term control of the upper gastrointestinal hemorrhage. Thus, emergency control with ligation proximally and distally of the bleeding gastroduodenal artery, with closure of the duodenal stump beyond the ulcer, and resection of the antrum with construction of gastrojejunostomy and truncal vagotomy will be subsequently described as the "gold standard" in the management of this patient.

With the patient supine, with indwelling nasogastric tube on suction and a Foley catheter in place, with an active transfusion of packed red blood cells and fresh frozen plasma through large-bore intravenous portals ongoing, general anesthesia is induced. The lower part of the chest and entire abdomen are prepared, draped as a sterile field from flank to flank. The abdominal cavity is entered through an upper abdominal left paramedian rectus-retracting incision.

Allen's method is a useful approach to control active bleeding from the gastroduodenal artery at the base of a duodenal ulcer. This is accomplished by rapidly clearing a small area along both curvatures of the stomach and placing Payr clamps across the stomach at this level to allow its division between them. Traction is placed on the distal Payr clamp to allow dissection to proceed rapidly down the greater curvature side, with division of the inflammatory adhesions at the pylorus. The distal Payr clamp is removed, and two long Kocher clamps are placed on the anterior wall of the stomach in its long axis, extending from the cut edge of the stomach to the pylorus. The stomach is divided between the clamps, and the left index finger is used to achieve digital tamponade of the bleeding within the ulcer. It is at this stage that the anesthesiologist should be permitted to resuscitate the patient from hypovolemia, while tamponade control is maintained.

The dissection is then carried along the common hepatic artery as it descends toward the stomach, and the right gastric and gastroduodenal arteries are divided between suture ligatures or clamped and tied if the vessels are not buried in inflammatory tissue. The common hepatic artery and common bile duct are the structures at risk during this stage of the procedure, and the surgeon should be cognizant that neighboring inflammation secondary to the ulcer may alter the usual relationships in the area. The distal end of the gastroduodenal artery immediately caudad to the duodenal bulb or its immediate branches is then controlled with a suture ligature placed no deeper than necessary to control the hemorrhage. Suture of the vessels within the ulcer bed can now be carried out, with minimum blood loss, with nonabsorbable suture material (Fig 14–1).

The management of the duodenal stump in the presence of active posterior duodenal ulcer disease may prove troublesome because of the accompanying inflammation. The dissection of the duodenum is facilitated by placement of the left index finger in the open duodenum, with dissection proceeding closely about the duodenum until an adequate length of cuff has been cleared to allow a reasonably secure closure. This may have to be done in part with a knife, suture-ligating bleeding points in turn as the dissection proceeds. If one is unsure of the relationship of the common bile duct to the area of dissection, the common duct may be cannulated with a firm catheter to serve as a guide (Lahey's method) for dissection and closed about a T-tube at the conclusion of the procedure.

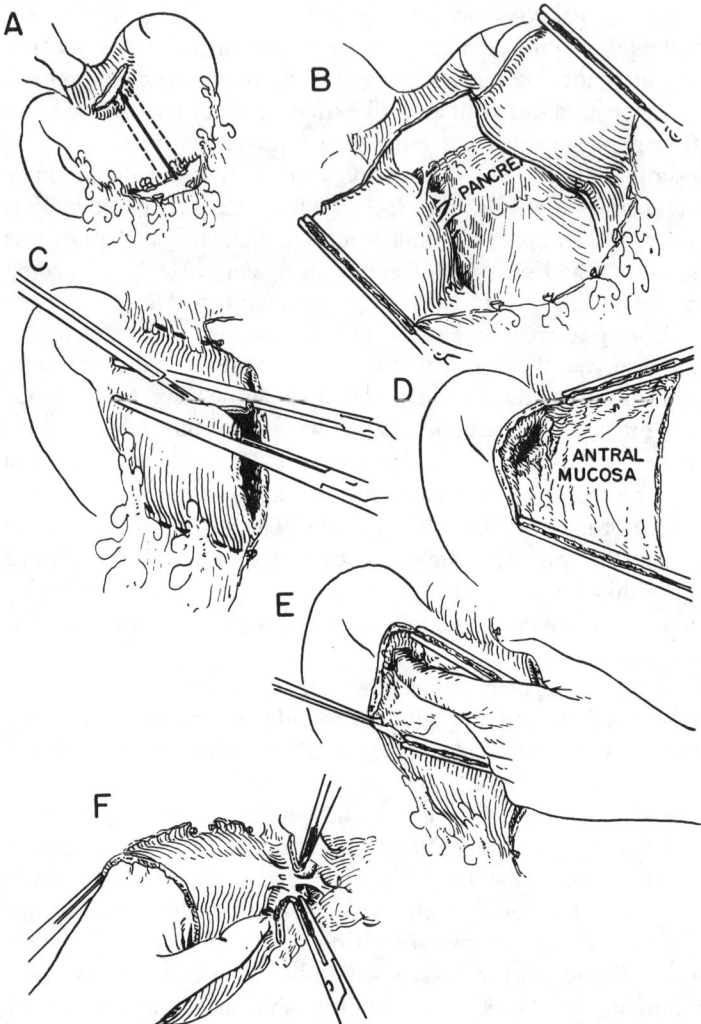

FIG 14–1.
Allen's method to control active bleeding from the gastroduodenal artery at the base of a duodenal ulcer is illustrated. *A*, a small area along both curvatures of the stomach is cleared and Payr clamps are placed across the stomach at this level. *B*, the stomach is divided between the Payr clamps. Traction is placed on the distal clamp to allow dissection to rapidly proceed down the greater curvature. *C*, the distal Payr clamp is removed, two long Kocher clamps are placed on the anterior wall of the stomach, in its long axis, extending from the cut edge of the stomach to the pylorus. *D*, the stomach is divided between the clamps. *E*,

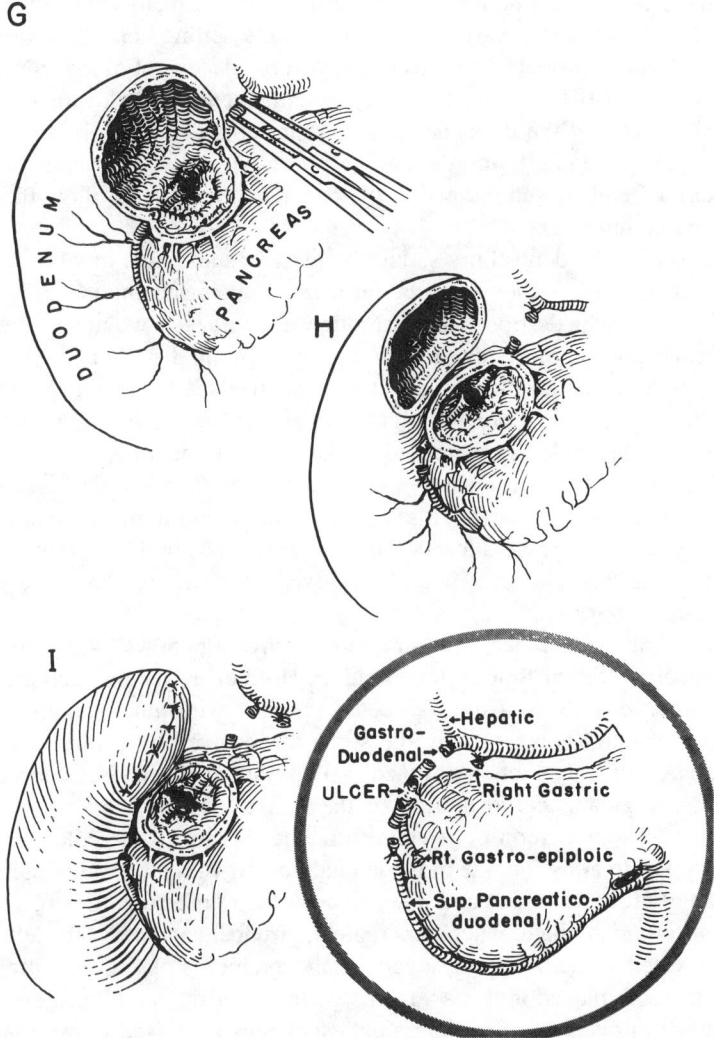

the left index finger tamponades the bleeding within the ulcer. F, dissection is carried along the lesser curve toward the pylorus and the right gastric artery is divided. G, the gastroduodenal artery is divided and tied at its origin. H, the distal end of the gastroduodenal artery, beyond the ulcer, is divided and tied. I, suture of vessels within the ulcer bed is completed and the duodenal stump is turned in. (From Welch CE: *Surgery of the Stomach and Duodenum*, ed 5. Chicago, Year Book Medical Publishers, 1973. Used by permission.)

In the presence of a relatively short cuff and inflammatory thickening of the duodenal wall, almost invariably present in this setting, open closure of the duodenal stump is probably best accomplished by placement of interrupted Connell sutures of 4-0 silk placed initially at either end, the closure proceeding toward the center of the duodenal stump. After completion of the first layer, a second layer of Lembert sutures may be placed. It may be necessary to place the posterior Lembert sutures within the pancreatic capsule to allow the second layer to be completed.

A side-tube duodenostomy should be placed in all cases in which the duodenal stump closure is thought to be insecure. This is accomplished by placing a No. 14 latex whistle-tip catheter through a small stab wound in the lateral distal second portion of the duodenum, the tip pointing distally and lying within the third portion of the duodenum. It is held in place by two circumferential purse-string sutures of chromic catgut and brought through omentum, exiting through the right flank. A cigarette drain is placed in the area, not touching the duodenum, and is brought through the same exit. (*Editor's note:* Most authors, including the Editor, advocate closed suction drains to minimize contamination and the possibility of abscess formation.) The side-tube duodenostomy is allowed to drain by gravity and is generally removed in 10 to 12 days; the drain is removed thereafter.

The author's preference for gastrojejunostomy, after 50% distal gastrectomy, is an antecolic afferent limb to lesser curve, Hofmeister reconstruction, closing the lesser curve portion of the transected stomach with inner running chromic catgut (hemostatic) and returning the stitch as an inverting suture to the point of origin. A third layer of interrupted 4-0 silk accomplishes seromuscular apposition. The greater curve portion of the transected stomach is anastomosed end-to-side to a short loop of jejunum brought anterior to the colon, the anastomosis approximating the size of the jejunal lumen, with inner running inverting (hemostatic) chromic catgut and outer interrupted Lembert sutures of fine silk.

To accomplish bilateral subdiaphragmatic truncal vagotomy, the left hepatic lobe is elevated with a retractor; a gauze handkerchief is placed over the spleen, and a retractor is placed in this area. The gastric remnant is retracted downward; the peritoneum overlying the abdominal esophagus is incised transversely, and the esophagus is encircled with a large Penrose rubber drain. The anterior and posterior vagal trunks are dissected free and a 4-cm segment of each resected, each end secured with a hemoclip. Any residual vagal fibers are divided. A headlight utilized by the operator facilitates accomplishing this portion of the procedure. (*Editor's note:* If bleeding is not massive, the vagotomy should be accomplished first, before the stomach is opened, to minimize contamination of the subdiaphragmatic area.)

ALTERNATE OPERATIVE APPROACH

Upon occasion, after entering the abdominal cavity, an inflammatory mass will be encountered in the area of the duodenum, necessitating an alternative approach to duodenal transection and closure beyond the ulcer. The alternative options include opening the anterior distal stomach and proximal duodenum in its long axis, obtaining digital tamponade of the bleeding. Suture ligation of the gastroduodenal artery proximally and distally outside the duodenum is accomplished, and thereafter residual bleeding within the ulcer bed is controlled with nonabsorbable sutures. This is followed by closure of the opening in the viscus as a pyloroplasty (Heineke-Mikulicz, if the gastroenterotomy is short; Finney, if it is long) and accomplishing a bilateral subdiaphragmatic truncal vagotomy. Placement of a gastrostomy tube for drainage is a useful adjunct to this procedure. In view of a higher incidence of recurrent hemorrhage in those patients undergoing this procedure, use of an H_2 antagonist postoperatively is wise.

PROGNOSIS

There is an increased incidence of postoperative subdiaphragmatic infected collections and wound infections in patients undergoing emergency procedures to control massive upper gastrointestinal hemorrhage, and early detection of this complication must be sought. The use of preoperative and intraoperative antibiotics, careful replacement of shed blood, and postoperative nutritional support are further helpful measures to ensure prompt recovery.

BIBLIOGRAPHY

1. Nyhus LM, Wastell C: *Surgery of the Stomach and Duodenum,* ed 4. Boston, Little Brown and Co, 1986.
2. Welch CE: *Surgery of the Stomach and Duodenum,* ed 5. Chicago: Year Book Medical Publishers, 1973.
3. Welch CE, Rodkey GV, von Ryll Gryska P: A thousand operations for ulcer disease. *Ann Surg* 1986; 204:454–467.

15

Management of Obstructing Duodenal Ulcer

A 67-year-old, recently retired truck driver has had intermittent epigastric distress for at least 25 years for which he has taken Tums, usually with good relief. During the past month, the distress has not been relieved by the Tums and has been accentuated by coffee and the occasional beer he consumes. For three weeks, he has felt full and uncomfortable after meals and has vomited at about 48-hour intervals; the vomitus consisted of food he had consumed 24 hours previously and was without blood. There has been no melena, but he has been constipated for two weeks. He has lost about seven or eight pounds in the last few weeks. There is a 40-pack-years of cigarette smoking. The abdomen shows some protrusion in the epigastrium and there is a succussion splash in the left upper quadrant. His tongue is dry and the skin has poor turgor. The x-ray films of the abdomen show an extremely large gastric shadow occupying most of the upper abdomen, with much debris (Fig 15–1).

Consultant: William Silen, M.D.

DIAGNOSIS

While the correct diagnosis of stenosing duodenal ulcer is readily made in the patient with long-standing history of duodenal ulcer who is unable to retain food, several pitfalls await the unwary. The term "gastric outlet obstruction," so readily and glibly given to any individual whose stomach appears dilated by radiologic assessment, is completely nonspecific and should be abandoned. When the stomach has been severely distended for a prolonged period and contains much food and debris, a contrast meal will often fail to distinguish between cancer and ulcer unless decompression has been in use for several days. The argument that the true state of affairs will be discovered at operation is not valid, since I have seen good surgeons confuse a small distal antral carcinoma with an obstructing peptic ulcer at the time of laparotomy, with dire consequences. For that reason, after suitable decompression, endoscopy and biopsy are almost always advisable unless the diagnosis has been clearly established previously.

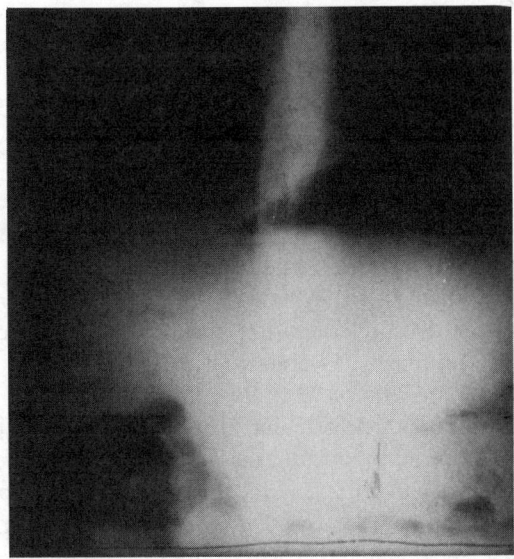

FIG 15–1.
The x-ray film of the abdomen showing an extremely large gastric shadow occupying most of the upper abdomen, with much debris.

It is not general knowledge that patients with completely obstructing duodenal ulcers usually vomit rather infrequently. Vomiting of large quantities of ingested food often occurs at 48- or 72-hour intervals, in contrast to the patient with a pyloric channel ulcer who may vomit small amounts of gastric content three or four times daily. The latter patient shows no radiologic or endoscopic evidence of obstruction and need not be considered further in the context of a piece on obstructing ulcer, except to attempt to dispel the prevalent notions that patients with channel ulcers who vomit frequently are obstructed and that patients with truly obstructing ulcers vomit after virtually every meal.

PREPARATION AND TRIAL OF NONOPERATIVE TREATMENT

Decompression

It is essential that adequate decompression of the stomach be achieved. In most patients with subacute or chronic obstruction, the usual 14 or 16 F nasogastric tube is simply too small to allow evacuation of the large amounts of food and solid debris that are usually present in the gastric lumen. It is usually necessary to empty the stomach by means of a large-bore orogastric Ewald tube, and even such a maneuver may require an hour or two of effort, using isotonic sodium chloride (NaCl) for irrigation in order to avoid overt washout of large amounts of potassium (K^+) and chloride (Cl^-) in a patient already depleted of these electrolytes. Once it is determined that the major portion of the solid debris has been removed, the Ewald tube can be replaced with the standard, reasonably sized nasogastric tube. Decompression should be continuously applied for at least 72 to 96 hours, during which time fluid and electrolyte repletion can be carried out.

If one is to have any chance at all of achieving resolution of the obstruction by nonoperative means, stuttering attempts to discontinue decompression for brief periods in less than 72 to 96 hours will serve only to prolong the time necessary to make the definitive decision whether operative treatment need be instituted at the 96-hour mark. My practice is to advise a saline load test of 750 ml of isotonic NaCl at the end of 72 to 96 hours of *continuous* decompression. A residual volume of more than 250 ml at the end of 30 minutes clearly indicates that operation will be required during this admission. Lesser residual volumes signify that the patient will tolerate oral feedings and that operation may be postponed for a more propitious time. During the important period of decision, at and around the 72-hour mark, I usually prefer to discontinue treatment with H_2-receptor blocking agents for six or eight hours since it is known that these drugs slow gastric emptying. However, intravenous H_2-blocker drugs should be given prior and subsequent to that time.

Fluid, Electrolytes and Nutrition

While one might on reflex consider the immediate institution of parenteral hyperalimentation in this clinical setting, I believe that this temptation should be resisted. First, the initial and subsequent requirements for replacement of volume and electrolyte deficits are usually large, and such correction may require as long as 72 hours during which time superimposition of hyperalimentation may seriously hamper precise interpretation of shifts in fluid and electrolytes. Second, the decision for or against operation should be made somewhere between 72 and 96 hours, at the end of which time either the patient will be able to accept adequate nutrition orally or operation will need to be done. In my opinion, if operation is mandatory, three or four days of preoperative hyperalimentation cannot be shown to have a beneficial effect. (*Editor's note:* This is by no means certain and is under active investigation. An educated guess based on current data as to the minimum preoperative duration of parenteral nutrition to be efficacious in improving outcome is probably five- to seven days.) Far more satisfactory and effective alimentation can be achieved by means of a jejunostomy placed at the time of operation in the *seriously* malnourished patient.

During the early periods of fluid and electrolyte repletion, the aspirated gastric juice should be replaced quantitively. Relatively low outputs of gastric juice even in the absence of H_2-blocking agents should not be misconstrued to indicate that the ulcer disease is "burnt out" (a comment often found in the older literature). It is well established that potassium deficiency can profoundly lower acid secretion, and it is the lack of understanding of this fact that led previously to this now discredited burnt out theory. Conversely, very high acid outputs should arouse suspicion that a gastrinoma or G-cell hyperplasia might be present. Consequently, serum gastrin determinations should be made on the day of admission so that the results are known at the time of operation.

SELECTION OF OPERATION

In the presence of hypergastrinemia, it is mandatory that the diagnosis of gastrinoma be established or refuted before operation is undertaken. It is not within the scope of this report to discuss the management of gastrinoma. On the other hand, if gastrinoma is excluded by a secretin test in a patient with an elevated level of serum gastrin, the surgeon should seriously consider antrectomy with truncal vagotomy as the operation of choice, with the view that one is dealing with antral G-cell hyperplasia, the presence of which cannot be conclusively established if the response of the serum gastrin to a meal cannot be tested. I prefer an antecolic gastrojejunostomy to a gastroduodenostomy under these circumstances because I believe that emptying, which must occur largely by gravity, is more effective after gastrojejunostomy. A wide Hofmeister or Mayo-Polya anastomosis is employed, with great care to place the afferent loop of jejunum to the lesser curvature side and the efferent loop to the greater curvature. I use a single-layer sutured anastomosis to turn in as little extraneous tissue as possible, since postoperative delay in emptying can be a serious problem. Feeding jejunostomy should be strongly considered, especially if preoperative weight loss and malnutrition are evident.

In the absence of G-cell hyperplasia, other surgical options are available. Some surgeons have carried out highly selective vagotomy and combined it with dilatation of the stenosed area at the pylorus of duodenum. I am extremely reluctant to do so if the patient has not resolved the obstruction preoperatively, because I greatly fear that inadequate gastric emptying will continue to be a problem in the postoperative period. This, of course, is the advantage of a trial of nonoperative treatment. The addition of pyloroplasty to highly selective vagotomy, as advocated by Holle, does not provide a good gravity-employing emptying procedure for an edematous flabby stomach and mitigates the tremendous advantage of highly selective vagotomy alone in avoiding undesirable postoperative digestive symptoms. Thus, unless the operation is being done at a time of election after a brief episode of subacute obstruction that is now resolved, I am afraid the patient is denied the opportunity of an excellent operation such as highly selective vagotomy.

Truncal vagotomy and posterior gastrojejunostomy is an excellent procedure for the aged or especially debilitated patient. It can be carried out expeditiously and with high expectation for rapid return of normal gastrointestinal function. I would strongly advise against the use of pyloroplasty in this circumstance because the elongated J-shaped stomach will not empty well against gravity, particularly when the antral pump has been denervated by the truncal vagotomy. (*Editor's note:* Liberal indications for the use of gastrostomy, if this procedure is carried out, although in my opinion gastric emptying is better with a posterior gastrojejunostomy.)

In the better-risk patient, the surgeon can choose between antrectomy and truncal vagotomy or gastroenterostomy and truncal vagotomy. The long-term outcome after either of these procedures is very good. The antrectomy, however, probably provides an added protection against an incomplete truncal vagotomy.

BIBLIOGRAPHY

1. Dunn DC, Thomas WEG, Hunter JO: Highly selective vagotomy and pyloric dilatation for duodenal ulcer with stenosis. *Br J Surg* 1981; 68:194–196.
2. Jordan PH Jr: A follow-up report of a prospective evaluation of vagotomy-pyloroplasty and vagotomy-antrectomy for treatment of duodenal ulcer. *Ann Surg* 1974; 180:259–264.
3. McMahon MJ, Greenall MJ, Johnston D, et al: Highly selective vagotomy plus dilatation of the stenosis compared with truncal vagotomy and drainage in the treatment of pyloric stenosis secondary to duodenal ulceration. *Gut* 1976; 17:471–476.
4. White CM, Harding LK, Keighley MRB, et al: Gastric emptying after treatment of stenosis secondary to duodenal ulceration by proximal gastric vagotomy and duodenoplasty or pyloric dilatation. *Gut* 1978; 19:783–786.

16

Pyloric Channel Ulcer

A 60-year-old male with a 45-pack-years of cigarette smoking and modest use of alcohol, plus chronic lower back pain, is admitted with epigastric pain that is only modestly relieved by antacids and food and aggravated by coffee and his infrequent meals. Upper gastrointestinal (GI) series and endoscopy reveal a pyloric channel ulcer. He had previously been treated with histamine H_2 antagonists with only modest relief.

Consultant: John L. Sawyers, M.D.

DISCUSSION

This patient has a symptomatic pyloric channel ulcer that has failed standard medical treatment with antacids and histamine H_2 blockers. These ulcers are notorious for being resistant to medical treatment and are characterized by a relentless progressive course. If they heal, pyloric channel ulcers (PU) tend to recur despite management with H_2-receptor antagonists and antacids. In about one half of patients with PU, pyloric obstruction becomes a significant problem.

In 1959, Texter and associates described the symptoms associated with pyloric ulcers and named this entity the "syndrome pylorique." The syndrome is characterized by nausea and vomiting, pain developing immediately after meals, early satiety, and weight loss. These patients usually do not have the typical pain of patients with duodenal ulcers (DU) that is characterized by epigastric pain relieved by food.

The diagnosis of PU may be made by an upper GI series or endoscopy, as was done in this patient. Endoscopy is preferred so that biopsy can be performed. While carcinoma is rarely found in PU, gastric cancer occurs in prepyloric ulcers (PPU) often enough that all PU and PPU should be biopsied. Our policy is to biopsy all gastric and pyloric ulcers. Radiologic evaluation is helpful in assessing the degree of pyloric obstruction, which has been reported by Murray et al. to occur in about 50% of patients with PU.

INCIDENCE

Pyloric channel ulcers account for about 5% of all peptic ulcers. Bonnevie, in an epidemiological study of peptic ulcer disease in Copenhagen, found PU in 56 (4%) of 1,444 patients. At Duke University Hospital, PU accounted for 4.3% of peptic ulcers seen by Murray et al. Brethwaite and associates reported that 6.6% of peptic ulcers were PU in a 1952 review.

Pyloric channel ulcers occur in an older age group than DU. Most patients with PU are between 40 to 70 years of age, while most patients with DU are from 30 to 50 years of age. The ratio of men to women is closer to 1:1 in patients with PU, although Murray et al. reported that 64% of the patients in their series were men.

ANATOMY

Is a pyloric channel ulcer a duodenal or a gastric ulcer? It took a long time for surgeons to realize that peptic ulcers should be classified as either duodenal ulcers or gastric ulcers. The pyloric ulcer was originally considered by most surgeons to be a duodenal ulcer. The increasing use of proximal gastric vagotomy (PGV) to treat DU has caused surgeons to reconsider the classification of PU. There has been an unacceptably high (25% to 35%) recurrent ulcer rate following PGV for PU, while the recurrence rate following PGV for DU ranges from 5% to 15% as reported by Goligher.

Recent morphological studies of PU by Muller et al. supply additional information. Pyloric channel ulcers are defined as ulcers occurring within the pylorus ± 0.5 cm. Prepyloric ulcers occur more than 0.5 to 2.0 cm proximal to the pylorus, while DU occur 0.5 cm distal to the pylorus. Many surgeons have considered PU and PPU as one group. This concept arises from Johnson's classification for gastric ulcers—a type 1 gastric ulcer occurs on the lesser curvature of the stomach near the antroparietal border; a type 2 ulcer is a type 1 gastric ulcer in association with a duodenal ulcer; and type 3 ulcers are prepyloric ulcers with or without a type 1 gastric ulcer or duodenal ulcer. Since the type 3 ulcer has many similarities to pyloric channel ulcer, some surgeons have considered PU to be gastric rather than DU. The type 1 gastric ulcer patient has the same number of acid-secreting parietal cells as a normal individual, while type 2 and 3 gastric ulcer patients are hypersecretors of gastric acid and have an increased parietal cell mass similar to duodenal ulcer patients.

Ornsholt et al. studied acid secretion in patients with PPU, PU, and DU. The pentagastrin-stimulated peak acid output was significantly high in patients with DU compared to patients with PPU, while patients with PU constituted an intermediary group.

Oi et al. studied the location of gastric ulcers in 307 patients. Only four patients had PU, which Oi and associates termed "justapyloric ulcer" since the ulcer was "adjacent to the pyloric gland area on its gastric margin and in the duodenal gland area on its duodenal margin." Oi and associates decided to classify these ulcers as DU. In a subsequent study, Oi and Sakurai studied the location of DU and described in detail the relationship between the pyloric sphincter and the border zone between the duodenal and pyloric gland area. In 110 patients, the site of the border zone was within 5 mm from the summit of the pyloric channel. In the majority of cases, the distance was only 1 mm. Again, these studies indicate that PU should be considered DU rather than gastric ulcers (GU).

It would appear that PU are a mixture of both GU and DU. The PU lie in the transitional zone between the pyloric gastric glands and the duodenal glands. Over a short distance (5 mm), both pyloric and duodenal glands merge together at the pyloric ring. The PU represent a transition from PPU to DU. The clinical significance is that patients with PU are usually gastric acid hypersecretors and should have some type of vagotomy for surgical management. Experience has shown, however, that PGV without drainage is insufficient to prevent recurrent ulcer in about one third of patients with PU.

The surgical group at Basel of Muller and associates has studied this problem by examining the gastric outlet in 119 stomachs, comparing patients with PU, PPU, and DU against controls. Significant thickening of the muscle layer of the pylorus and antrum was found in patients with PU and PPU compared to that found in normal controls and patients with DU. This thickness appears to be due to hypertrophy of the muscle cells. Edema, fibrosis, and migration of mast and eosinophil cells were quantitatively increased in patients with PU compared to patients with DU. Acid secretion was reduced by PGV in both patients with DU and PU. The higher ulcer recurrence rate in patients with PU treated by PGV without drainage is due to an irreversible "antropyloric dystrophy" according to Muller and associates. This results in (or from) the morphological changes in the antrum and pylorus in patients with PU and PPU.

TREATMENT

Few reports are available of medical or surgical treatment results with patients having PU. Most reports consider patients with juxtapyloric ulcers, which include patients with PU, but usually combine these results with patients who have PPU and, in some reports (Rehnberg), combine results of patients with DU, PU, and PPU. The report of Murray and associates in 1967 is one of the few articles devoted exclusively to PU patients. They state that PU patients respond poorly to intensive medical therapy, but this report appeared before cimetidine was available. Strom et al. reported in 1984 the results of a prospective, randomized cimetidine vs. PGV study in patients with juxtapyloric ulcers. In that study, patients with PU and PPU were considered together. The relapse rate for patients treated with cimetidine was 57%, while patients with DU had relapse rates of 17%. The PGV-treated patients had a relapse rate of 32%, which is similar to the 35% ulcer recurrence rate after PGV for patients with PU reported in 1987 by Muller et al. In both series, PGV resulted in a profound decrease in both basal and peak acid output after operation, indicating that the operation was technically correct.

The high ulcer recurrence rate following juxtapyloric ulcers treated by medical measures emphasizes the need for correctly identifying the ulcer location in these patients. While patients with DU may be expected to respond favorably to the receptor antagonist drugs, such is not the response in patients with PU.

Since patients with PU respond poorly to medical treatment, surgical intervention should be considered early for these patients. The report by Murray et al. included a variety of operations for patients with PU. The only recommendation from that study was that vagotomy and pyloroplasty be done for perforated pyloric channel ulcer. Ten years later (1976), in a report from the Mayo Clinic, Davis et al. stated that the recurrence rate for patients with "channel ulcers" was 8.5% after partial gastrectomy and 3.8% after partial gastrectomy with vagotomy. Follow-up extended from 1 to 14 years.

The truncal technique of vagotomy was used in both reports. With the introduction of selective gastric vagotomy (SGV) and PGV, reports have appeared with the use of these procedures for patients with PU. Andersen et al. compared selective gastric vagotomy with pyloroplasty (SGV + P) with PGV in patients with PU and PPU. The ulcer recurrence rate with PGV was 33%; with SGV + P, 14%. The recurrence rate had no relation to preoperative gastric acid secretion levels. This study showed no significant difference in recurrent ulcer rates in patients with DU when comparing PGV with SGV + P, unlike the higher recurrence rate with PGV in patients with PU and PPU.

Rehnberg found that patients with PU and PPU treated by antrectomy alone had an ulcer recurrence rate of 18% within five years of operation. When vagotomy was added to antrectomy, the ulcer recurrence rate dropped to 2%. The two patients who developed a recurrent ulcer underwent a second vagotomy and had no further recurrence of their ulcer. The median reduction in peak acid output was reduced to 82% after vagotomy and antrectomy, but to only 57% after antrectomy alone. This report also showed that patients could not be preselected for operation on the basis of preoperative gastric acid secretion studies.

Andersen et al. reported no recurrent ulcers in 54 patients treated by vagotomy-antrectomy for PU and PPU. These studies would suggest that vagotomy and antrectomy should be done for patients with PU since these patients appear to have an aggressive type of ulcer. Studies in patients with DU, as reported by Herrington et al., have shown that vagotomy-antrectomy results in lower re-

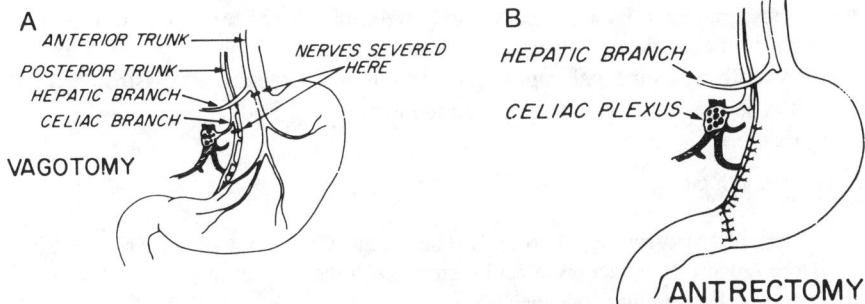

FIG 16-1.
Recommended operation for pyloric channel ulcer. **A,** selective gastric vagotomy. **B,** antrectomy: Billroth-I gastroduodenostomy reestablishes alimentary tract continuity.

currence rates (1% or less) than any other operative procedure for DU. The trade-off has been a higher incidence of postgastrectomy sequelae characterized by dumping, reflux gastritis, and diarrhea that occurs in about 25% of patients after vagotomy-antrectomy but is severe in only 2% to 3% of patients. While PGV is acceptable as a safe operation for patients with DU with minimal postgastrectomy sequelae, it cannot be used for patients with PU because of the high ulcer recurrence rate (approximately 33%). Yet, vagotomy is necessary in patients with PU. Could PGV + P be an acceptable operation for PU? Andersen's study of SGV + P resulted in a 14% ulcer recurrence rate. It seems logical to anticipate a similar recurrence rate with PGV + P.

It is my opinion that vagotomy and antrectomy (V-A) is the preferred operation for patients with PU, and studies report an ulcer recurrence rate of 2%. Vagotomy eliminates the cephalic phase of gastric secretion, while antrectomy obliterates the gastric phase. Alimentary reconstruction can be done by the Shoemacher modification of the Billroth-I gastroduodenostomy (Figure 16–1).

The type of vagotomy may be truncal or SGV. The latter results in a lower incidence of postvagotomy diarrhea, but not of dumping or reflux gastritis. By sparing the hepatic and celiac vagal branches, SGV has an advantage over truncal vagotomy, since it obviates the adverse effects of extragastric vagotomy on the biliary tract, pancreas, and small intestine.

SUMMARY

Pyloric channel ulcer constitutes about 5% of all peptic ulcers. These unique ulcers are notoriously resistant to medical management. Patients with PU are gastric-acid hypersecretors, but they also have anatomical changes in the antropyloric segment, with thickening of the pyloric and antral muscle layer. Patients with PU have high ulcer recurrence rates when treated surgically by vagotomy alone (PGV) or by antrectomy alone (35% and 18%, respectively). Patients with

PU are best managed by vagotomy and antrectomy, since this operation reduces acid secretion and removes the area of antropyloric dystrophy. I prefer selective gastric vagotomy to truncal vagotomy, but either is acceptable. Gastrointestinal continuity is reestablished by gastroduodenostomy.

BIBLIOGRAPHY

1. Andersen D, Hostrup H, Amdrup E: The Aarhus County Vagotomy Trial: II. An interim report on reduction in acid secretion and ulcer recurrence rate following parietal cell vagotomy and selective gastric vagotomy. *World J Surg* 1978; 2:91–100.
2. Andersen D, Amdrup E, Hostrup H, et al: The Aarhus County Vagotomy Trial: Trends in the problem of recurrent ulcer after parietal cell vagotomy and selective gastric vagotomy with drainage. *World J Surg* 1982; 6:86–92.
3. Bonnevie O: The incidence of duodenal ulcer in Copenhagen County. *Scand J Gastroenterol* 1975; 10:385–393.
4. Brethwaite S, Weintrub S, Skoog-Smith WA: Pyloric canal ulcer: An analysis of 86 cases. *Proceedings of the 53rd Annual Meeting of the American Gastroenterological Association.* Atlantic City, NJ, May 2–3, 1952. Baltimore, Williams & Wilkins Co, 1952, pp 40–41.
5. Davis Z, Verheyden CN, Van Heerden JA, et al.: The surgically treated chronic gastric ulcer: An extended follow-up. *Ann Surg* 1977; 185:205–209.
6. Goligher JC: Proximal gastric vagotomy without drainage, in Scott HW, Sawyers J (eds): *Surgery of the Stomach, Duodenum and Small Intestine.* Boston, Blackwell Scientific Publications, 1987, pp 627–650.
7. Herrington JL, Sawyers JL, Scott HW Jr: A 25-year experience with vagotomy-antrectomy. *Arch Surg* 1973; 106:469–474.
8. Johnson HD: Gastric ulcer: Classification, blood group characteristics, secretion patterns and pathogenesis. *Ann Surg* 1965; 162:996–1004.
9. Muller C, Liebermann-Meffent D, Allgower M: Pyloric and prepyloric ulcers. *World J Surg* 1987; 11:339–344.
10. Murray GF, Ballinger WF, Stafford ES: Ulcers of the pyloric channel. *Am J Surg* 1967; 113:199–203.
11. Oi M, Oshida K, Sugimura S: The location of gastric ulcer. *Gastroenterology* 1959; 36:45–56.
12. Oi M, Sakurai Y: The location of duodenal ulcer. *Gastroenterology* 1959; 36:60–64.
13. Ornsholt J, Amdrup E, Andersen D, et al.: Aarhus County Vagotomy Trial: Acid secretory patterns in patients with prepyloric, pyloric, and duodenal ulcer. *Digestion* 1983; 26:146–152.
14. Rehnberg O: Antrectomy and gastroduodenostomy with or without vagotomy in peptic ulcer disease: A prospective study with a 5-year follow-up. *Acta Chir Scand (Suppl)* 1983; 515:1–63.
15. Strom M, Lindhagen J, Bodemar G, et al: Cimetidine or parietal-cell vagotomy in patients with juxtapyloric ulcers. *Lancet* 1984; 2:894–897.

16. Texter EC Jr, Smith HW, Bundesen WE, et al: The syndrome pylorique: Clinical and physiologic observations. *Gastroenterology* 1959; 36:573–579.

17

Recurrent Marginal Ulcer

A 55-year-old male longshoreman with a long history of duodenal ulcer disease had undergone truncal vagotomy and hemigastrectomy for chronic duodenal ulcer. Following this, he had a satisfactory result initially, with only a 10-lb weight loss, his postoperative weight stabilizing at 210 pounds. Over the next months, however, he gradually develops symptoms that are similar to those for which he was operated on: epigastric pain, only sometimes relieved by food and antacid. A trial of histamine H_2 antagonists gives initial relief, but finally symptoms persist. Upper gastrointestinal (GI) series reveals no ulceration, but endoscopy reveals a marginal ulceration in the gastrojejunostomy.

Consultant: David C. Carter, M.D.

On the face of it, our task seems simple. The history clearly suggests recurrence of ulceration, a major disappointment to the patient and his surgeon that occurs in 5% to 10% of patients after surgery for peptic ulcer disease. Recurrence is approximately six times more common in males than in females, and after duodenal ulcer surgery it occurs in 3% to 10% of patients as opposed to only 2% after operation for gastric ulcer. Much, of course, depends on the nature of the original operation and, particularly when vagotomy is performed, on the ability of the surgeon. For example, gastroenterostomy alone was once practiced widely as an operation for uncomplicated peptic ulceration, but it is now discredited, given that ulceration recurred in one in three patients. After gastric resection the reported rate varies from 1% to 15%, much depending on the amount of stomach removed. Perhaps the greatest variation is reported following truncal vagotomy and drainage and after the newer operation of highly selective vagotomy (also known as parietal cell vagotomy or proximal gastric vagotomy), after which recurrence rates vary from low single figures to as high as 30%. Surgical seniority is no guarantee of ability and it is well recognized that surgeons vary greatly in their ability to achieve complete vagotomy.

Of all the operations available for treatment of duodenal ulceration, vagotomy combined with resection is accepted universally as carrying the lowest rate of recurrence by virtue of its dual assault on acid secretion. Not only is the parietal cell mass deprived of its vagal drive to H^+ secretion, but removal of the antrum eradicates the major source of production of the hormone gastrin. In the large Veterans Administration Cooperative study reported by Postlethwait, operative mortality and five-year recurrent ulcer rates following vagotomy and gastric resection were both beneath 1%.

Thus, recurrence is somewhat surprising in our patient and we need reassurance about the confidence of the diagnosis. The history is certainly consistent with recurrence, and the failure of an upper GI series to display an ulcer certainly does not exclude ulceration. The upper GI series has a much lower yield (50% to 60%) in diagnosing recurrence than diagnosing primary ulcer disease, and an ulcer crater is notoriously difficult to define at a gastrojejunostomy stoma. On the other hand, endoscopy carried out by an experienced endoscopist will confirm the presence of recurrent ulceration in approximately 90% of cases. This is not to say than an upper GI series is of no value. In addition to revealing the ulcer crater in over 50% of patients, the investigation may imply ulceration by showing spasm around the stoma. Anatomical relationships can be defined, the adequacy of gastric drainage can be assessed, and occasionally unsuspected problems such as afferent loop obstruction and the rare retrograde jejunogastric intussusception are detected.

CAUSES OF RECURRENT ULCERATION

Given that the diagnosis of ulceration is secure, attention must now focus on its cause and the following factors must be considered: (1) Has there been inadequate surgery? (2) Does the patient have an endocrine basis for recurrence? (3) Are there any other contributing factors?

Inadequate Surgery as a Factor in Ulcer Recurrence

Measurement of gastric acid secretion in response to insulin-induced hypoglycemia six months after surgery suggests that gastric vagotomy is incomplete in up to 40% of cases, as reported by Fawcett et al. This does not mean that 40% of patients develop recurrent ulceration, as "enough" vagal fibers may have been divided to bring acid secretion down to levels that are no longer ulcerogenic. However, virtually all recurrent ulcers develop in patients with positive insulin tests and, as studies of patients undergoing revagotomy (as reported by Stabile and Passaro) have shown, it is usually a substantial vagal trunk rather than small strands that have been left intact—54% posterior trunk, 24% posterior and anterior trunk, 7% anterior trunk, 15% no definite major trunk. However, in our patient the combination of vagotomy with hemigastrectomy usually compensates for any shortcomings in the performance of vagotomy, and alternative explanations must be excluded.

If vagotomy is not performed, resection of 30% to 50% of the stomach is followed by recurrence in a third of patients, whereas resection of 50% to 70% of the stomach drops the recurrence rate to around 10%. Reading the operation note in conjunction with assessment of stomach remnant size on the upper GI series and endoscopy should provide reassurance on this score. The information provided implies that our patient has undergone a Billroth-II type of resection, in that the recurrence is located at the gastrojejunostomy stoma rather than at the gastroduodenal anastomosis, which would have been performed in a Billroth-I resection. This opens the possibility that failure to take the resection line distal to the pylorus may have resulted in inadvertent retention of part of the gastric antrum with the duodenal stump. In the absence of luminal gastric acid, such antral mucosa is freed from any inhibitory check, and continuous hypersecretion of gastrin may occur. The prevalence of retained antrum in collected series of patients with recurrence after gastrectomy is estimated to be almost 10% (as reported by Stabile and Passaro). The levels of serum gastrin and of gastric acid secretion in these patients may mimic those found in patients with the Zollinger-Ellison syndrome. In this context, it should be remembered that antral mucosa may extend for some 0.5 cm beyond the pylorus and that an approximate cuff of duodenum must be removed with the stomach at the time of gastrectomy. (*Editor's note:* Information about the adequacy of the distal resection margin may be available from the pathology specimen report. It is unfortunate that some pathologists do not make an attempt to be specific about this information.)

Other technical factors that can occasionally contribute to ulcer recurrence are poor gastric drainage due to anastomotic hold up and inadvertent anastomosis of the stomach to distal small bowel at the time of gastrectomy. (*Editor's note:* The human counterpart of the Mann-Williamson experimental ulcerogenic preparation.) This latter mistake favors ulcer recurrence in that the environment at the stoma may be less alkaline than after anastomosis to the proximal jejunum.

Endocrine Basis for Ulcer Recurrence

While the Zollinger-Ellison syndrome is rare, the possibility of a gastrin-secreting tumor must always be borne in mind, particularly when an ulcer recurs after vagotomy and hemigastrectomy. (Full consideration of the Zollinger-Ellison syndrome is beyond the scope of this case discussion and is provided in another section by Dr. Zollinger.) It is also worth mentioning that a link is generally accepted between hypercalcemia and peptic ulcer disease, particularly when hypercalcemia is the result of hyperparathyroidism. The relationship between hyperparathyroidism and hypergastrinemia is controversial, and most patients with this association probably have an occult gastrinoma as part of a type I multiple endocrine neoplasia.

Other Contributing Factors in Ulcer Recurrence

A number of drugs, notably nonsteroidal anti-inflammatory drugs (such as indomethacin, salicylates, and phenylbutazone), corticosteroids, and reserpine may occasionally be implicated in the causation or exacerbation of recurrent ulceration.

INVESTIGATION

Given a firm diagnosis of recurrent ulcer, what further investigations are needed? Measurement of serum gastrin levels on fasting blood samples is certainly worthwhile as a screening test for the rare Zollinger-Ellison syndrome and as a means of detecting a retained antrum. Gastrin levels may be extremely high in both conditions, whereas they are normally reduced markedly after antrectomy. (*Editor's note:* Serum gastrin level may be elevated to 200 to 300 pg/ml by prior vagotomy.) Additional use of the secretin provocation test may distinguish between patients with Zollinger-Ellison syndrome and those with a retained antrum. Technetium pertechnetate scans can be used to detect antral retention, and cuffs as small as 1 cm have been defined as an abnormal "hot spot" in the right upper quadrant. Serum calcium levels should also be determined to detect patients with hyperparathyroidism who may also prove to be suffering from multiple endocrine neoplasia.

Considerable controversy surrounds the use of acid secretory studies, as the days have gone when no self-respecting surgical unit would submit all peptic ulceration patients to routine testing before (e.g., histamine, betazole, or pentagastrin tests) and after (e.g., pentagastrin or insulin tests) gastric surgery. In the present context, the Hollander insulin test was used most widely as a test for completeness of vagotomy but was at best an imperfect instrument. In most centers the test was considered positive when there was a rise in acid concentration of at least 20 mmole/L when the basal and peak periods of acid secretion were compared. However, as mentioned earlier, positivity was far from synonymous with ulcer recurrence, while occasional patients developed recurrence despite a negative test. In addition, the test was unpleasant for the patient and potentially dangerous because of the associated hypoglycemia. While completeness (or otherwise) of vagotomy can probably be informed from the less dangerous pentagastrin or betazole tests of maximal acid output, there is now a general feeling that isolated postoperative acid secretory tests add little to the management of the patient with suspected or proved recurrent ulceration.

On the other hand, raised levels of serum pepsinogen-I can be detected reliably by radioimmunoassay, as reported by Samloff and Liebman. Basal levels may be raised in patients with recurrent ulcer, and after betazole injection they rise. In contrast, levels decrease paradoxically in patients who have had a complete vagotomy and who have no recurrence of ulceration.

TREATMENT

Patients with recurrent ulcer respond less well to histamine H_2-receptor antagonists than those with primary ulceration. Although as many as 90% of patients may show an early response while receiving full-dose therapy, maintenance doses often permit relapse and current reports suggest a relapse rate of some 70% once the patient stops taking the drug. One must also remember that recurrent ulcers are frequently complicated by bleeding and perforation, and that gastro-jejunocolic fistula may develop in patients, such as that discussed here, in whom a gastrojejunal anastomosis has been performed. This means that surgery is indicated for recurrent ulceration unless there are overwhelming contraindications.

Given that incomplete vagotomy is by far the most likely cause of failure, surgery must include a careful search for intact vagal fibers and, in particular, for the posterior vagus. The objective should be to skeletonize the lower 5 cm of esophagus, but adhesion formation often means that great care is needed to remobilize the esophagus without perforating it. Some surgeons prefer to use a transthoracic approach, arguing that morbidity is lower and completeness of vagotomy more likely. My own preference is for the abdominal route, as it is important to check that part of the antrum has not been retained in the duodenal stump. If no large vagal trunks are found after clearing the esophagus, a 70% gastrectomy is indicated. Ensuring complete vagotomy and adequate gastric resection should prevent further recurrence in as many as 95% of patients. Some surgeons advocate Roux-en-Y reconstruction to minimize the possibility of troublesome alkaline reflux gastritis, although this is not routine practice. Total gastrectomy should be reserved for the 5% of patients who develop a second recurrence in the absence of any defined cause and as an option for the treatment of the Zollinger-Ellison syndrome.

SUMMARY

Recurrent ulceration is a major cause of failure in the surgery of peptic ulceration. Its incidence may be reduced by skilled surgery and appropriate choice of operation. The diagnosis is not necessarily a source of gloom and despair, as recurrent ulceration is arguably an easier complication of gastric surgery to treat than, for example, dumping and diarrhea. With prompt and accurate diagnosis, coupled with management by skilled surgeons, good-to-excellent results can be achieved in 85% of patients at the expense of an operative mortality of 1% to 2%.

BIBLIOGRAPHY

1. Fawcett AN, Johnston D, Duthie HL: Revagotomy for recurrent ulcer after vagotomy and drainage for duodenal ulcer. *Br J Surg* 1969; 56:111–116.
2. Gillespie G, Elder JB, Gillespie IE, et al: The long term stability of the insulin test. *Gastroenterology* 1970; 58:625–632.
3. Postlethwait RG: Five year follow-up results of operations for duodenal ulcer. *Surg Gynecol Obstet* 1973; 137:387–392.

4. Samloff IM, Liebman WM: Radioimmunoassay of group I pepsinogens in serum. *Gastroenterology* 1974; 66:494–502.
5. Stabile BE, Passaro E: Recurrent peptic ulcer. *Gastroenterology* 1976; 70:124–135.

18

Giant Duodenal Ulcer

A 64-year-old man presented to the emergency room with acute onset of hematemesis and melena. His past history is significant for peptic ulcer disease treated previously with cimetidine. Recently he has been experiencing epigastric pain with nausea and radiation to his back that is more severe than his previous "ulcer pain" and is not relieved by food or antacids. Esophagogastroduodenoscopy reveals a widened pylorus and a large duodenal ulcer, approximately 2.5 cm in diameter, involving the entire duodenal bulb with fresh clot adherent posteriorly.

Consultant: Michael S. Nussbaum, M.D.

Giant duodenal ulcer is a variant of peptic ulcer disease. It is defined as a full-thickness ulcer in the first part of the duodenum, accurately measured to be greater than 2 cm in diameter. These ulcers are four to five times larger than normal duodenal ulcers and are significantly more dangerous, with a greater propensity for perforation, massive hemorrhage, and obstruction. In addition, the overwhelming majority of these patients come to surgery. In the event of an acute perforation, definitive surgery for ulcer disease, not just patching of the duodenum, must be carried out. Giant duodenal ulcers are very different entities, with an entirely different life history than "garden variety" duodenal ulcers.

Since Brdiczka first described giant duodenal ulcer in 1931, over 200 cases of this disease have been reported in the literature, the majority since 1960. The incidence is probably more common than originally thought, due to a high level of suspicion and more accurate diagnosis utilizing modern roentgenologic techniques as well as the widespread use of endoscopy. Diagnosis is often elusive unless specific diagnostic and roentgenologic criteria are followed. Typically, these are penetrating ulcers involving more than 80% of the duodenal bulb. Successful noninvasive treatment is rare. The chances of retaining normal physiologic function when such extensive duodenal involvement occurs have been seriously questioned. Although the morbidity and mortality rates have decreased markedly since giant duodenal ulcer was initially described, the condition is commonly fatal unless accurate diagnosis is made and treatment implemented.

CLINICAL PRESENTATION

The majority of patients reported in the literature are men (approximately 80%), with an average age of 55 to 60 years old. They commonly present with a history of long-standing ulcer symptoms that respond poorly to medical management. Because of the anatomical location, perforation usually occurs as a slow penetration so that adjacent structures or organs wall off the area of destroyed duodenal wall. Most patients present with chronic illness, weight loss, and abdominal pain, with the epigastric pain often more intense than in the "usual" ulcer patient. As the ulcer burrows into the pancreas and adjacent structures, the pain may be referred more to the right upper quadrant or posteriorly into the back. The pain is generally not relieved by food or antacids, which is understandable in view of the size and penetration of the ulcer. The most common emergency presentation in these patients is massive gastrointestinal hemorrhage. The gastroduodenal artery has often been found in the middle of the ulcer bed, actively hemorrhaging at operation. Partial or complete obstruction of the duodenum distal to the ulcer crater may occur, leading to vomiting, weight loss, and malnutrition. The cachexia can be so prominent with the association of an inflammatory mass in the epigastrium that carcinoma may be the preliminary diagnosis in these patients.

INVESTIGATION

The highest mortality occurs in giant duodenal ulcer patients who remain undiagnosed. Mortality is decreased in those patients diagnosed intraoperatively and is lowest in patients accurately diagnosed preoperatively. Therefore, a high index of suspicion and early accurate diagnosis are crucial in achieving an optimal outcome. The upper gastrointestinal series, in conjunction with endoscopic confirmation and biopsy, is the most important tool for making the diagnosis of giant duodenal ulcer. A major problem is that giant duodenal ulcers are commonly misdiagnosed. They are so large that they may resemble a normal or slightly abnormal duodenal bulb, which might be considered a deformity rather than a giant ulcer. However, as awareness of this lesion has increased, certain diagnostic criteria have been established that have not only led to earlier diagnosis but have also demonstrated that the disease is not as rare as initially believed. The radiographs of this lesion have been so deceptive to radiologists and other physicians that the number of unreported cases must be quite large.

The radiologic diagnosis is subtle, with the salient points being: (1) fixation of the duodenal bulb and lack of normal peristaltic waves; (2) constancy in size and shape of the ulcer; (3) loss of the mucosal pattern around the crater; (4) a tendency to stand out as the duodenum empties barium (Fig 18–1); (5) multiple filling defects resembling polypoid tumors (these represent either necrotic pan-

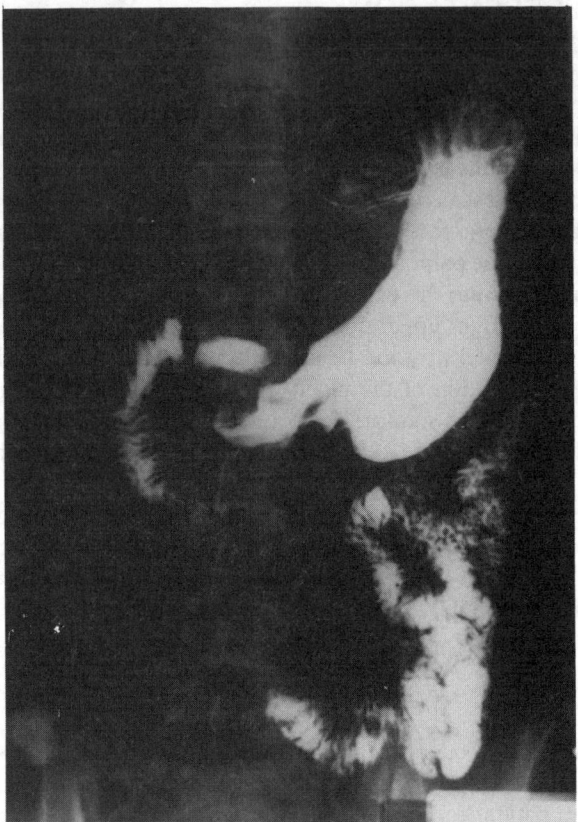

FIG 18–1.
The ulcer has a tendency to stand out as the duodenum empties the barium. (From Nussbaum MS, Schusterman MA: *Am J Surg* 1985; 149:359. Used by permission.)

creas, granulation tissue, or blood clots); (6) air-fluid level in the crater; (7) a patulous or partially destroyed pylorus (Fig 18–2); and (8) obstruction or spasm of the duodenum distal to the ulcer due to inflammation and edema (Fig 18–3). These criteria have been refined and developed over 30 years and are the mainstays of early diagnosis.

During endoscopy the pyloric spincter is widened, edematous, and hyperemic. In addition, it is often less mobile than normal. The ulcers are so large that they can be clearly seen through the pyloric sphincter. On passage through the pylorus, soft necrotic slough is seen extending circumferentially around the entire bulb and virtually replaces the duodenal wall.

The major differential diagnosis of giant duodenal ulcer is pseudodiverticulum of the bulb or a true diverticulum of the postbulbar area, gastric ulcer, and a carcinoma or lymphosarcoma of the duodenum. The diverticulum can be diagnosed by observation of the changing size and shape of the crater. Gastric ulcer can be distinguished at endoscopy. While neoplasms are extremely rare, the distinction can be made at the operating table or by endoscopic biopsy.

CASE SCENARIO

Following initial stabilization and transfusion of 2 units of packed red blood cells, the patient was admitted to the intensive care unit and therapy with histamine H_2 blockers and antacids instituted. On the second hospital day, he developed recurrent bleeding, a precipitous fall in hematocrit reading from 31% to 24%, and orthostatic hypotension. Blood transfusion was initiated and he was taken to the operating room for an emergent laparotomy. At operation, a distal gastrotomy was made and extended across the pylorus. The ulcer had completely eroded through the entire posterior wall of the duodenum into the head of the pancreas. An actively bleeding vessel in the depth of the crater was controlled with several silk sutures and the duodenum was lifted up off of the pancreas, leaving the ulcer bed in situ. The duodenal stump was closed in two layers and a duodenostomy tube was placed. A truncal vagotomy and antrectomy with a

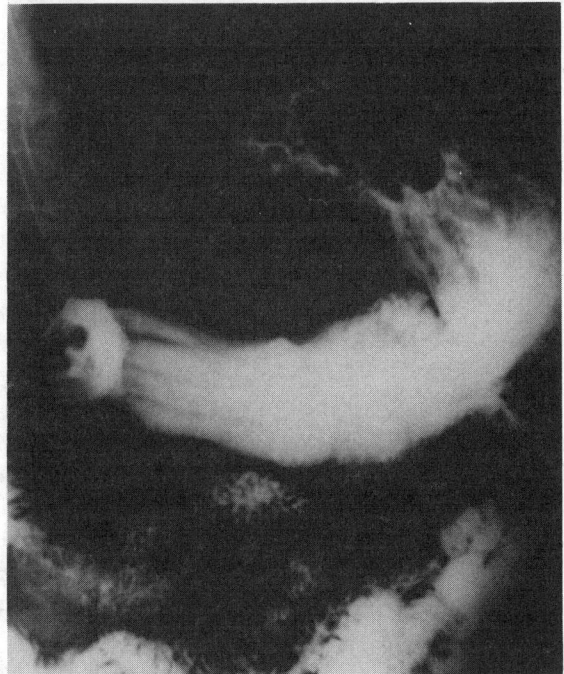

FIG 18–2.
The pylorus appears patulous or partially destroyed.

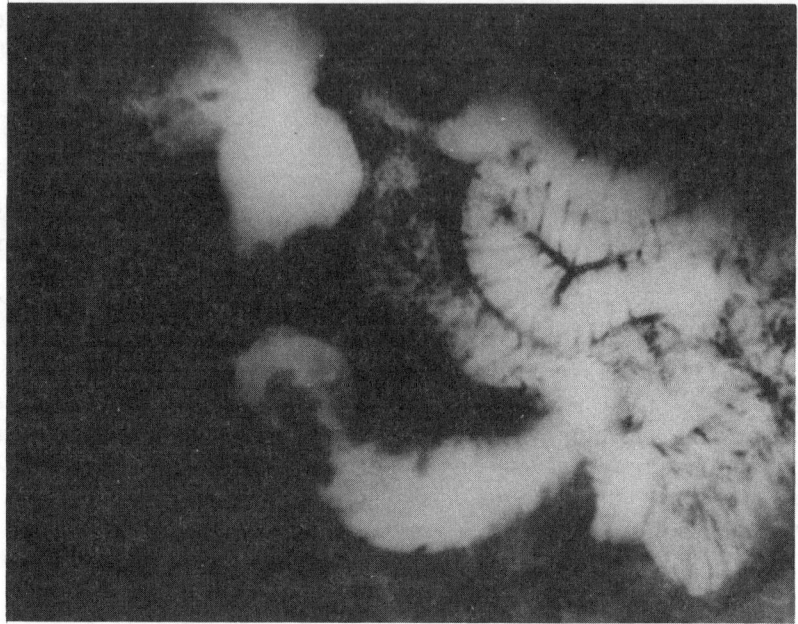

FIG 18–3.
Obstruction or spasm secondary to inflammation or edema of the duodenum distal to the ulcer may be noted.

Billroth-II gastrojejunostomy was then performed. A needle catheter jejunostomy was inserted for postoperative enteral nutrition, a closed suction drain was placed in the region of the pancreatic head; the incision was closed, and the patient was returned to the intensive care unit for continued organ system support.

TREATMENT

Early diagnosis and surgical management are the mainstays of treatment for giant duodenal ulcer. Successful medical treatment has been the exception in the past, and there are many reports of patients initially treated medically who died from sudden massive hemorrhage or required emergency operations for bleeding or free perforation. Since the ulcer is literally a walled-off, through-and-through perforation and involves the majority of the duodenal bulb, the long-term ability of the duodenum to function adequately after healing must be questioned, if indeed the patient does not die from the complications. In addition, surgical morbidity and mortality is significantly increased if these patients require emergency operation. Medical therapy does play an adjunctive role as a prelude to surgery, its aim being to improve the patient's general condition and allow time for any inflammatory swelling around the ulcer to subside. Many of these patients are malnourished, and total parenteral nutrition may be indicated. Antacids, H_2-receptor blockers, and antibiotics are also helpful in reducing the inflammation and edema so that safe resection can be carried out.

Surgical treatment of this condition is not without complications. The death rate in the 1940s and 1950s was extremely high. Since 1966 the overall mortality has gradually declined from 41% to 7% in the most recent reports. The progressive reduction in mortality can be attributed to numerous factors. Improvements in radiologic equipment (such as image intensification), the advent of fiberoptic endoscopy, improved perioperative nutritional support, better antibiotics, and improved surgical and anesthetic techniques have led to earlier diagnosis, prompt surgical intervention, and improved management of these patients.

A definitive acid-reduction operation is the procedure of choice. Truncal vagotomy and gastric resection, with removal of the involved duodenum, should be considered whenever possible. If the inflammation and edema are markedly decreased, a Billroth-I reconstruction can occasionally be safely performed. A Billroth-II gastrojejunostomy, however, is the most frequent method of reconstruction utilized in these patients. Frequently, the mass is so inflamed and indurated that duodenal dissection becomes hazardous. Because of the size of the ulcer bed and proximity to vital structures (i.e., pancreas, common bile duct, liver) in some of these patients, the ulcer bed may be left in situ, resecting the duodenum around the ulcer bed, oversewing the duodenum, and decompressing it with a duodenostomy tube. It has been our experience that the use of tube duodenostomy is a safe, rapid, and effective means of managing the difficult stump so often encountered in giant duodenal ulcer disease. In the severely debilitated patient, another option is truncal vagotomy and gastroenterostomy or pyloroplasty if the duodenum is manageable.

BIBLIOGRAPHY

1. Brdiczka JG: Das grosse ulcus duodeni in rontgenbild. *Fortschr Geb Rontgenstr* 1931; 44:177–181.
2. Dawson J: Giant duodenal ulcer. *Br J Radiol* 1958; 31:666–668.
3. Klamer TW, Mahr MM: Giant duodenal ulcer: A dangerous variant of a common illness. *Am J Surg* 1978; 135:760–762.
4. Lumsden K, MacLarnon JC, Dawson J: Giant duodenal ulcer. *Gut* 1970; 11:592–599.
5. Mistilis SP, Wiot JF, Nedelman SH: Giant duodenal ulcer. *Ann Intern Med* 1963; 59:155–164.
6. Morrow CE, Mulholland MW, Dunn DH, et al: Giant duodenal ulcer. *Am J Surg* 1982; 144:330–331.
7. Nussbaum MS, Schusterman MA: Management of giant duodenal ulcer. *Am J Surg* 1985; 149:357–361.

19

Alkaline Reflux Gastritis

A 35-year-old woman with a chronic history of duodenal ulcer underwent successful vagotomy and antrectomy for chronic, unremitting, intractable duodenal ulcer. Over the next two years, she gradually developed epigastric pain not relieved, but in fact made worse, by food. Occasional vomiting occurred; the vomitus was described as green and not tinged with blood. Vomiting partially relieved the symptoms. In addition, she reported heartburn not relieved by milk or antacid. She has lost 15 lb and is unable to eat as she had in the past.

Consultant: Wallace P. Ritchie, Jr., M.D., Ph.D.

OVERVIEW

All operations for peptic ulcer disease have a common and compelling rationale: To achieve a sufficient reduction in the secretion of acid and pepsin to permit healing of the ulcer and to prevent recurrence. At the same time, however, the untoward sequelae that can result from the procedures employed to achieve this end must be minimized. These sequelae are known collectively as the postgastrectomy syndromes—a group of conditions, each with distinctive pathophysiologic and clinical features that result from loss of the gastric reservoir, from ablation or bypass of the pylorus, or from parasympathetic denervation of the stomach (perhaps also of the small intestine), either alone or in combination. The essential problem encountered by the surgeon is that those procedures with the greatest potential to cure the disease are also those that are most likely to produce undesirable side effects.

The clinical problem of epigastric pain and bilious vomiting following gastric resection is as old as gastric surgery itself; Billroth reported a case in 1885. Three quarters of a century later, the pathophysiology of chronic intermittent obstruction of the afferent limb following gastrectomy with gastrojejunostomy was delineated. Thereafter, most patients with this combination of symptoms were believed to suffer from the afferent loop syndrome. Approximately 20 years ago, however, reports began to appear in the surgical literature that suggested that excessive reflux of upper intestinal content into the residual stomach might, in and of itself, be responsible for a unique postgastrectomy syndrome, so called alkaline reflux gastritis. Symptoms allegedly specific for this syndrome included burning mid-epigastric pain unrelieved by antacids, often exacerbated by eating, and worse at night. Vomiting frequently relieved the pain and was usually bilious in nature. Nausea was a frequent accompaniment. Signs included a diminished capacity to secrete acid, endoscopic evidence of bile reflux, endoscopic and histologic "gastritis," weight loss, and a hypochromic microcytic anemia. Patients undergoing gastric resection with reconstruction as a Billroth II gastrojejunostomy seemed to be at greatest risk. These same clinical reports indicated that following shunting of upper intestinal content away from the residual gastric pouch with a long-limb Roux-en-Y gastrojejunostomy, good-to-excellent results were regularly achieved in 80% to 90% of patients.

As is so often the case, early uncritical acceptance has gradually been replaced by healthy skepticism, not only about the postulated pathophysiology of the syndrome, i.e., excessive enterogastric reflux, but also about its very existence. Such skepticism seems quite justified. More recent and more carefully analyzed series clearly indicate that when operation is undertaken on the basis of symptoms alone, a poor result can be anticipated in anywhere from 30% to 50% of patients. These reports also indicate that reliable symptomatic, endoscopic, or histologic predictors of success or failure are extremely difficult to identify; indeed, in some series the outcome seems almost random. Furthermore, it has become increasingly apparent that the preferred therapy, the creation of a Roux limb, may itself produce problems, specifically, marked delays in gastric emptying (the Roux syndrome). This is thought to be the consequence of Roux limb dysmotility, the result perhaps of interrupting the duodenal pacemaker. Anecdotal clinical reports suggest that patients undergoing concomitant truncal vagus section and those with delayed gastric emptying of solids preoperatively are at great risk. The combination of unpredictable results and a corrective operative procedure that is far from innocuous have served to dampen considerably the early enthusiasm concerning the existence of the syndrome and its appropriate treatment.

The basic problem, of course, is that no clear understanding of the pathophysiologic consequences of enterogastric reflux exists. While it appears quite certain that prolonged exposure of acid peptic secreting mucosa to upper intestinal content results in a specific type of gastritis (foveolar hyperplasia, cystification of the glands), the specific components of content responsible are largely undefined. Furthermore, the mechanisms by which reflux might produce symptoms are also unknown. For these reasons, the problem of selecting patients who will predictably benefit from a diversion is a major one. Thus, the cautious surgeon should approach patients such as the one illustrated with considerable circumspection, perhaps even a bit of trepidation.

DIAGNOSTIC EVALUATION

There are two features of this patient's history that are consistent with (but hardly diagnostic of) excessive enterogastric reflux. First, the vomitus is bilious. In my experience, this is the symptom found more frequently in symptomatic postgastrectomy patients with excessive enterogastric reflux relative to other dyspeptic postgastrectomy patients without excessive reflux. Second, the patient reports heartburn unrelieved by alkali, suggesting an alkaline rather than acid esophagitis. The evaluation of the patient should proceed with the realization that, if it exists, the syndrome of alkaline reflux gastritis is, at a minimum, a diagnosis of exclusion. Specifically, it is important to rule out cholelithiasis, recurrent ulcer, the afferent loop syndrome, efferent limb obstruction, and idiopathic gastroparesis as alternative causes of symptomatology.

The first step in evaluation should be an endoscopic examination of the esophagus, stomach, and anastomosis. In experienced hands, this is the most accurate way to rule out anastomotic ulcer. The severity of the esophagitis can also be assessed. At the same time, it is important to evaluate the extent of erythema seen in the residual gastric pouch; it is becoming increasingly apparent that a reddened, friable, and edematous mucous membrane involving more than the perianastomotic area may well be a specific consequence of enterogastric reflux. Biopsies of the residual stomach can also be obtained and examined for evidence of foveolar hyperplasia and glandular cystification, as noted above. Finally, stomal patency can also be assessed.

An upper gastrointestinal series is also of importance. The postgastrectomy anatomy can be demonstrated—review of the previous operative notes is also helpful in this regard; the position of the anastomosis with respect to the colon can be determined; a dilated afferent limb can be searched for, and anastomotic or efferent loop obstruction can be assessed. Finally, an abdominal ultrasound should be performed to evaluate the gallbladder, extrahepatic biliary tree, and pancreas.

If, at this point, no condition other than putative alkaline reflux gastritis has been identified as a cause of the patient's epigastric pain and bilious vomiting, quantitation of the magnitude of enterogastric reflux should be accomplished. Reflux is not a constant phenomenon; it is most pronounced postprandially and in the early morning hours. Therefore, studies to quantitate reflex should be performed under rigorously standardized conditions; we prefer the fasting state and early after arising from sleep. A nasogastric tube is passed and positioned under fluoroscopy to lie in the mid-portion of the residual gastric pouch. With the patient in the upright position, the gastric contents are aspirated and the stomach gently lavaged. The tube is then clamped and the patient placed in the recumbent position for one hour. At the end of this time, an aliquot is withdrawn and saved for subsequent analysis of total bile acid concentration. Following this, a small amount of isosmotic mannitol solution containing polyethylene glycol (PEG) as a nonabsorbable marker is instilled and rapidly mixed. An aliquot is then withdrawn and subsequently analyzed for PEG concentration. The residual volume in the stomach can then be calculated, which, in turn, permits calculation of net bile acid reflux per unit time.

On a subsequent day, again early in the morning, the patient is transported to the scintography suite. With the patient positioned supine under the detector of a gamma camera, 5 mCi of ^{99m}Tc-labeled HIDA is administered intravenously and count rates are recorded continuously over the hepatobiliary tree for 45 minutes or until the ^{99m}Tc activity is maximal in the gallbladder. The patient is then given 0.04 μg/kg of purified cholecystokinin (CCK) intravenously. At 15-minute intervals for the next two hours, ^{99m}Tc activity is monitored over liver, gallbladder, biliary tree, small bowel, and residual stomach. An enterogastric reflux index (EGRI) can then be calculated. In essence, the EGRI measures the fraction of activity initially in the hepatobiliary tree that ultimately is found in the gastric pouch. It should be noted that, although noninvasive, scintigraphic assessment of reflux may be less sensitive and less specific than assessment using the intubation techniques described.

The values obtained for recumbent bile acid concentration, net bile acid reflux per hour, and EGRI are used as quantitative markers of reflux magnitude. All have been shown to extremely reproducible. Those obtained in a given patient are then compared to similar values obtained in asymptomatic postgastrectomy patients (Table 19–1). If the patient demonstrates reflux indices that fall more than 2 SD beyond the mean of the control values in two of the three tests that directly or indirectly quantitate reflux, excessive enterogastric reflux more than likely exists. If these criteria are fulfilled, a useful adjunctive test (indeed, a necessary one prior to operative diversion) is to assess the rate of gastric emptying of solids using ^{99m}Tc-labeled sulphur colloid injected into the white of an egg that is then ingested by the patient. The normal half-time of gastric emptying of solids, i.e., that found in asymptomatic postgastrectomy patients, is also illustrated (see Table 19–1).

TABLE 19–1.

Reflux Values and Gastric Emptying in Asymptomatic Postgastrectomy Patients

	BA* (mM/L)	Net BA/hr* (uM)	EGRI† (%)	Emptying (t ½ min)‡
Mean	0.8	20	22	42
+2 SD	2.2	72	42	70

*BA = bile acid.
†EGRI = enterogastric reflux index.
‡t½ min = time required to supply the test meal.

An additional diagnostic maneuver involves provocative testing. Instillation of autologous intestinal content or 0.1 N sodium hydroxide into the intact stomach has been reported to reproduce typical symptomatology in putatively afflicted patients, but not in controls. It has been claimed, therefore, that these relatively simple tests are quite sensitive, specific, and accurate, and, therefore, useful in establishing a correct diagnosis. Whether or not this is actually the case remains to be seen.

NONOPERATIVE THERAPY

A variety of nonoperative therapies have been proposed to treat patients with excessive enterogastric reflux. These include the use of aluminum antacids to bind bile salts, the use of cholestyramine to accomplish the same goal, and the use of metoclopramide to enhance clearance of refluxate from the stomach. None of these approaches has proved salutory in the vast majority of patients. However, one recent report suggests that treatment with ursodeoxycholic acid (1,000 mg, orally, every day) results in a profound decrease in the intensity and frequency of epigastric pain and a virtual elimination of nausea and vomiting. The reasons for this circumstance are unclear, but they may relate to an alteration in the composition of refluxate such that the relative proportion of the more damaging secondary bile acids is diminished. Unfortunately, this drug is not available for general use in the United States at the present time. Despite the relative inefficacy of nonoperative treatment regimens, a trial of several months (with added prokinetic agents in the presence of delays in gastric emptying) is warranted if only to convince both patient and surgeon that all alternative therapies have been exhausted prior to undertaking operation.

OPERATIVE APPROACH

If operation is elected, one additional study is of extreme importance. Diversion of upper gastrointestinal content away from the residual gastric pouch using a Roux limb is potentially an extremely ulcerogenic procedure, as it is a variant of the Mann-Williamson operation. Recent experience suggests, however, that marginal ulceration is very infrequent if cholinergic denervation (vagotomy) of the stomach is complete. In most patients, vagotomy has been attempted as part of the original operative procedure. It is important, therefore, to test for its completeness because, if incomplete, revagotomy will be necessary at the time of reoperation. Such testing can be accomplished using a variation of the Hollander test (sham feeding). A nasogastric tube is positioned in the midportion of the stomach with the patient in the upright position; a fasting acid output is measured, and the pH of intragastric content is assessed. The patient is then instructed to smell, taste, chew, and expectorate a meat meal. Measurement of acid output and pH continues at 15-minute intervals over the subsequent two hours. It is highly probable that previous vagotomy is incomplete if the fasting pH is less than 3.5, if the concentration of acid increases by more than 20 mEq/ L, or if the pH falls to 3.5 or less following sham feeding, irrespective of its initial level.

The extent of the operative procedure to be performed depends upon three factors: (1) whether or not previous vagotomy has been undertaken and is found complete; (2) whether or not the patient demonstrates significant delays in gastric emptying; and (3) whether or not the previous gastric resection has been adequate (i.e., at least 50%). In those patients in whom vagotomy is demonstrably complete, who demonstrate normal postgastrectomy gastric emptying, and in whom resection has been adequate, it has been our practice simply to divide the afferent limb close to the stomach, oversew the distal end, and reimplant the proximal end 45 cm distally in the jejunum (end-to-side jejunojejunostomy). Even though gastric emptying is prolonged under these circumstances, in our experience this usually is of no clinical consequence.

On the other hand, in those patients in whom no previous vagotomy has been attempted, in those whose previous vagusection is demonstrably incomplete, in those with more than 50% of residual stomach in place, or, most importantly, in those who demonstrate significant delay in gastric emptying of solids preoperatively, the operative procedure required is more extensive if the Roux syndrome is to be avoided. Under these circumstances, we prefer to resect the entire anastomosis, to perform an 80% to 90% gastrectomy, and to use an end-to-side (polya) gastrojejunostomy for reconstruction. Additional technical maneuvers that may facilitate the effect of gravity on emptying of the residual pouch include placing the limb in a retrocolic position and fashioning the anastomosis in such a way that the blind end is at the lesser curvature and the efferent limb at the greater curvature. Some feel that the Roux syndrome is less frequent if the Roux is fashioned as a Tanner 19 (i.e., the afferent limb is divided, the proximal line of transection is anastomosed 45 cm distally to the jejunum, and the distal line is placed end-to-side into the existing efferent jejunal limb). The data to suggest that this procedure promotes better gastric emptying than the more standard Roux are completely anecdotal; nevertheless, the approach appears deserving of further clinical investigation.

Conversion to a 45-cm Roux limb gastrojejunostomy results in complete, permanent elimination of enterogastric reflux, irrespective of the methodology employed to assess this parameter. Concomitantly, gastritis improves markedly, fasting intragastric pH falls, and the capacity to secrete acid increases modestly. The erythema of the residual gastric pouch also disappears rapidly. As already indicated, delays in gastric emptying are common in the early postoperative period. With time, however, emptying tends to normalize to pre-Roux levels.

The reasons for this circumstance are unclear, but they may relate to reconstitution of a pacesetter in the proximal portion of the Roux limb.

PROGNOSIS

The early symptomatic results observed in subjects who have had operations have been gratifying. Continuous burning mid-epigastric pain and bilious vomiting are eliminated in almost all patients, and nausea and vomiting are relieved in most. On late follow-up, however, despite the complete absence of reflux, symptomatic deterioration is not uncommon; epigastric pain can recur in as many as 20% of patients, and recurrent or persistent nausea and vomiting can be experienced by up to one third. Bilious vomiting is the only symptom that appears to be permanently eliminated. The other side of the coin, of course, is that two thirds of patients have a satisfactory result lasting at least three years. Whether this circumstance will persist for longer periods is unknown. In my opinion, these outcomes are sufficiently salutory that the existence of a syndrome based on excessive enterogastric reflux should not be rejected out of hand. Conversely, in view of the numerous unresolved vagaries surrounding the syndrome and the occasional severe problems related to its surgical treatment, and prudent surgeon will undertake remedial operative therapy only after excessive enterogastric reflux has been convincingly documented and all other causes of postgastrectomy "dyspepsia" have been thoroughly excluded.

BIBLIOGRAPHY

1. Malagelada JR, Phillips SF, Shorter RG, et al: Postoperative reflux gastritis: Pathophysiology and long-term outcome after Roux-en-Y diversion. *Ann Intern Med* 1985; 103:178–183.
2. Ritchie WP Jr: Alkaline reflux gastritis: A critical reappraisal. *Gut* 1984; 25:975–987.
3. Ritchie WP Jr: Alkaline reflux gastritis: Late results of a controlled trial of diagnosis and treatment. *Ann Surg* 1986; 203:537–544.

PART III

Liver, Biliary, Pancreas

20

Sclerosing Cholangitis

A 29-year-old woman had previously undergone total proctocolectomy and a sphincter-preserving continence procedure for ulcerative colitis. Before operation, the transaminase level was elevated; the value for alkaline phosphatase was slightly elevated, and the bilirubin level was normal. Recovery from the operative procedure was satisfactory. Over the next several years, however, she noted intermittent epigastric pain and occasional dark urine and relatively light stools. For the few weeks before admission, she felt poorly and had right upper quadrant pain without fever. Two days before admission, she was icteric. Light stools and dark urine had been present for approximately ten days. Endoscopic retrograde cholangiopancreatography revealed multiple sclerotic areas in the common hepatic and common bile ducts that terminated near the bifurcation. Bilirubin level was 7 mg/dl; alkaline phosphatase value was 620 mg/dl, and serum glutamic oxaloacetic transaminase (SGOT) was 45 international units (IU)/L.

Consultant: Kenneth W. Warren, M.D.

DISCUSSION

Primary sclerosing cholangitis is a rare disease characterized by total or partial involvement of the extrahepatic and intrahepatic biliary ducts. Synonyms include primary sclerosing cholangitis, primary stenosing cholangitis, chronic fibrous choledochitis, sclerosing pericholedochitis, and chronic obliterative cholangitis. It is characterized by a progressive inflammatory sclerosing and obliterative process that may result in chronic biliary obstruction followed by secondary biliary cirrhosis and eventually liver failure. Not infrequently, portal hypertension and bleeding esophageal varices herald the terminal phase of the disease.

The clinical course is highly unpredictable, and this has led to many controversial and diverse opinions regarding the natural course of the disease and, in turn, its proper treatment. The extremes of clinical behavior can vary from frequent attacks and relentless progression, to an interval of 19 years between an operation to relieve biliary obstruction and a reoccurrence with rapid progression to combined biliary and portal cirrhosis associated with bleeding esophageal varices and progressive liver failure and death.

A major controversy surrounds the definition and criteria for diagnosis of this disease. The term sclerosing cholangitis implies nontraumatic, nonmalignant fibrosis occurring in the submucosal portion of the bile ducts, causing thickness of the walls with consequent narrowing of the lumens. The external diameter of the ducts undergoes little change.

The precise criteria necessary for diagnosis are controversial. Myers et al. proposed the most stringent criteria for the diagnosis of primary sclerosing cholangitis, suggesting that the following features are essential: (1) progressive jaundice of the obstructive type, (2) absence of biliary calculi, (3) no prior biliary surgery, (4) generalized thickening and stenosis of the walls of the biliary ductal system, (5) absence of biliary tract malignancy as determined by reasonable long-term follow-up, (6) no evidence of primary biliary cirrhosis as determined by liver biopsy, and (7) absence of associated disease such as ulcerative colitis, regional enteritis, or retroperitoneal fibrosis.

These criteria are obviously too rigid for most physicians and surgeons who have had considerable experience with patients with sclerosing cholangitis. Indeed, most of my patients would be eliminated by accepting these rigid criteria. To begin with, 70% to 80% of the patients I have cared for with sclerosing cholangitis have had an operation before coming to see me. Many of these patients will have associated gallstones, but gallstones can be present at the early manifestation of biliary ductal stenosis, as demonstrated in Figure 20-1. The entire ductal system does not have to be involved simultaneously. It is much more likely that the disease starts in a segment of the common bile duct or common hepatic duct. Furthermore, the disease is frequently associated with ulcerative colitis and less frequently with Crohn's disease. Indeed, 12 of the 42 patients whose cases I reported in 1966 had ulcerative colitis. Since the pathologic characteristics of the disease when associated with chronic inflammatory bowel disease are identical to the idiopathic variety, the inclusion of these patients in any consideration of this disease is justifiable.

The present case report has some important features that deserve attention. It is noteworthy that this 29-year-old woman had undergone total proctocolectomy before the clinical manifestations of sclerosing cholangitis developed. In my experience, most patients with sclerosing cholangitis who have associated chronic ulcerative colitis or Crohn's disease have biliary manifestations for a year or more after the recognition of the chronic inflammatory bowel process. Since sclerosing cholangitis does not develop in most patients with chronic inflammatory bowel disease, it is difficult, when the two diseases appear in sequence or in concert, to assess the etiologic factors involved. It can be theorized that in chronic inflammatory bowel disease the portal venous system is constantly or intermittently flooded with bacteria from the involved segment of the intestine, but this theory would not explain why sclerosing cholangitis develops in some persons with inflammatory bowel disease and not in the majority.

This case also demonstrates that total colectomy does not affect (except in

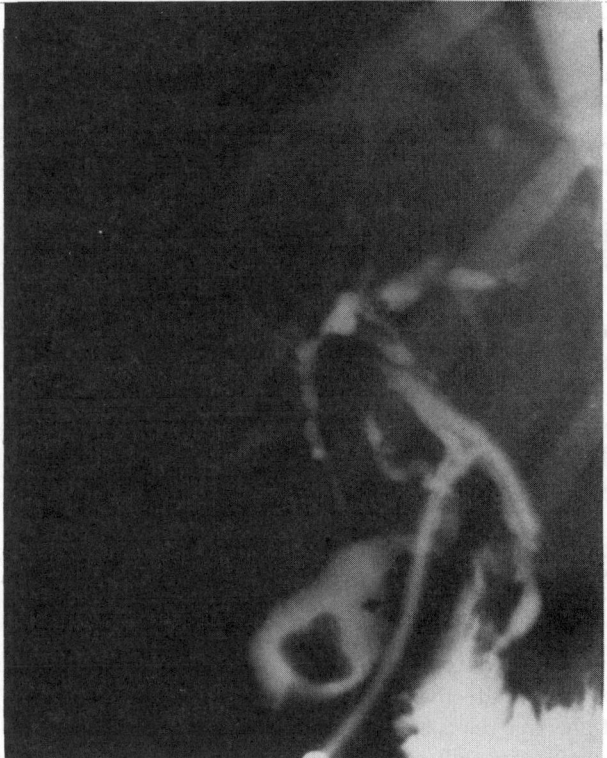

FIG 20–1.
T-tube cholangiogram showing characteristic narrowing and beading of the ductal system. Note stones in the gallbladder.

rare instances) the course of sclerosing cholangitis. It would appear that this patient had total colectomy before any clinical manifestations of sclerosing cholangitis were found. It is also interesting that the severity of chronic inflammatory bowel disease, when present in these patients, varies from mild involvement to the most severe type of ulcerative colitis. It is still my conviction that the decision regarding surgery on the colon or the small bowel in chronic inflammatory bowel disease associated with sclerosing cholangitis should be made on the basis of what one would do in the management of the inflammatory bowel disease if the patient did not have sclerosing cholangitis. (*Editor's note:* Agreed. Most authorities believe that once sclerosing cholangitis is present, colectomy does not affect the subsequent course. On the other hand, to argue for colectomy as a prophylaxis against sclerosing cholangitis does not appear to me to be reasonable.)

INCIDENCE

The incidence of sclerosing cholangitis is unknown. While it is a rare disease, the increasing frequency of reports in the literature indicates that the condition is being recognized more commonly. With the increasing application of endoscopic retrograde cholangiopancreatography and with the use of percutaneous transhepatic cholangiography, this disease will be recognized more often and perhaps at an earlier stage in its development.

Men are more frequently affected than women. In 1966, I reported that the ratio of males to females was 1:1 when sclerosing cholangitis was associated with ulcerative colitis; 7:4, without a history of gallstones; and 1:2, with a history of gallstones or previous biliary operation.

With a multitude of conflicting theories, the suggestions of Peck et al. that sclerosing cholangitis represents a reaction of the biliary tree (perhaps immunologically based) to a group of heterogenous agents or stimuli may be the most logical approach to the cause of this disease.

PATHOLOGY

The affected extrahepatic bile ducts are palpably indurated and pale, with greatly thickened walls and reduced lumens. The overall diameter of the duct is usually not increased. While the characteristic microscopic appearances of the intrahepatic and extrahepatic ducts are not consistent, some features are usually present. The ductal mucosa is usually normal, particularly in the early phase of the disease. Squamous metaplasia, proliferative changes, atrophy, patchy mucosa, and microscopic ulcerations may be observed. Microscopically, the walls of the ducts are characterized by dense fibrosis. Some patients have pericholangitis, which has led authorities to speculate that in some patients pericholangitis apparently progresses to sclerosing cholangitis.

Wellwood and I reported the following operative findings in 84 patients. Diffuse extrahepatic and intrahepatic ductal involvement was seen in 45 patients (54%); both hepatic ducts and intrahepatic ducts, 7 patients; both hepatic ducts only, 7 patients; all extrahepatic ducts, 5 patients; distal common duct only, 5 patients; all common ducts and one hepatic duct, 4 patients; intrahepatic ducts only, 4 patients; proximal common duct only, in 3 patients; both hepatic ducts and proximal common duct, 1 patient; and gallbladder only, 3 patients.

CLINICAL FEATURES

The clinical features of sclerosing cholangitis are those of obstructive jaundice, which may initially be intermittent but is usually progressive. When sclerosing

TABLE 20–1.
Clinical Manifestations of 84 Patients With Sclerosing Cholangitis Treated at Lahey Clinic*

Clinical Features	No. of Patients	Percentage of Series
Historical features		
Jaundice	78	93
Pain	58	69
Weight loss	53	63
Anorexia and malaise	50	59
Chills and fever	42	50
Pruritus	41	48
Nausea and vomiting	40	45
Colitis	27	32
Physical findings		
Jaundice	48	57
Liver enlargement	37	44
Local tenderness	29	34
Ileostomy	5	6

*From Warren KW, Williams CI, Tan GC, in Schiff L, Schiff ER (eds): *Diseases of the Liver, ed 6.* Philadelphia, JB Lippincott Co, 1987, pp 1289–1335. Used by permission.

cholangitis and ulcerative colitis are related, the symptoms of sclerosing cholangitis are usually preceded by those of ulcerative colitis by a number of years. On occasion, however, the ulcerative colitis or chronic inflammatory bowel disease may occur after sclerosing cholangitis is well established. The onset is usually insidious. Epigastric pain or pain in the right hypochondrium may be present, but the pain is usually less severe than that associated with biliary calculi. Pain may precede, accompany, or follow the development of jaundice or pruritus. Malaise, anorexia, nausea, vomiting, and accompanying weight loss are also features of the disease. Occasionally, patients may be febrile and may have chills. The disease usually progresses, but long periods of latency may occur. Ultimately, many of the patients have progressive biliary cirrhosis and then combined biliary and portal cirrhosis leading to liver failure, portal hypertension, and massive hemorrhage from esophageal varices. The major clinical manifestations of sclerosing cholangitis are shown in Table 20–1.

Two striking features of the progress of the disease are worthy of comment. First is the long interval that may elapse between an operation that has accomplished its primary purpose of overcoming the obstructive jaundice and the onset of rapid and relentless progression of the disease. The initial response may have resulted from dilatation and intubation of the stenosed ducts or to a biliary enteric bypass at an appropriate level. In some patients without any intervening attacks and without any apparent provocation, the symptoms of the disease characterized by chills, fever, distress, malaise, and jaundice may occur. Under these circumstances, the course may be rapid and may lead to liver failure, manifestations of portal hypertension, hemorrhage, and death. The longest such interval I have observed was 19 years. I saw the patient periodically during those years, and the results of liver function tests were only slightly disturbed. When the symptoms recurred, the patient was evaluated again for surgical relief of the jaundice, but it was discovered that he had severe coronary artery disease, for which a triple bypass was performed. Although he recovered from this operation, he was never considered a reasonable risk for major biliary surgery. He had frequent episodes of variceal hemorrhage and died of a combination of hemorrhage and liver failure.

Recently, a patient who had sclerosing cholangitis for 16 years and who had multiple operations to relieve the obstructive jaundice, with satisfying results extending over periods of three to four years, had a sudden massive hemorrhage due to varices with rapid progression of jaundice. He was hospitalized for evaluation for liver transplantation. He continued to have massive and recurrent episodes of severe hemorrhage from the varices and had a reverse splenorenal shunt performed by Dr. Roger Jenkins, Chief of the Liver Transplant Program at the New England Deaconess Hospital in Boston. He survived this procedure and hopefully will not require an early operation for sclerosing cholangitis.

The second striking feature is the tendency in some patients who have had a relatively mild course of the disease to have startling progression of signs and symptoms suggesting an approaching terminal phase of the illness. The condition then stabilizes at a plateau of moderate severity, and these patients live a reasonable life for many years.

DIAGNOSIS

A history of ulcerative colitis, Crohn's disease, or other associated conditions should alert the physician to the possibility of sclerosing cholangitis when a patient with intermittent jaundice, epigastric pain, and fever is being treated. Laboratory tests are nonspecific but reflect the pattern of obstructive jaundice. More than half of these patients have elevated serum bilirubin levels at the time of hospital admission. Alkaline phosphatase levels are elevated in more than 80% of the patients.

Ultrasonography may be misleading in sclerosing cholangitis in not demonstrating a dilated ductal system in the presence of obstructive jaundice. Percutaneous transhepatic cholangiography is technically difficult because of the small caliber of the ducts but, if successful, will demonstrate areas of stenosis and ductal attenuation. Endoscopic retrograde cholangiopancreatography is the most helpful and the safest method of demonstrating the changes in the extrahepatic and intrahepatic ductal system. Because of the irregular narrowing of the ducts, it is important that the endoscopist inject sufficient contrast medium into the peripheries of the ducts (Figs 20–2 and 20–3). Since endoscopic retrograde cholangiopancreatography is less invasive, it is the preferred method of evaluating sclerosing cholangitis.

It is important to have a proper visual pattern of the ducts preoperatively if this can be obtained safely. If endoscopic retrograde cholangiopancreatography is not successful, I rarely resort to transhepatic percutaneous cholangiography. If a patient has clinical evidence of jaundice supported by appropriate laboratory data, negative results on ultrasonography may be highly suggestive of the presence of sclerosing cholangitis. Obviously, the surgeon feels better if endoscopic retrograde cholangiopancreatography is successful, as it will show the characteristics of the disease, its location and extent, and will be helpful in planning the surgical procedure.

Differential Diagnosis

Sclerosing cholangitis must be differentiated from other diseases that have, as a major clinical feature, the presence of jaundice. In the past, consideration had

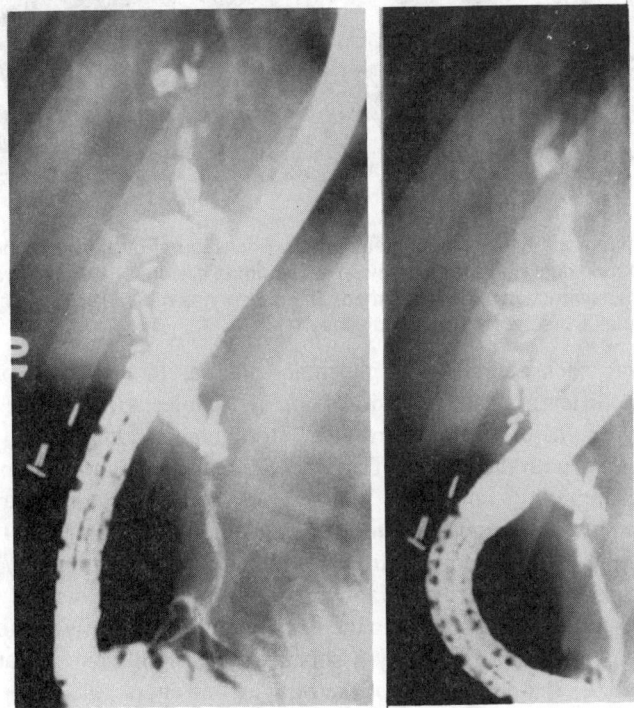

FIG 20–2.
Endoscopic retrograde cholangiography showing marked involvement of most of the biliary ductal system. Currently, the patient is being managed by periodic endoscopic stenting after transduodenal sphincteroplasty.

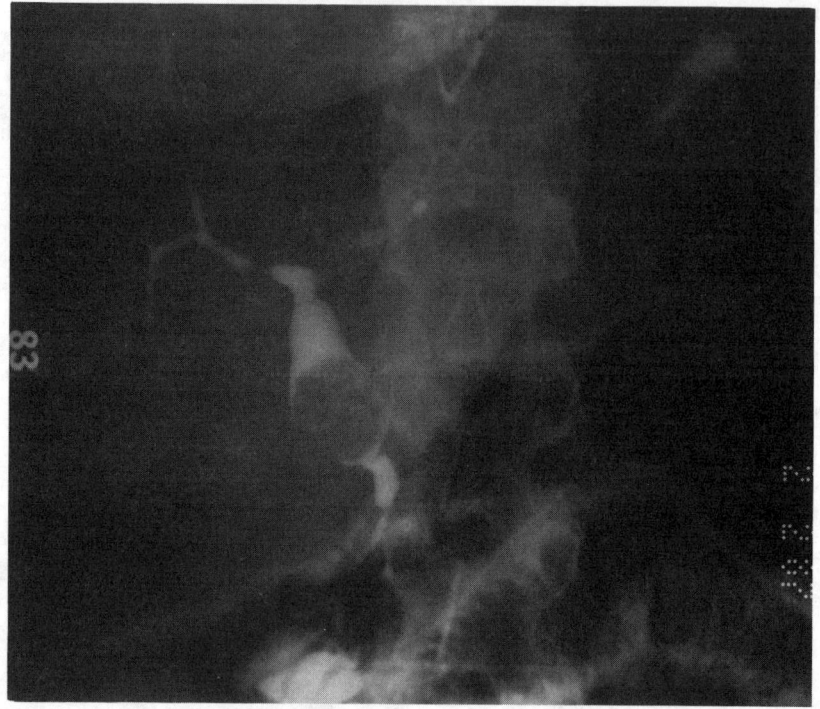

FIG 20–3.
Endoscopic retrograde cholangiopancreatography showing narrowing of intrahepatic ducts and distal common duct with a large stone in the common bile duct. The stone was removed, and choledochojejunostomy was performed. The patient has had multiple segmental resections of the small intestine for Crohn's disease.

to be given to such diagnoses as gallstones and carcinoma of the pancreas. It still must be differentiated from viral hepatitis, cholestatic jaundice secondary to a drug hypersensitivity, and particularly to cholangiocarcinoma.

Fortunately, with the advent of endoscopic retrograde cholangiopancreatography, ultrasongraphy, computed tomography, and percutaneous transhepatic cholangiography, the diagnosis can be made with greater certainty. Indeed, the graphic findings by endoscopic retrograde cholangiopancreatography or by percutaneous transhepatic cholangiography may be typical of the disease. However, cholangiocarcinoma can also mimic the disease radiographically. While it is true that cholangiocarcinoma is usually associated with significant dilatation of the biliary tree above the obstruction of the bile duct or ducts, this is not uniformly true. Cholangiocarcinoma may be associated with narrowing, irregularity, and beading of the intrahepatic ducts. The differential diagnosis may be extremely difficult even at surgery, and multiple biopsies are often necessary. If the disease is primarily intrahepatic, the confusion is compounded because it is difficult to obtain an appropriate biopsy of the most suspicious duct or ducts.

With the relentless progress by interventional radiologists, the diagnosis and treatment of patients with sclerosing cholangitis have been improved.

TREATMENT

Unfortunately, no satisfactory medical treatment for this condition exists. Most physicians and surgeons dealing with patients with sclerosing cholangitis do not stress any dietary restrictions. I believe a simple bland diet with 85 gm of fat is helpful to the patient's general nutrition and perhaps in some degree to their natural resistance.

Some reports in the literature indicate that steroid therapy may lower the bilirubin level and reverse to some extent the abnormal radiographic pattern seen in bile ducts. This has not been my experience. Most patients I have treated surgically have been taking steroids administered in a wide variety of doses and over varying periods of time. If steroids were effective, surgeons would rarely be operating on patients with sclerosing cholangitis.

Kaplan and his associates reported results with two patients with sclerosing cholangitis who responded to treatment with low doses of methotrexate. This is an interesting report; however, the authors stated that although the response was dramatic and, to the best of their knowledge, unique, they do not encourage its use in such patients. These authors plan to conduct a carefully controlled study of low-dose methotrexate and a placebo in patients with sclerosing cholangitis.

The use of a broad-spectrum antibiotic that is excreted in high concentrations in the bile may be of value in two ways: (1) attacks of ascending cholangitis may be treated or prevented, which has been the main reason for their use; and (2) theoretically, their antibacterial action might be of value if the cause of sclerosing cholangitis is infective.

Formerly, we used a choluretic (Zanchol) in the hope that it would minimize or delay recurrent attacks of cholangitis, but we have no scientific evidence that the choluretic was effective. Zanchol is no longer available.

The search for satisfactory medical treatment of the disease continues, but the mainstay of treatment remains surgical decompression of the bile ducts whenever possible. The early surgical approach to the treatment of patients with sclerosing cholangitis involved procedures to decompress the biliary tree and included dilatation of the ducts and the insertion of an appropriate stent, such as a T-tube or Y-tube or other transhepatic latex or Silastic tubing. In this era, it was my practice to leave the stents in for prolonged periods of time. The buried Y-tube was left in until the patient had recurrent attacks of cholangitis that required removal of the stent. I subsequently modified the Y-tube so that the stent had the advantage of the Y-tube and the further advantage that the stent could be removed in the office.

Recently, more aggressive surgical approaches to the management of sclerosing cholangitis have been pursued.

Biliary Enteric Bypass

Patients who have an accessible point above the major obstruction in the extrahepatic ductal system may be treated best by a Roux-en-Y choledochojejunostomy. During the procedure, the intrahepatic ducts are gently and progressively dilated. The biliary enteric bypass may thus be combined with a variety of stents. The frustrating part of the surgical management of this condition is the fact that often no part of the biliary system is suitable for an appropriate biliary enteric anastomosis.

Cameron has advocated resection of the extrahepatic ductal system including the bifurcation of the right and left hepatic ducts followed by Roux-en-Y hepaticojejunostomy, implanting both the right and left hepatic ducts independently into the Roux-en-Y limb. Cameron also dilates the stenotic areas within the hepatic ducts and routinely inserts a transhepatic Silastic tube through the right and left ducts. The Silastic tubes traverse the anastomosis of the ducts to the jejunum and exit from the dome of the liver. This is a reasonable approach when the bifurcation is involved and when the caliber of the right and left hepatic ducts at the point where they are to be divided is sufficient to permit adequate anastomosis and appropriate intubation. I have used a similar technique in repairing high common-duct strictures, as shown in Figure 20–4. In many of these patients, the right and left hepatic ducts have been anastomosed to the jejunum separately. I have employed both latex and Silastic transhepatic tubes and have observed no difference in their behavior. These tubes should be changed over a guidewire every three or four months.

Role of Interventional Radiologist

In recent years, interventional radiologists have developed many interesting, innovative, and successful techniques to manage various intrahepatic and extrahepatic ductal pathologic conditions. Initially, the approach was commonly through a choledochostomy tube tract. Subsequently, percutaneous transhepatic manipulation was used. The manipulation was carried out through transhepatic tracts in patients in whom external transhepatic tubes had been placed surgically. Recently, percutaneous manipulation has been initiated in patients who have had no transhepatic or T-tubes in place. It has been possible for radiologists to cannulate and dilate points of obstruction located in both intrahepatic and extrahepatic ductal segments in both benign and malignant disease.

Sclerosing cholangitis, because of the nature of its clinical course and a tendency for the areas of ductal stenosis to be progressive, should be a fertile field for the radiologist. One of the technical difficulties with the percutaneous technique when no stent has been placed surgically is the small caliber of the ducts. Experienced interventional radiologists have become adept at cannulating these ducts.

The patient whose radiography is shown (see Fig 20–2) has been managed by the endoscopist and radiologist for a period of six years with excellent results. The patient whose radiograph is shown in Figure 20–5 with diffuse extreme narrowing of the ductal system has been managed by Dr. Ernest Ring in the Department of Radiology, University of California at San Francisco, for many years. My most recent communication indicates that the patient is doing well clinically, with his bilirubin level at or near normal. He has had chronic ulcerative

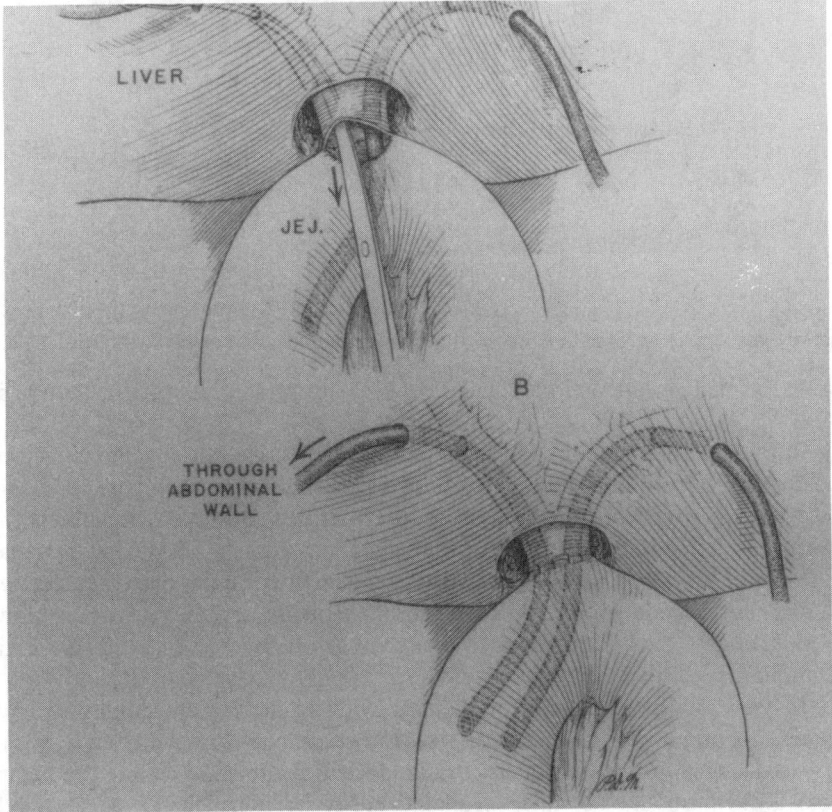

FIG 20–4.
Bilateral transhepatic latex tube stents for high hepaticojejunostomy. (From Warren KW, Jefferson M: *Surg Clin North Am* 1973; 53:1169–1190. Used by permission.)

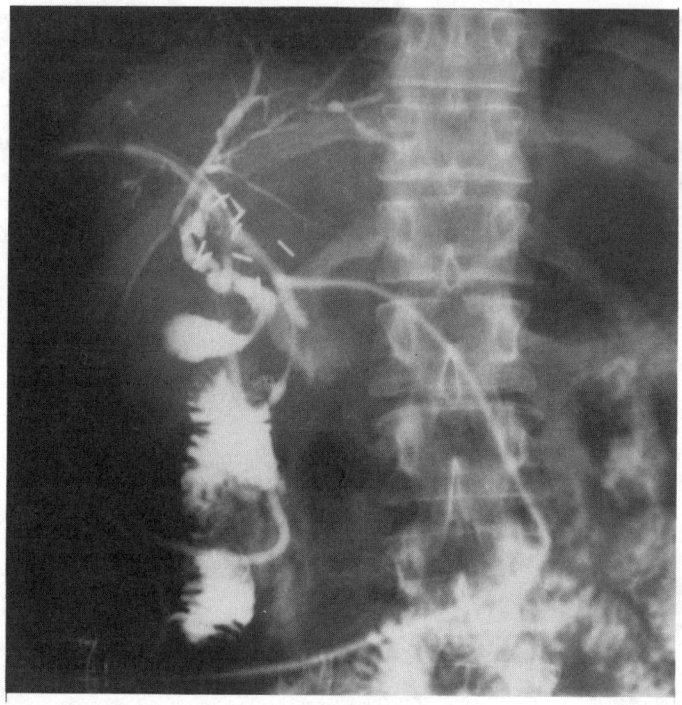

FIG 20-5.
Cholangiogram through U-tube traversing the right hepatic duct and T-tube in the common duct reveals diffuse stenosis and beading of the intrahepatic and extrahepatic bile ducts.

colitis for many years and had choledochojejunostomy at another institution in 1979.

In a recent publication, Maroney and Ring described an ingenious method of cannulating the biliary ducts by way of a percutaneous transjejunal approach. These authors performed this procedure in 11 patients. Seven of the patients had sclerosing cholangitis. One patient had pyogenic cholangiohepatitis; two had anastomotic strictures, and one had recurrent cholangiocarcinoma. They pointed out that the procedure was successful in all patients, and they experienced no complications. That report indicates the extent to which interventional radiologic techniques have advanced.

In view of the tendency for patients with sclerosing cholangitis to have frequent recurrent attacks of cholangitis and commonly to have relentless progressive stenosis of the bile ducts, it would seem that easy access to the biliary ductal system should be made available either by transhepatic or retrograde insertion of straight tubes into the intrahepatic ductal system at the time of surgery when the disease is primarily intrahepatic and into the common bile duct when the disease is essentially in the distal portion of the duct. Placing the blind end of the Roux-en-Y jejunal limb in the subcutaneous area or just beneath the rectus sheath simplifies identifying the segment of jejunum attached to the biliary ducts during recurrent operations and can permit the endoscopist and the interventional radiologist to have easier access to the ductal system.

Liver Transplantation

Since a considerable number of patients with sclerosing cholangitis will progress to hepatic failure, not infrequently associated with esophageal varices and massive hemorrhage, it is only natural that liver transplantation has been employed in the management of patients in the terminal phase of this disease. Unfortunately, in the early experience of liver transplantation in sclerosing cholangitis, the extent of liver damage and particularly the profound deficiencies in the clotting mechanism reflected in prolonged prothrombin time and partial thromboplastin time have accounted for the high mortality in these patients. Consequently, efforts must be made to refer these patients to surgeons for transplantation before they reach this desperate condition. When these patients receive a transplant at an early stage, the mortality is similar to that for liver transplantation for other conditions.

CONCLUSIONS

Sclerosing cholangitis is a rare disease, but one that tends to be progressive, although long intervals of apparent remission may occur. With current imaging techniques, the diagnosis can be made with relative certainty, but radiographically it can be confused with cholangiocarcinoma. Although no satisfactory medical treatment exists, steroid therapy has almost always been given. Evaluation of other medications, including methotrexate, is being pursued.

Aggressive surgical procedures are indicated in the management of this condition, and interventional radiologists have a great deal to contribute to the management of patients with sclerosing cholangitis. Ultimately, more patients are going to need liver transplantation in the later phase of the disease. A consideration of liver transplantation should not be delayed until serious and irreversible defects in the clotting mechanism have developed.

BIBLIOGRAPHY

1. Cameron JL: Managing wound infection: Transhepatic stents in biliary stricture. *Confronting Infection* 5, No. 1, April 1987.
2. Kaplan MM, Arora S, Pincus SH: Primary sclerosing cholangitis and low-dose oral pulse methotrexate therapy. *Ann Intern Med* 1987; 106:231–235.

3. Maroney TP, Ring EJ: Percutaneous transjejunal catheterization of Roux-en-Y biliary-jejunal anastomoses. *Radiology* 1987; 164:151–153.
4. Myers RN, Cooper JH, Padis N: Primary sclerosing cholangitis: Complete gross and histologic reversal after long-term steroid therapy. *Am J Gastroenterol* 1970; 53:527–538.
5. Peck JJ, Kern WH, Mikkelsen WP: Sclerosis of extrahepatic bile ducts. *Arch Surg* 1974; 108:798–800.
6. Warren KW, Athanassiades S, Monge JI: Primary sclerosing cholangitis: A study of 42 cases. *Am J Surg* 1966; 111:23–38.
7. Warren KW, Williams CT, Tan GC: Diseases of the gallbladder and bile ducts, in Schiff L, Schiff ER (eds): *Diseases of the Liver,* ed 6. Philadelphia, JB Lippincott, 1987, pp 1289–1335.
8. Wellwood J, Warren KW: Sclerosing cholangitis, in Smith R, Sherlock S (eds): *Surgery of the Bile Ducts.* London, Butterworths, 1981, pp 455–478.

21

Klatskin Tumor

A 53-year-old man in good health presents with the gradual onset of jaundice. Stools are light and urine is dark. He has had no previous history suggesting cholelithiasis. Ultrasound reveals dilated intrahepatic ducts with a normal gallbladder. The computerized tomography scan confirms the sonographic findings and demonstrates a normal, nondilated common bile duct.

Consultants: Charles J. Yeo, M.D.
John L. Cameron, M.D.

The presentation described is typical of a patient with a proximal biliary tumor. This entity was first reported by Altemeier in 1957 and subsequently described in 13 patients by Klatskin in 1965. Approximately 13,000 new cases of liver and biliary tract cancer are diagnosed annually in the United States, with roughly 10% of these cases being Klatskin tumors. Proximal biliary tumors by definition are adenocarcinomas occurring at or near the hepatic duct bifurcation. Grossly, the lesions are usually small, firm, nodular, scar-like strictures. Klatskin tumors are often slow-growing, and the majority are localized to the hepatic hilus at presentation.

In the past, the diagnosis and management of patients with proximal biliary tumors were entirely unsatisfactory. Diagnosis was usually not made until postmortem examination, and most patients died from liver failure or sepsis without having satisfactory biliary decompression. With current diagnostic techniques, however, these patients can be quickly and accurately diagnosed. In addition, using both percutaneous and intraoperative biliary stents, many of these tumors can be resected and the biliary tree can be successfully reconstructed.

CLINICAL PRESENTATION

A broad age distribution for Klatskin tumors has been noted, with most patients being in their fifth to seventh decade. However, patients in their 20s with Klatskin tumors have been reported. A slight male predominance exists. Patients typically present with progressive jaundice; pruritus, weight loss, anorexia, and nonspecific gastrointestinal complaints are common. Pain is usually absent or mild, and characterized as a dull right upper quadrant ache. Cholangitis rarely occurs prior to invasive biliary tract manipulation, and thus biliary sepsis is an unusual mode of initial presentation.

DIAGNOSIS

Initial diagnostic evaluation generally follows the usual guidelines for any jaundiced patient; evaluation consists of either abdominal ultrasound or computerized tomography (CT). If the patient is young and without weight loss or back pain, sonography is favored. In older patients with weight loss or back pain, CT scan is preferred as it may provide substantive evidence to support alternative diagnoses such as pancreatic or periampullary neoplasms. Findings at ultrasound or CT scan suggestive of a Klatskin tumor include a dilated intrahepatic biliary tree, a normal or collapsed gallbladder and extrahepatic biliary tree, and a normal pancreas. Only rarely does ultrasound or CT scan demonstrate a tumor mass in the hepatic hilum.

Following documentation of intrahepatic bile duct dilatation, the biliary anatomy is visualized using either endoscopic retrograde or percutaneous transhepatic cholangiography. The latter technique is favored because it defines the extent of the proximal tumor involvement at the hepatic hilus and allows for the preoperative placement of percutaneous transhepatic Ring catheters into both the right and left hepatic ducts. If possible, at the time of initial placement, the Ring catheters are advanced through the obstructing neoplasm into the duodenum. Even if the initial attempt at Ring catheter manipulation through the tumor is unsuccessful, a subsequent effort several days later will usually allow for Ring catheter advancement through the tumor into the duodenum. The Ring catheters are not placed to provide for long-term preoperative biliary tract decompression, as currently available data do not support this use in a patient in a nonseptic state. However, advantages of preoperative transhepatic Ring catheter placement that support its use include (1) assistance in the technical aspects of hilar dissection by allowing palpation of the Ring catheter within the biliary tree at the time of surgery, and (2) facilitation of Silastic transhepatic stent placement.

Prior to surgery, all patients with Klatskin tumors are staged by cholangiography and angiography. The finding of extensive bilobar hepatic parenchymal involvement by cholangiography indicates unresectability, as does the finding of tumor encasement or occlusion of the portal vein or the hepatic artery by angiography. The use of magnetic resonance imaging holds promise as a noninvasive tool in assessing tumor extent and invasion of major portal vascular structures. In all, approximately 75% of patients are judged to be operable by preoperative staging. Those patients with extensive bilobar hepatic involvement or major hepatic arterial or portal venous involvement are not surgical candidates, and they are managed nonoperatively with percutaneous transhepatic catheters for biliary decompression. Of the operable patients, one half are found to be resectable at the time of surgery, and the remaining one half have grossly unresectable tumors.

Prior to percutaneous cholangiography and exploration, the patient's coagulation status is assessed in the face of obstructive jaundice and possible resultant hepatocellular injury. Hypoprothrombinemia is corrected by the administration of parenteral vitamin K or fresh frozen plasma. Nutritional assessment is performed, and appropriate nutritional support is initiated. (*Editor's note*: The place of preoperative nutritional resuscitation in this and other malignant diseases of the pancreas and biliary tract is controversial. However, recent evidence suggests that a combination of preoperative biliary decompression together with parenteral nutrition may improve outcome.) Prophylactic antibiotics are utilized in the perioperative period.

OPERATIVE MANAGEMENT

Dissection

The abdomen is entered through a right subcostal incision that can be extended onto the left side. Dissection of the hepatic duct bifurcation is facilitated by two maneuvers. First, early mobilization of the gallbladder assists greatly in exposing the bifurcation, which can be palpated using the preoperatively placed Ring catheters as guides. Second, early division of the distal common bile duct aids in the technical aspects of proximal hepatic duct dissection and tumor resection (Fig 21–1). The distal common duct is sutured closed and then the proximal segment is reflected cephalad, using the preoperatively placed transhepatic Ring catheters as handles. This maneuver allows progressive cephalad dissection along the common bile duct, common hepatic duct, and hepatic duct bifurcation, freeing the biliary tree from the portal vein and hepatic artery under direct visualization. This dissection is carried out circumferentially into the hepatic hilus, beyond all gross tumor. Should gross tumor extend along either the left or right hepatic duct into the hepatic parenchyma, appropriate hepatic lobectomy can be considered. The right and left hepatic ducts are then divided above the gross extent of the Klatskin tumor, leaving the Ring catheters in place, exiting through each lobar hepatic duct (Fig 21–2, A).

Stent Insertion

The insertion of two Silastic transhepatic biliary stents is performed following resection of the hepatic duct bifurcation, using the previously placed Ring catheters present in the right and left hepatic ductal systems. With the 8 F Ring

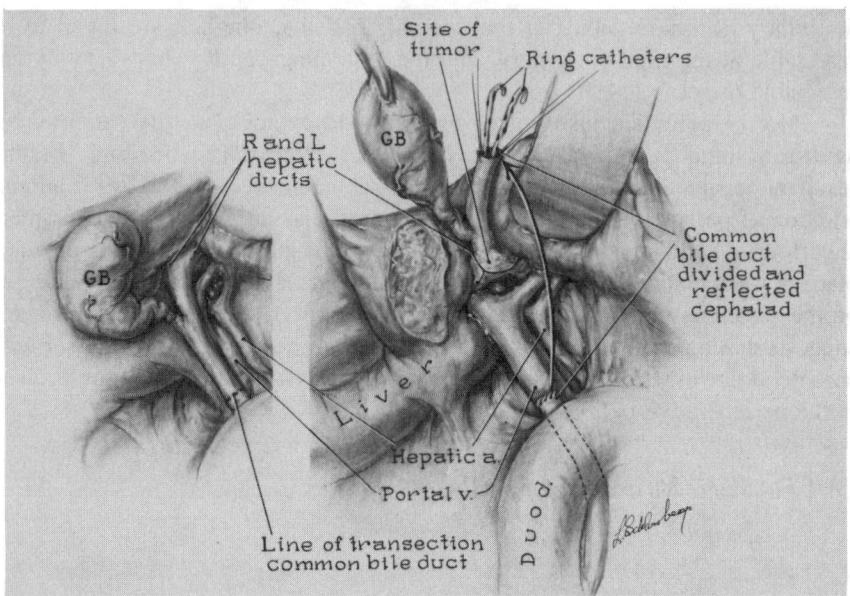

FIG 21-1.
During exploration and resection of a Klatskin tumor, early gallbladder mobilization and transection of the distal common bile duct are recommended. This allows cephalad reflection of the common bile duct, using the preoperatively placed transhepatic Ring catheters as handles, and facilitates hilar dissection of the common hepatic duct and tumor off the portal vein. (From Broe PJ, Cameron JL: *Advances in Surgery*, vol 14. Chicago, Year Book Medical Publishers Inc, 1981, pp 47–91. Used by permission.)

catheters protruding from the individual proximal hepatic ducts, a 14 F Coudé catheter is passed over and sutured to each Ring catheter. The Coudé catheters are then positioned in the preexisting intrahepatic Ring catheter tracts by withdrawing the Ring catheters upward through the liver (see Fig 21–2, B). A Silastic transhepatic stent (8-mm outside diameter, 70-cm length) is then secured to each Coudé catheter, and the stents are appropriately positioned by withdrawing the Coudé catheters upward through the liver. Occasionally, a third Silastic transhepatic stent is inserted if a third major hepatic duct is identified and defined in the hepatic hilus following resection of the Klatskin tumor. The Silastic transhepatic stents are in proper position when all of their sideholes reside in the intrahepatic biliary tree and the upper portion of the Roux-en-Y jejunal loop that is to be used for the biliary enteric anastomoses.

Biliary-Enteric Anastomoses

The biliary-enteric anastomoses are performed between the right and left hepatic ducts and a 60-cm long retrocolic Roux-en-Y loop (Fig 21–3). The end of the

Roux loop is closed using surgical staples or manual suturing techniques. Intestinal continuity is reestablished 60 cm from the end of the Roux loop, using an end-to-side jejunojejunostomy. Two separate end-to-side hepaticojejunostomies are then performed over the Silastic transhepatic stents exiting from the porta hepatis. A gap of 2 to 3 cm is left between the sites of the two hepaticojejunostomies on the Roux-en-Y loop. Interrupted 4-0 or 5-0 Polypropylene sutures are used for the hepaticojejunal anastomoses, since the Silastic stents are left in place permanently. After completion of the biliary-enteric anastomoses, the Roux-en-Y loop can be sutured to the undersurface of the liver to avoid tension on the anastomoses. The free ends of the stents are brought out directly through separate stab wounds in the upper abdomen. The stents are secured to the skin of the anterior abdominal wall by stainless steel wires and are attached to extension tubing and a bile bag for dependent gravity drainage. Closed suction or Penrose drains are left to drain the biliary-enteric anastomoses. Closed suction drains are left at each site on the hepatic diaphragmatic surface where the transhepatic stents exit from the liver.

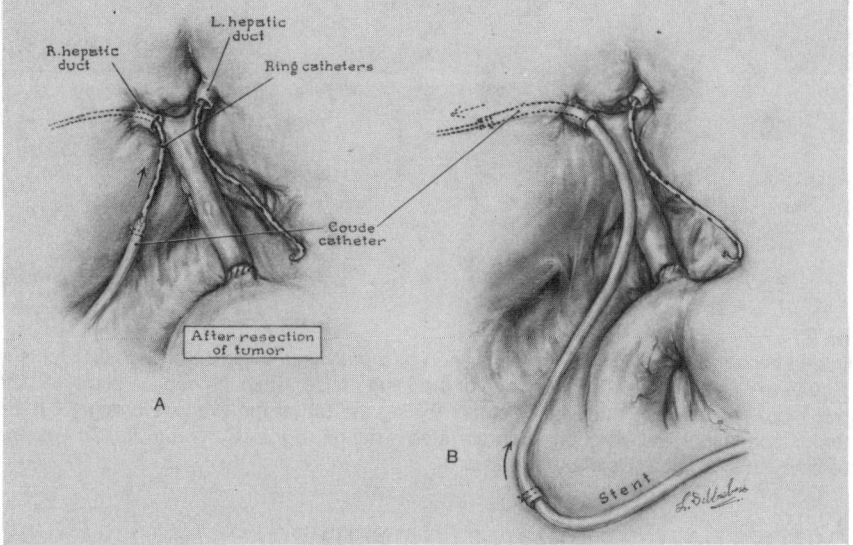

FIG 21-2.
A, after resection of the tumor at the hepatic duct bifurcation, the Ring catheters are used in placing the Silastic transhepatic stents. A 14 F Coudé catheter is first sutured to the 8 F Ring catheter, and the Ring catheter is withdrawn out the top of the liver, leaving the Coudé catheter in transhepatic tract. This dilates the size of the transhepatic tract and corrects the size discrepancy between the 8 F Ring catheter and the 18 F Silastic transhepatic stent. **B,** an 18 F Silastic transhepatic stent is sutured to the widened flange of the Coudé catheter, and the stent is pulled into position by pulling the Coudé catheter out the top of the liver. (From Crist DW, et al: *Surg Gynecol Obstet*, 1987; 165:421-424. Used by permission.)

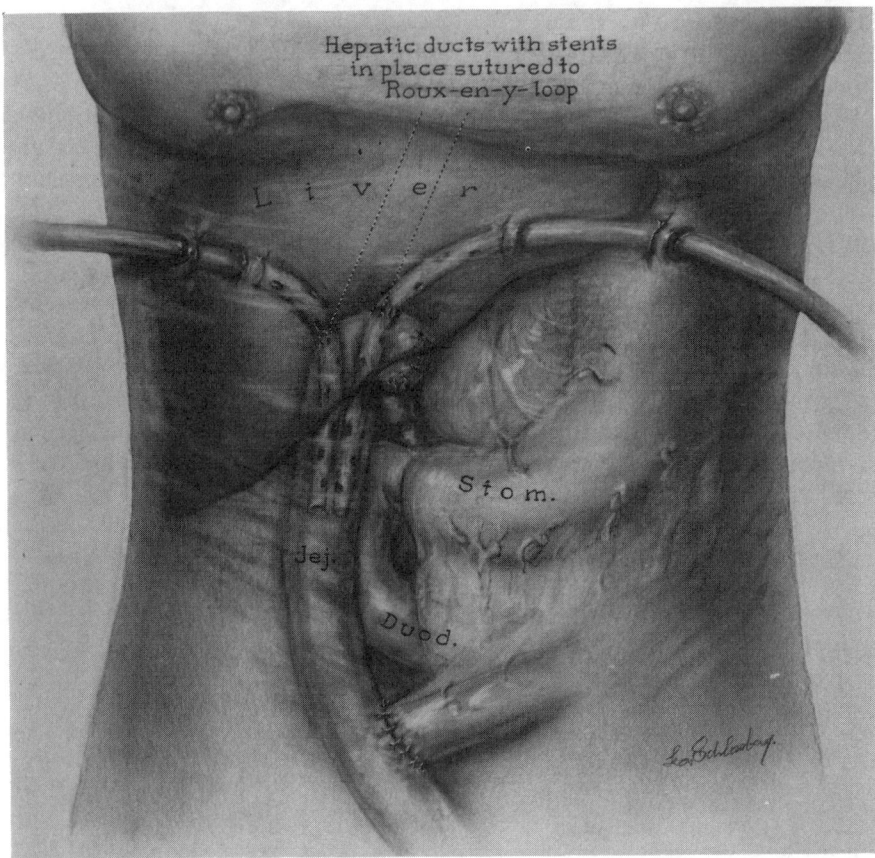

FIG 21-3.
Bilateral hepaticojejunostomies are performed over individual Silastic transhepatic stents to a Roux-en-Y jejunal loop. The sideholes of the stent reside within the hepatic ducts and the Roux loop. The ends of the Silastic stents exiting the top of the liver are brought out the anterior abdominal wall through separate stab wounds. (From Cameron JL: *Confronting Infection* 1987; 5:1-12. Used by permission.)

POSTOPERATIVE CARE AND RADIOTHERAPY

The Silastic transhepatic stents are left to drain dependently to bile bags for five to seven days. At this time, cholangiography is performed through the stents to evaluate for bile leakage and biliary decompression. In the absence of demonstrable leakage, the bile bag and extension tubing are removed, and the biliary drainage is internalized using a three-way stopcock or heparin lock. If no bile leakage to the operatively placed closed-suction or Penrose drains occurs after internalization of biliary drainage, then the drains are removed. The patient is instructed to irrigate each stent twice a day with 20 cc of normal saline. If postoperative cholangiography demonstrates a bile leak, then dependent bile bag drainage is continued until complete healing is demonstrated.

Approximately 6 to 12 weeks following surgery, adjuvant radiotherapy is instituted. External beam radiation totaling 5,500 rads is delivered to the hepatic hilus, and an additional boosting dose of 2,000 rads can be delivered to the site of tumor or tumor resection by lowering iridium-192 seeds down the Silastic stents.

Over time the sideholes of the Silastic transhepatic stents become occluded by biliary sludge. In order to prevent sidehole occlusion, poor hepatic drainage, and subsequent infection, the stents are exchanged every two to four months over guidewires using fluoroscopy. This stent exchange is a simple procedure performed on an outpatient basis in the radiology suite.

OPTIONS FOR UNRESECTABLE TUMORS

At the time of surgical exploration, if the porta hepatis is unapproachable due to extensive tumor mass, two operative approaches to palliation exist. First, the common bile duct distal to the tumor mass is opened and divided, and the malignant stricture is dilated using Bakes dilators. Following luminal dilatation, the preoperatively placed Ring catheter is used to place Silastic transhepatic stents as previously discussed. A second alternative that can be utilized, if the malignant stricture is undilatable from below, is to intubate the left hepatic duct above the tumor. The left hepatic duct can frequently be identified transversing the undersurface of the left lobe of the liver 4 to 5 cm from the bifurcation, before entering the liver parenchyma. The duct can be intubated using a Silastic transhepatic stent at this location. Following either of these two methods, a biliary-enteric anastomosis is performed to a Roux-en-Y jejunal loop, as previously described. In patients who cannot undergo resection or biliary decompression at the porta hepatis, continued percutaneous decompression with the preoperatively placed Ring catheters is the best available treatment option. Following biliary decompression, postoperative radiotherapy is utilized.

RESULTS

The inhospital mortality for resection or palliation of patients with Klatskin tumors is less than 5%. Following resection and radiotherapy for operable Klatskin tumors, the mean survival is greater than two years, with some patients surviving more than five years. When the tumor is unresectable and operative palliation of biliary obstruction is accomplished followed by radiotherapy, the mean survival exceeds 12 months, with good palliation achieved in some patients for up to 3 years. Nonoperated patients with extensive tumor involvement, who undergo only percutaneous transhepatic Ring catheter placement, have a mean survival averaging less then six months.

The use of Silastic transhepatic biliary stents in the operative management of a Klatskin tumor prevents the recurrence of biliary obstruction and avoids the onset of hepatic failure or biliary tract sepsis. An aggressive surgical approach to the evaluation and treatment of patients with a diagnosis of carcinoma of the hepatic duct bifurcation is recommended. If no evidence of unresectability is found at preoperative workup, the first exploration should be in a setting where resection and biliary reconstruction, if feasible, can be undertaken.

BIBLIOGRAPHY

1. Altemeier WA, Gall EA, Zinninger MM, et al: Sclerosing carcinoma of the major intrahepatic bile ducts. *Arch Surg* 1957; 75:450–461.
2. Cameron JL, Broe P, Zuidema GD: Proximal bile duct tumors: Surgical management with Silastic transhepatic biliary stents. *Ann Surg* 1982; 196:412–419.
3. Cameron JL, Gayler BW, Zuidema GD: The use of Silastic transhepatic stents in benign and malignant biliary strictures. *Ann Surg* 1978; 188:552–561.
4. Crist DW, Kadir S, Cameron JL: Proximal biliary tract reconstruction: The value of preoperatively placed percutaneous biliary catheters. *Surg Gynecol Obstet* 1987; 165:421–424.
5. Klatskin G: Adenocarcinoma of the hepatic duct at its bifurcation within the porta hepatis: An unusual tumor with distinctive clinical and pathologic features. *Am J Med* 1965; 38:241–256.
6. Ottow RT, August DA, Sugarbaker PH: Treatment of proximal biliary tract carcinoma: An overview of techniques and results. *Surgery* 1985; 97:251–262.
7. Yeo CJ, Cameron JL: Transhepatic biliary stents and high benign and malignant biliary tract obstructions, in Nyhus LM, Baker RJ (eds): *Mastery of Surgery*, ed 2. Boston, Little Brown & Co, in press.

22

Asymptomatic Gallstones

A 21-year-old woman, gravida 2, para 2, undergoes an elective second cesarean section. At operation, exploration of the abdomen by the obstetrician reveals several gallstones. She is asymptomatic and, even in retrospect, does not have a history of fatty food intolerance.

Consultant: Charles K. McSherry, M.D.

The management of patients with silent gallstones has been controversial since the subject was initially discussed in the early years of this century. The core of this dispute centers around the question: Does the frequency of eventual symptoms and the complications of gallstone disease justify the known morbidity and mortality of cholecystectomy in this subset of patients with calculous biliary tract disease?

The brief case report cited above is quite unusual and not at all representative of the vast majority of patients with silent gallstones. How many of you know of obstetricians that carefully explore the abdomen in the course of a cesarean section? Indeed, most patients with silent stones are in the older age group and have various and sundry medical problems that prompt diagnostic studies, especially roentgenograms of the abdomen that identify radiopaque calculi in the right upper quadrant. In 1985 my co-workers and I reported cases of 135 patients with asymptomatic gallstones; the mean and standard deviation age was 73.6 ± 13.9 years and there were no postpartum patients.

The recommendations to any particular patient with silent gallstones must be based on a knowledge of the natural history of the disease and the risks and benefits of interventional therapy such as cholecystectomy or chemical dissolution. Although broad recommendations are possible for the group, each patient must be considered in the light of his/her own status.

Shortly after the turn of the century, Lord Moynihan warned of the consequences of silent stones. Mayo, in 1911, wrote that the "innocent" gallstone was a myth. From a practical point of view, however, there were no detailed accounts of the fate of patients with silent stones until 1948, when Comfort et al. reported that 46% of patients with silent stones developed symptoms when followed up for 10 to 20 years. However, dyspepsia was considered to reflect gallbladder disease and, therefore, these authors may have overstated the true incidence of symptoms in their patients. The next report on this subject appeared in 1960, when Lund reported cases of 562 patients with cholelithiasis observed for 5 to 20 years. In this group of patients, 50% of the women and 30% of the men had symptoms of biliary calculous disease, usually within five years of diagnosis. Serious sequelae of gallstone disease, such as acute cholecystitis and common duct obstruction, occurred in 25% of the patients. In 1966, Wenckert and Robertson reported on 781 patients with gallstones followed up for 1 to 11 years. Symptoms appeared in one third of these patients and 18% had jaundice or pancreatitis and 5% had acute cholecystitis.

Based upon the above reports, surgeons were confident in their recommendation to most patients with silent gallstones that they should undergo elective cholecystectomy. This conviction was reinforced by a knowledge of the relatively low mortality and morbidity of cholecystectomy performed in patients for nonacute disease vs. acute cholecystitis with or without common bile duct exploration. In 1980, we reported a mortality of 0.5% in over 7,000 patients operated upon for chronic cholecystitis. Patients less than 50 years old had a mortality of 0.1% and those more than 50 years old had a mortality rate of 0.8%. The incidence of nonfatal complications was 6.9%. In contrast, the mortality for cholecystectomy in 2,347 patients with acute cholecystitis was 3.8%. Once again, the mortality was largely age-dependent. Patients less than 65 years old had a mortality rate of 1.6% and those more than 65 years old had a mortality of 9.7%. The combination of both acute cholecystitis and common duct stones was especially lethal and had a mortality of 7.7% in 351 patients.

The need to take a new look at patients with silent gallstones was prompted by the 1982 article by Gracie and Ransohoff who reported on 123 faculty members at the University of Michigan with asymptomatic gallstones. None of these individuals died because of gallstone disease or as a result of the operations performed after the onset of symptoms or complications related to the biliary calculi. The 15-year cumulative probability of the development of biliary symptoms or complications was only 18%.

The conclusions derived from the study by Gracie and Ransohoff are obvious, namely, that there is very little risk to patients with silent gallstones and that, for many, prophylactic cholecystectomy would have been unnecessary. Acceptance of these recommendations was not prompt or universal. The study group consisted almost entirely of white American males; only 13 of the 123 subjects were female. Most surgeons greeted this report with a good deal of skepticism. Indeed, there are very few surgeons that enjoy a patient population of this degree of intelligence, attainment, and selectivity.

The University of Michigan study stimulated us at the Beth Israel Medical Center in New York to seek out a population group with silent gallstones that was more heterogeneous and representative of middle-class Americans. In order to accomplish this goal, the medical records of subscribers to a large, nonprofit HMO in New York City (Health Insurance Plan of New York) were examined for evidence of calculous biliary tract disease and its sequelae that were confirmed and documented by such evidence as reports of ultrasound or radiographic examinations as well as pathology and operative reports. In all of these patients, at least six months had elapsed from the date of diagnosis to operation or, in the nonoperated patients, follow-up visits. Of the 691 patients who fulfilled the entry criteria for this study, 135 (19.5%) were asymptomatic.

In comparison to symptomatic patients with gallstones, asymptomatic patients were older and included a disproportionately higher number of men than women. Moreover, they were much more likely to have radiopaque calculi (64.4%) as opposed to the radiolucent variety. The incidence and severity of their associated medical problems were also significantly higher than in the symptomatic group. Indeed, only 4 of the 135 patients with silent gallstones were free of complicating medical illnesses such as heart disease, hypertension, diabetes, etc.

Cholecystectomy was recommended to only 7 (5.2%) of the 135 asymptomatic patients at the time of diagnosis, and none of these patients accepted this recommendation. In the course of their follow-up, the mean duration of which was 58 ± 50.2 months (median, 46.3 months), only 14 (10.4%) of the patients developed symptoms. Three of these 14 patients experienced acute cholecystitis and one choledocholithiasis. Fifteen of the 135 asymptomatic patients underwent biliary tract operations during the time span of this study. Five of these procedures consisted of incidental cholecystectomy performed *en passant* to other intra-abdominal operations. Eight patients had a planned cholecystectomy and one each had cholecystostomy and cholecystectomy plus common bile duct exploration. Six patients who developed symptoms of chronic cholecystitis and cholelithiasis were not operated on. Thus, the proportion of patients with asymptomatic stones that were operated on for biliary tract disease was 7.4% (10 of 135 patients), and there were no operative deaths. However, in the course of this same period of follow-up, there were 25 (18.5%) deaths due to nonbiliary causes in the asymptomatic group. This high mortality reflected their advanced age and poor general health.

The specter of carcinoma is often raised in the context of the treatment of patients with silent gallstones. Epidemiologic studies of the incidence of cancer in relation to the prevalence of gallstones and the operative mortality attendant to cholecystectomy indicate that there would be no benefit provided by a policy of routine cholecystectomy for all patients with silent stones.

On the basis of our study, one would have to agree with the recommendation of Gracie and Ransohoff that elective "prophylactic" cholecystectomy is unwarranted in the vast majority of patients with silent gallstones. Returning to the present case that initiated this discourse, one must confess that the experience with silent stones in relatively young people is poorly defined and that life-table analysis of the development of symptoms is lacking for someone at age 21 years and with a presumed life expectancy of approximately 55 years. Given the weight of the evidence cited above, I would be inclined to advise the patient to adopt a "wait-and-see" attitude.

BIBLIOGRAPHY

1. Comfort MW, Gray HK, Wilson JM: The silent gallstone: A ten to twenty year follow-up study of 112 cases. *Ann Surg* 1948; 128:931–937.
2. Glenn F, McSherry CK, Dineen P: Morbidity of surgical treatment for nonmalignant biliary tract disease. *Surg Gynecol Obstet* 1968; 126:15–26.
3. Gracie WA, Ransohoff DF: The natural history of silent gallstones: The innocent gallstone is not a myth. *N Engl J Med* 1982; 307:798–800.
4. Lund J: Surgical indications in cholelithiasis: Prophylactic cholecystectomy elucidated on the basis of long-term follow-up on 526 nonoperated cases. *Ann Surg* 1960; 151:153–162.
5. Mayo WJ: "Innocent" gallstones a myth. *JAMA* 1911; 56:1021–1024.
6. McSherry CK, Glenn F: The incidence and causes of death following surgery for nonmalignant biliary tract disease. *Ann Surg* 1980; 191:271–275.
7. McSherry CK, Ferstenberg H, Calhoun F, et al.: The natural history of diagnosed gallstone disease in symptomatic and asymptomatic patients. *Ann Surg* 1985; 202:59–63.
8. Moynihan BGA: An address on inaugural symptoms. *Br Med J* 1908; 2:1597–1601.
9. Wenckert A, Robertson B: The natural course of gallstone disease: Eleven year review of 781 nonoperated cases. *Gastroenterology* 1966; 50:376–381.

23

Acute Cholecystitis

A 29-year-old woman, 5 ft 7 in. tall and weighing approximately 160 lb, is admitted with a five-hour history of right upper quadrant pain, a temperature of 100° F, and vomiting. Previous history reveals a fairly classic history for intolerance to fatty foods and cabbage. There is no suggestion of any ulcer history. Urine is light and stool is normal in color, and she is not icteric. On physical examination, she is moderately tender in the right upper quadrant, with pain radiating through to her back.

Consultant: Robert E. Hermann, M.D.

The presentation of this patient is a common problem seen by surgeons. The patient has a history of fatty food intolerance and this, taken with her clinical presentation, should immediately raise the suspicion that she has either acute cholecystitis, acute pancreatitis, or some other acute inflammatory process in the right upper abdomen. Certainly, if consulted about this patient, my first response would be to recommend hospitalization.

Biliary disease is one of the most common problems encountered in the adult population of the United States, and cholecystectomy is now the most frequently performed abdominal operation in most acute-care hospitals in this country. It is estimated that 15% to 20% of the adult population of the United States (i.e., almost 20 million Americans) may have gallstones.

Of this entire group of potential patients with gallstones, several studies have indicated that more than half (perhaps 60%) have no symptoms, and a somewhat lesser number (perhaps 40%) are symptomatic. Of the group of patients with symptoms, office practice and hospital admission statistics indicate that roughly 20% of patients with symptomatic biliary disease develop acute cholecystitis. An additional increment of patients (5% to 10%) will develop a complication such as jaundice, cholangitis, or pancreatitis. Those factors that increase the overall risk of cholecystitis include: (1) the presence of acute inflammation or infection, (2) common bile duct stones with jaundice, (3) age more than 65 years, (4) pancreatitis, and (5) the coexistence of other illnesses such as cardiovascular, pulmonary or renal disease, or cirrhosis of the liver. Recent evidence shows that diabetes is not a risk factor. (*Editor's note:* This is not universally held; many authors still consider diabetes a cause for concern in patients with gallbladder disease.) There is some evidence that patients with small stones in the gallbladder are more likely to develop complications of cholecystitis, since these stones may pass into the common bile duct.

In the patient presented, there is no evidence of these increased risk factors, except for the probable diagnosis of acute cholecystitis with fever. The patient is moderately obese, but she is young and has no evidence (on the history given) of any other complicating illnesses. She does not appear to be jaundiced on physical examination, and her urine and stool colors appear to be normal. She does have pain radiating through into the back, a symptom typical of cholecystitis but one that should also raise the suspicion of possible pancreatitis.

MEDICAL THERAPY AND DIAGNOSIS

As mentioned above, I would admit this patient to the hospital and, during the first 24 hours after admission, begin medical therapy to modify the inflammatory aspects of this disease, replace fluids lost by vomiting or into the area of inflammation, and begin testing to confirm the diagnosis and to rule out coexisting illnesses. Intravenous fluids are begun using crystalloid solutions; pain relief is obtained by the use of analgesics administered intramuscularly (my preference is meperidine (Demerol), 100 mg every four hours), and a nasogastric tube should be passed to decompress the stomach since the patient has been vomiting.

Basic diagnostic studies should include a complete blood cell count, SMA-16 profile (to include serum electrolytes and basic determinations of liver and renal function), serum amylase level, chest x-ray film, plain x-ray film examination of the abdomen (KUB film), an ultrasound scan of the biliary system and pancreas, and a technetium-99 scan (DISIDA or PIPIDA scan).

If this patient has an elevated white blood cell count to go along with the fever of 100° F, I would begin antibiotic therapy, using either a third-generation cephalosporin or piperacillin, both of which are excreted in bile and cover the mixed flora of bacteria seen in biliary tract inflammation. The chest x-ray film, along with the patient's clinical examination, is utilized to rule out a pneumonic process in the right lung that can cause fever and upper abdominal pain. The abdominal x-ray film is utilized to look for evidence of calcified gallstones, air in the biliary system, free air in the peritoneal cavity, gastric distention, renal or ureteral calculi, or evidence of abnormally dilated loops of intestine or other lesions. The ultrasound scan is carefully assessed for the presence of gallstones, a dilated or thick-walled gallbladder, dilated bile ducts, pancreatic swelling, a liver lesion, or some other upper abdominal abnormality (Fig 23–1).

The technetium-99 scan is obtained to confirm that there is no visualization of the gallbladder while the liver, common bile duct, and duodenum are visualized (Fig 23–2). A nonvisualized gallbladder confirms the diagnosis of acute cholecystitis, indicating cystic duct obstruction or inflammation with passive dilation of the gallbladder. With the rapidity and safety of ultrasound and technetium-

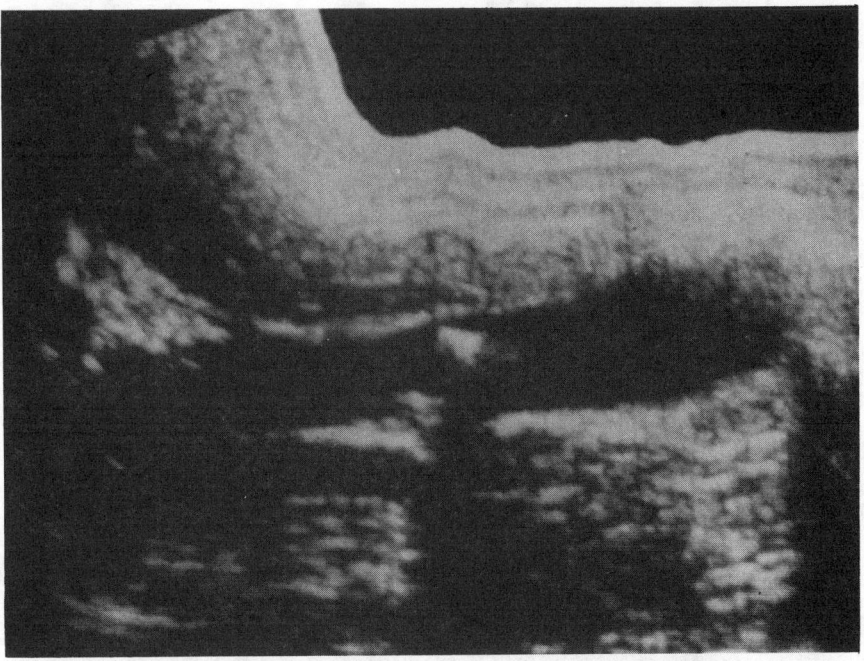

FIG 23–1.
Ultrasound study shows a nondilated gallbladder that contains at least one stone. Note the echogenic shadow behind the stone.

99 scans, confirmation of the diagnosis of acute cholecystitis can be obtained within a matter of hours. There is no longer any reason to use the oral cholecystogram in patients with acute cholecystitis.

If this patient were older or if the clinical history suggested other risk factors, further studies such as an electrocardiogram, pulmonary function tests, renal function studies, or other tests should be performed as deemed appropriate.

If an elevated serum amylase level is found, this may indicate pancreatitis or only hyperamylasemia in association with acute cholecystitis. The medical therapy for both acute pancreatitis and acute cholecystitis is similar, that is, the treatment given above. Further studies to identify the presence or severity of pancreatitis would include ultrasound scan or, if this is unclear, a computed tomography (CT) scan of the pancreas to look for pancreatic edema or inflammatory swelling, as well as serum calcium determinations, elevation of serum glucose, serum lipase, and measurements of the urinary excretion of amylase. The treatment of acute pancreatitis and acute gallstone pancreatitis is discussed elsewhere in this text.

TIMING OF OPERATION

Provided no other complicating illness or severe risk factor is identified in this patient, and having confirmed the diagnosis of acute cholecystitis, I would plan to perform a cholecystectomy as an elective procedure on (most likely) the day after admission to the hospital or the day following. I believe there is no harm in delaying removal of this inflamed organ for 24 to 48 hours, during which time the patient's general condition can be improved, fluid losses replenished, antibiotic therapy begun, diagnostic studies completed, and the patient's overall risk assessment evaluated.

If the patient had a palpably dilated gallbladder (hydrops of the gallbladder) or showed evidence of increasing toxicity, infection, or systemic sepsis during the first 48 hours, I would schedule cholecystectomy as an urgent or emergency procedure. Conversely, if severe risk factors such as a recent myocardial in-

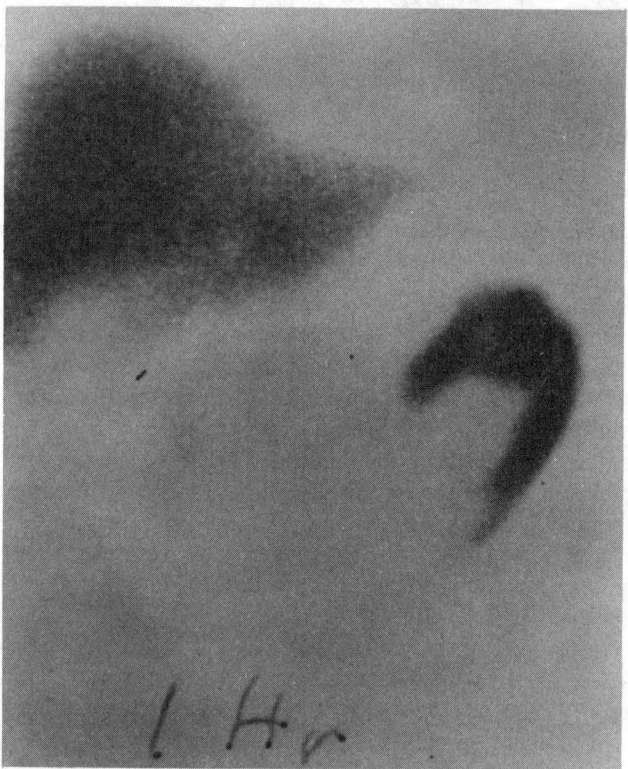

FIG 23–2.
DISIDA scan shows no visualization of the gallbladder at one hour. Radioactive contrast is seen in the duodenum-jejunal flexure.

farction, renal failure, severe pneumonia, or acute pancreatitis are present that might not be quickly or easily corrected, medical therapy should be continued and the operative procedure delayed so long as the patient continues to show improvement. If the high-risk patient has continuing or worsening pain or sepsis, cholecystostomy can be performed as an urgent procedure (under either general, epidural, or local anesthesia) to drain the gallbladder and remove the gallstones.

My own philosophy in regard to the patient with acute gallstone pancreatitis, depending upon the severity of the pancreatitis, is to go ahead with cholecystectomy within the first 48 hours after admission, provided the patient has evidence of cholecystitis and does not have overly severe pancreatitis with shock, hypocalcemia, or other evidence of toxicity. In the presence of this degree of pancreatitis, it may be wiser to continue medical therapy until the patient's condition stabilizes, then to perform cholecystectomy and common bile duct exploration, and perhaps endoscopic sphincterotomy if a gallstone has failed to pass and is impacted in the ampulla of Vater.

Cholecystectomy is a safe operative procedure when performed within the first 48 to 72 hours after the onset of acute cholecystitis, provided all risk factors are identified and appropriately treated. The technical aspects of the operation are not unusually difficult during the early period of edema and inflammatory swelling. However, once the inflammatory process has gone on for five or more days, the procedure becomes technically more difficult as chronic induration, vascularity, and fibrosis progress. Early cholecystectomy for acute cholecystitis, performed electively on the first or second day after admission (24 to 48 hours), after the diagnosis is confirmed and medical therapy has been instituted to moderate the disease, is, in my opinion, the safest and most cost-effective way to manage the patient with acute cholecystitis.

Recent studies from other centers confirm the fact that delaying the operation for a longer period of medical treatment increases the risk of morbidity and mortality from potential gangrene and perforation of the gallbladder, and that delaying the definitive operation to another, later hospital admission increases the risk of another episode of cholecystitis prior to definitive operation, thus increasing the cost of treatment.

OPERATIVE PROCEDURE

As cholecystectomy is a commonly performed operation, it must be performed safely. I prefer a subcostal incision for most patients, especially an obese patient as in the case presented. A midline longitudinal incision is used only in thin patients or those with a narrow costal margin. After opening the peritoneal cavity, protective drapes are used to line the operative incision in order to prevent contamination of the incision and subcutaneous tissue. A general abdominal examination should always be performed initially to rule out other disease in the abdomen. I place several large intra-abdominal laparotomy pads in the right

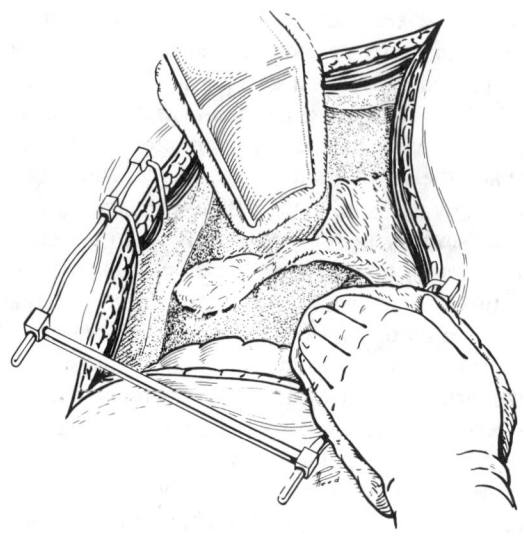

FIG 23–3.
Drawing showing exposure of gallbladder and bile ducts through a subcostal incision.

upper abdomen to depress the hepatic flexure of the colon and to isolate the right upper abdomen from contamination during the dissection. Large, flat-bladed retractors are used to elevate the liver and expose the subhepatic space, while the first assistant's hand is used on another laparotomy pad to retract the duodenum inferiorly and expose the gallbladder, bile duct, and portal area (Fig 23–3).

In all patients with acute cholecystitis, the dissection of the gallbladder should be undertaken from the fundus toward the junction of the cystic duct and common bile duct. I believe this is the safest technique for cholecystectomy in all patients, but especially in patients with acute inflammation when inflammatory edema may obscure some of the usual landmarks, this dissection diminishes the likelihood of injury to other structures. The dissection is carried down, with traction on the gallbladder, until the cystic artery is exposed. The artery can then be clamped, divided, and ligated with a silk ligature. As the gallbladder is dissected from the liver bed, the electrocautery unit is used to control small bleeding vessels and to provide a dry field.

After division of the cystic artery, the ampulla of the gallbladder and cystic duct can be carefully dissected down to the junction of the cystic duct with the common hepatic duct. At this point, any stones in the cystic duct should be milked back into the gallbladder, a ligature tied around the upper cystic duct, and the lower cystic duct partially divided and opened for placement of a flexible catheter or tubing for intraoperative cholangiography (Fig 23–4). In my practice, operative cholangiography is a routine part of all cholecystectomies. It provides visualization of the entire biliary system so that the surgeon can be certain that he/she has not missed any unsuspected pathology (e.g., bile duct stones, tumors, sclerosing cholangitis, congenital abnormalities) in the common bile duct. In a review of our routine operative cholangiograms, an unsuspected stone or other disease was found in 7% of patients having a cholecystectomy.

After completion of the operative cholangiogram, the cystic duct is clamped close (0.5 to 1.0 cm) to the common bile duct, divided, and the gallbladder specimen removed. After removal of the gallbladder, we open it and obtain cultures of the bile. The cystic duct stump is tied with a 2-0 silk ligature. The subhepatic space is irrigated with sterile saline, the gallbladder bed on the liver is inspected for any further bleeding, and the common bile duct and porta hepatis area are palpated and examined for any evidence of a palpable mass, bile duct stones, or other problems.

After the operative cholangiograms have been returned and reviewed, if they are normal, preparation for closure of the abdomen is undertaken. If the operative cholangiogram shows a bile duct abnormality or if palpation and inspection of the bile duct or liver shows any additional problems, the bile duct should be opened and explored or a biopsy obtained of the additional lesion.

POSTOPERATIVE COURSE

In patients having cholecystectomy for acute cholecystitis, I continue to drain the right upper abdomen and subhepatic space for one to two days postoperatively, using a multiperforated, closed-system suction drain.

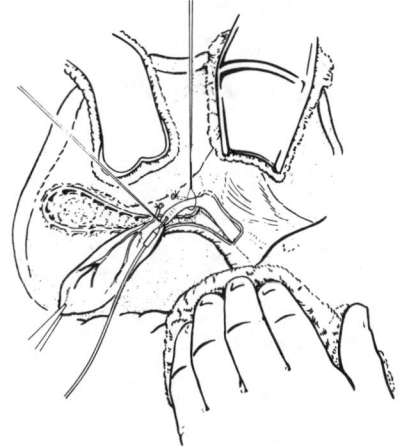

FIG 23–4.
Drawing of an operative cholangiogram catheter being placed into the cystic duct. The gallbladder has been dissected from the liver and the cystic artery has been divided and ligated.

Antibiotic therapy, which was started preoperatively, is continued for approximately 24 hours after the operative procedure and then discontinued unless there is continuing evidence of infection. In patients with a continuing fever, elevated white blood cell count, or other signs of infection, antibiotics may be continued for five to six days postoperatively.

After cholecystectomy most patients are discharged from the hospital four to five days postoperatively. Although the mortality for patients having cholecystectomy with acute cholecystitis in all age groups is approximately 3.5%, if one analyzes these studies, it becomes apparent that this mortality occurs predominantly in patients over 50 years of age or in patients with other severe risk factors. For a 29-year-old woman without other identifiable risk factors, the mortality of cholecystectomy for acute cholecystitis should be almost zero.

BIBLIOGRAPHY

1. Hermann RE, Broughan TA: Intraoperative radiology, in Blumgart LH (ed): *Surgery of the Liver and Biliary Tract*. New York, Churchill Livingstone Inc, 1988, pp 361–371.
2. Jarvinen HJ, Hastbacka J: Early cholecystectomy for acute cholecystitis: A prospective randomized study. *Ann Surg* 1980; 191:501–505.
3. Ransohoff DF, Miller GF, Forsythe SB, et al: Outcome of acute cholecystitis in patients with diabetes mellitus. *Ann Intern Med* 1987; 106:829–832.

24

Postcholecystectomy Syndrome

A 33-year-old woman with persistent right upper quadrant pain radiating through to the back, made worse by certain types of food and exercise, is operated on elsewhere for a presumed cholelithiasis despite a negative ultrasound and negative Graham-Cole test. The gallbladder is not inflamed and no stones are found. After the operation, her pain is relieved for approximately three months; following this, however, it recurs. In addition, she reports intermittent diarrhea with foul-smelling floating stools. Right upper quadrant and epigastric pain radiating through to the back is present. This has progressed to the point where it has interfered with her function at work.

Consultant: George L. Nardi, M.D.

DIAGNOSTIC CONSIDERATIONS

With or without gallstones, this patient's recurrent symptoms after cholecystectomy places her into that diagnostic wastebasket known as the postcholecystectomy syndrome. If gallstones had been present originally, the first diagnostic consideration would be retained common duct stone. However, her prior negative evaluation, a normal gallbladder, and a presumably normal exploration rule out the biliary system as the cause of her symptoms. Her continuing symptoms, the presence of food intolerance, and the development of foul-smelling stools suggests pancreatic insufficiency with recurrent pancreatitis as the cause of her symptoms.

The patient's history should be carefully reviewed. Does she really have intolerance to some foods? What kind of food? Does she have intolerance or "allergies" to medications such as codeine or opiate derivatives that might cause sphincter spasm? The occurrence of unexplained abdominal pain and surgery in a family member may suggest hereditary pancreatitis, a rare but frequently overlooked condition with a greater than normal incidence of carcinoma. Has she been taking any chronic medication? At her age, she may have been taking birth-control pills. Estrogens can cause episodes of recurrent pancreatitis. Chlorothiazides may occasionally be implicated. Cessation of therapy with such medication usually results in relief of symptoms.

A therapeutic trial of oral pancreatic enzymes would be diagnostic. Relief of the diarrhea would provide evidence for pancreatic exocrine insufficiency and pancreatitis. Blood tests should be performed for hyperlipidemia and to determine serum calcium level. The former would suggest a possible lipid disorder as the basis for her symptoms, and an elevated fasting calcium level would indicate hyperparathyroidism. Cure of the hyperparathyroidism by excision of the offending adenoma will almost always relieve the abdominal symptoms. For screening purposes the serum calcium determination is quicker, less complicated, and less expensive than a parathormone assay and is equally reliable. I would next perform endoscopic retrograde cholangiopancreatography (ERCP). This would detect many of the conditions to be considered in the postcholecystectomy syndrome such as hiatus hernia, bile gastritis, peptic ulcer, and other esophagogastroduodenal abnormalities. It also permits evaluation of the papilla of Vater for hypertrophy and stenosis of the orifice and, when available, permits pressure measurements of the pancreatic and biliary systems. In addition, ERCP will demonstrate two very important anatomical details: (1) dilated ducts, and (2) pancreas divisum.

Dilated Ducts

If the duct is dilated (large duct disease), this is proof positive of pancreatitis with fibrosis. Decompression should be performed and is most commonly done with a Roux-y pancreatojejunostomy. It must be recognized that while this procedure will frequently provide relief for a prolonged period of time, the intrinsic pathology will continue to progress with eventual exocrine and endocrine insufficiency.

Pancreas Divisum

Should normal-sized ducts be demonstrated (small duct disease), their configuration should be examined for the presence of "pancreas divisum," a failure of fusion of the ducts of Wirsung and Santorini. This is the most common congenital anomaly of the pancreas and is estimated to occur in about 5% of the population. It is thought by some that patients with pancreas divisum have an increased incidence of recurrent pancreatitis on the basis that the small minor papilla is inadequate for the volume of pancreatic secretion, and back pressure and partial obstruction results. Others, however, have provided evidence that the incidence of pancreas divisum is the same in patients with pancreatitis and other pancreatico-biliary disease. Nevertheless, stenosis of the accessory papilla

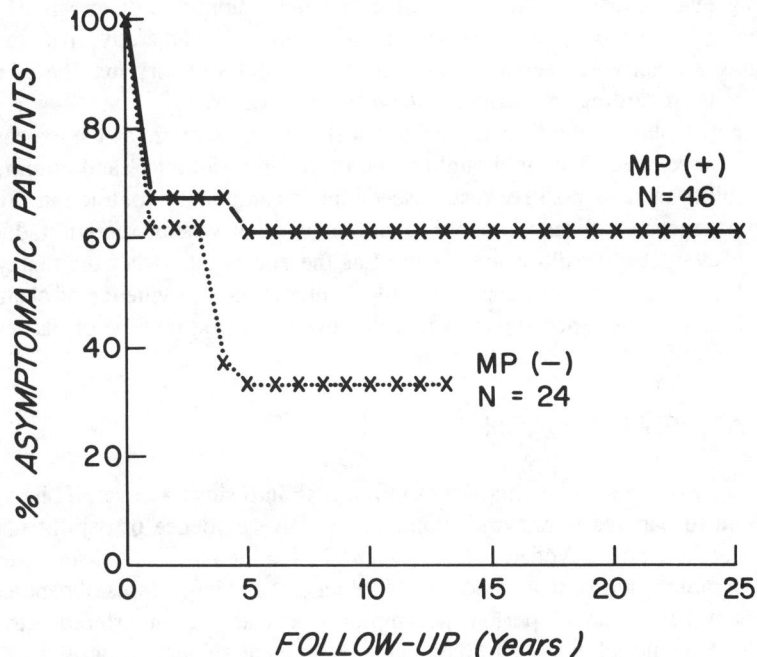

FIG 24–1.
A positive evocative test doubles the chance for surgical relief.

is of particular significance since pancreatic secretions have no alternative egress route (via the major papilla) in this condition.

EVOCATIVE TESTS

Further evidence for obstructive pancreatopathy may be obtained by evocative tests. The oldest of these is the Morphine-Prostigmine Evocative Test (Fig 24–1), wherein 8 to 10 mg of morphine and 1 mg of prostigmine is injected intramuscularly, and serum amylase and lipase are obtained at serial intervals. The morphine produces some degree of ampullary contraction and the prostigmine stimulates the pancreas to produce a scanty, viscid, enzyme-rich juice. Reproduction of the patient's pain frequently occurs. Elevation of levels of serum amylase and lipase are considered a positive test, indicating obstruction to pancreatic outflow. As can be seen in Table 24–1, patients with a positive enzyme response had a 60% or better chance of a good result from sphincteroplasty, whereas a history of alcoholism coupled with a negative enzymatic response predicted that surgery would be of no benefit. While this test is not a reliable screening test for pancreatitis, a positive test may support a diagnosis of obstruction and help patient and surgeon in deciding on surgical therapy. In addition, combining a positive or negative test with the patient's history may be of predictive value regarding the efficacy of proposed surgery.

In recent years, a modification of this test utilizing secretin as the evocative agent has developed. This is thought to be more "physiologic" and eliminates the possibility of false-positive results secondary to ampullary contraction. Since secretin produces a low-enzyme, high-bicarbonate, high-volume secretion, ductal dilatation evaluated by ultrasound is used as the end point, rather than enzyme assays. It is believed that dilatation could be interpreted as evidence of obstruction. A limited experience suggests that this evocative test may be of particular use in patients with pancreas divisum.

OPERATIVE APPROACH

In a young woman such as this, I would not rush into surgery, even if she were to respond to pancreatic enzyme supplements, have evidence of papillitis, and demonstrate a positive evocative test. I would be inclined to treat her for a period of several months with antispasmodics, H_2 blockers, and large doses of pancreatic supplements. After such a period, if symptoms persisted and interfered with her life-style, I would advise her to have a transduodenal sphincteroplasty.

In the presence of pancreas divisum, the procedure is performed on the minor papilla. This is frequently difficult to locate. However, intravenous administration of 1 to 2 units of secretin per kg of body weight will usually identify the tiny orifice by characteristic spurts of pancreatic juice. The stenotic orifice is incised over a probe, carefully opened with fine scissors, and the cut edges sutured with fine interrupted sutures.

With normal ductal anatomy, the major papilla is dilated with lacrimal probe dilators and incised for a distance of about 2 cm. This procedure unroofs the

TABLE 24–1.
Clinical Results of Sphincteroplasty

	M - P Test	
	(+)	(−)
Good result	60%	35%
History of		
Drug abuse	65%	30%
Diarrhea	65%	15%
Abdominal surgery	75%	15%
EtOH	65%	0

common duct and exposes the small orifice of the duct of Wirsung in the floor of the common duct. This orifice is now sectioned for 1 cm or more so that a No. 3 Bakes dilator can be passed freely into the pancreatic duct.

POSTOPERATIVE COURSE

Failure to relieve pain by drainage procedures of this type is not uncommon, but the probability of success and the low morbidity justify the attempt. Occasionally, recurrence after years of relief results from restenosis, and reoperation is justified.

Most failures, I believe, result from the patient having chronic recurrent, rather than acute recurrent, pancreatitis. Unfortunately, the two cannot be easily distinguished. Chronic pancreatitis is a progressive, fibrosing disease that requires total pancreatectomy. The pain of chronic pancreatitis is one that does not yield to sympathectomy or nerve blocks. Total pancreatectomy should be performed sooner rather than later if it is to be effective. The quality of life for patient and family is far superior with controlled exocrine and endocrine insufficiency than with chronic pain and narcotic dependence.

BIBLIOGRAPHY

1. Nardi GL, Michelassi F, Zannini P: Transduodenal sphincteroplasty: 5 to 25 year follow-up of 89 patients. *Ann Surg* 1983; 98:453–461.
2. Nardi GL: Surgery for chronic pancreatitis, in Malt RA (ed): *Surgical Techniques Illustrated*. Philadelphia, WB Saunders Co, 1985, pp 361–434.
3. Sugawa C, Walt AJ, Nunez DC, et al.: Pancreas divisum: Is it a normal anatomic variant? *Am J Surg* 1987; 153:62–67.
4. Warshaw AL, Popp JW Jr, Schapiro RH: Long-term patency, pancreatic function, and pain relief after lateral pancreaticojejunostomy for chronic pancreatitis. *Gastroenterology* 1980; 79:289–392.

25

Cancer of the Gallbladder

A 67-year-old man is operated on for symptoms suggesting cholelithiasis; a positive ultrasound and a negative upper gastrointestinal series had been obtained. On exploration, cholelithiasis is found, but there is a mass within the gallbladder that appears adherent to the liver. On attempting a cholecystectomy, the mass appears to invade the gallbladder wall and the liver. A Trucut needle biopsy reveals adenocarcinoma.

Consultant: James H. Foster, M.D.

The presentation of this patient is perhaps the most common way in which gallbladder cancer is diagnosed, in spite of all of the recent improvements in radiologic imaging. Symptoms more typical of benign than malignant disease often precede the diagnosis by many years. It may well be that this patient's symptoms, and those of most patients with cancer, are mostly due to the gallstones rather than the malignancy.

Gallbladder cancer is a disease of older people and is more common than generally recognized. It ranks fifth in the list of gastrointestinal cancers in the United States (just behind rectum, colon, pancreas, and stomach), but because many cases are diagnosed at autopsy, this frequency may not be apparent to most surgeons. In patients over 70 years of age, as many as 10% of gallbladders removed for presumed benign disease may contain cancer. The only atypical aspect of this case is the patient's gender; women predominate in most series, just as they do with cholelithiasis.

Most patients with gallbladder cancer have stones. Is this because stones and chronic inflammation predispose to malignant change, or because the biochemical factors common to gallstone formation also lead to cancer? No answer is yet possible, but it is interesting that implanted foreign bodies potentiate the carcinogenic potential of chemical agents in the gallbladders of experimental animals.

Will removal of stone-containing gallbladders prevent the subsequent development of cancer?—Certainly, since no one has ever developed a gallbladder cancer after cholecystectomy. However, calculations made to investigate the reasonable suggestion to remove all stone-containing gallbladders to prevent cancer work out, on the basis of incidence and mortality figures, to rule against the removal of asymptomatic stones. Certainly, cancer prophylaxis can be added to the reasons to recommend cholecystectomy to patients with symptomatic stones. Whether alternative ways to handle stones (e.g., chemical dissolution or lithotripsy) will reduce the subsequent risk of gallbladder cancer remains to be seen. An exception to the general rule to avoid elective operation solely to prevent gallbladder cancer is afforded by the patient with a calcified gallbladder, the so-called "porcelain" gallbladder. Cancer may be found in up to 30% of these unusual cases.

Gallbladder cancer has a well-deserved bad reputation. The vast majority of patients are dead within one year of diagnosis. The disease is very aggressive locally, with early spread to adjacent nodes and other structures. Distant spread is uncommon, and many patients die with disease confined to the right upper quadrant. Most gallbladder malignancies are adenocarcinoma, although as many as 4% to 5% may be squamous or adenosquamous. Only the papillary form carries with it a better prognosis.

Nevin and associates have staged gallbladder cancer. Stage I is defined as intramucosal or in situ disease; stage II, as microinvasive (not through gallbladder muscle); stage III, as locally invasive through gallbladder wall (with or without cystic duct node involvement); and stage IV, as extension into liver, other adjacent viscera, lymph node involvement beyond bile duct nodes, or metastatic spread. Our patient is already in stage III on the basis of the information given to us. Almost all of the long-term cures of patients with gallbladder cancer occur in patients with stage I and II disease, and most follow the discovery by a pathologist of a small focus of cancer unrecognized at operation to remove presumed benign gallbladder disease—the so-called "occult" cancer.

Can a patient with stage III disease ever be cured? Will extension of the resection beyond cholecystectomy alone make any difference in long-term survival? Do chemotherapy and/or radiotherapy have anything to add? Unfortunately, there is little solid evidence to justify a clear affirmative answer to any of these questions.

Given 100 patients with a story and findings similar to ours, less than 10% would survive one year unless the histology showed a papillary pattern. Anecdotal reports of palliation or even prolonged survival after radiotherapy for gallbladder cancer exist, but they are few and far between. Chemotherapy with 5-fluorouracil, either alone or in combination with other agents, has had little reported success. I know of no controlled series that demonstrates any survival advantage to the use of any of the currently available adjuvant therapies, which brings us back to resection.

To place either limited or extended operation in perspective, we need to look at the characteristics of long-term survivors and at patterns of failure. In 1970, Vaittinen of Finland summarized the world's reported experience up to that date in an encyclopedic article.

TABLE 25-1.
Extended Operations for Gallbladder Cancer*

	Liver Resection†		Lymphadenectomy Without Liver Resection	Overall
	Wedge	Lobectomy		
Patients	46	23	3	72
Operative deaths	4	9	0	13 (18%)
DWD < 3½ yr††	31	12	3	
AFD < 5 yr††	4	1	0	
AWD < 1 yr††	3	0	0	
Lost to follow-up	1	0	0	
5-yr survivors	3§	1§	0	4 (6%)

*Adapted from Foster JH: Carcinoma of the gallbladder, in Way LW, Pellegrini CA (eds): *Surgery of the Gallbladder and Bile Ducts*. Philadelphia, WB Saunders Co, 1987.
†Liver resection was combined with regional lymphadenectomy in some of these cases.
§One patient after wedge resection and one patient after lobectomy died with disease after 5 yr.
††DWD = dead with disease; AFD = alive free of disease; and AWD = alive with disease

A more recent review that I completed adds to the experience. Ninety-two patients who survived five years or more after operation were found in this literature review. The extent of therapy was known for 78 patients, 73 of whom had cholecystectomy alone; three others had extended resection, and two received adjuvant radiotherapy. In 36 of 43 five-year survivors for whom sufficient information was available, the surgeon was *not* aware of the cancer during operation.

Survival of patients with disease confined to the gallbladder wall (i.e., stages I and II) ranges from 25% to 100%. Thirty-four percent of patients with papillary cancer in one series lived five years, while less than 10% of patients with other histologic types lived one year. Clearly, the patients with early disease have a fairly good prognosis after cholecystectomy alone. When a pathologist finds an "occult" carcinoma without invasion through the gallbladder wall, there is no current justification for reoperation for wider excision.

Patients who had recurrence usually did so within one year. Direct extension into liver; invasion of adjacent duodenum, stomach, or colon; and intraductal spread (particularly with papillary tumors) are common, as is embolic metastasis to the liver. Diffuse peritoneal seeding or dissemination to lungs, brain, and bone is rare and late. Vaittinen, analyzing 1,611 patients, found at the time of the first operation and diagnosis regional and retroperitoneal lymph node spread in 65% of patients, embolic spread to liver in 51% of patients, and direct invasion of liver in 52% and of bile ducts in 42% of patients.

These findings would suggest that an aggressive local resection combined with regional lymphadenectomy might have merit. However, Vaittinen found only seven five-year survivors after 187 extended operations. Table 25-1 attempts to document the reported experience with liver resection and/or lymphadenectomy in 72 patients with more recently reported cases. Note that operative mortality was three times the five-year survival rate in this small series. However, the occurrence of nine deaths after 23 liver lobectomies is much higher than we should expect today, given modern refinements in technique and greater experience.

Does hepatic lobectomy have any place in the treatment of patients with gallbladder cancer? I think not—on both anatomical and pathologic grounds. The gallbladder lies in the central (interlobar) plane of the liver, and one could argue as well for left as for right lobectomy. I know of no report of curing a patient with disease spread into the liver beyond the immediate vicinity of the gallbladder. Perhaps cure is possible with the resection of a few satellite nodules resulting from reflux into adjacent portal venules, but wedge excision of the gallbladder bed should accomplish this as well as extended lobectomy. For similar reasons, I doubt that liver transplantation will ever provide an answer for this disease.

Thirty-five years ago, Glenn and Hayes recommended wedge excision of the gallbladder bed and regional lymphadenectomy. More recently, Adson has reported results after this operation in three patients with stage I and II disease, and in four who had microinvasion outside of the gallbladder wall. The three with early disease were still alive three to ten years later. Of the four patients with disease outside of the gallbladder wall, two are dead with disease at 3 1/2 and 6 years, and two are alive at the time of reporting, apparently free of disease at less than 1 year and at 13 years.

A position that cholecystectomy alone is the only rational operation for gallbladder cancer could be strongly defended. Cholecystectomy will probably cure the vast majority of the "curable" patients. There simply is not yet enough evidence to recommend more radical operation. In fact, the reported experience would seem to recommend against such a course. However, the patient under consideration here pushes us into a corner. An astute surgeon has recognized the disease during cholecystectomy and has documented its local invasion into adjacent liver. The surgeon should continue exploration, with particular attention to the rest of the liver and the regional lymph nodes. If intraoperative ultrasonography is available, the surgeon should use it to explore the liver, particularly in the area immediately adjacent to the gallbladder. If embolic disease is found in the liver or in a node beyond the bile duct, no further resection should be done. I would hold radiation therapy until a symptomatic recurrence was obvious, and I would advise the patient to get his affairs in order.

If no embolic disease is found, in spite of the lack of supporting scientific evidence, I would recommend a wedge excision of the gallbladder bed and a limited regional lymphadenectomy. The wedge excision should include a 2-cm margin of normal liver, which can usually be teased out using blunt suction technique without hilar control of vessels and ducts. The lymph nodes around the cystic duct, Calot's triangle, and along the common bile duct should be taken down to where the bile duct disappears into the duodenum, avoiding circumferential dissection of the common bile duct. A Kocher maneuver will assist this dissection, but the additional exposure should not tempt the surgeon to extend the lymphadenectomy to include peripancreatic nodes.

Other alternatives would be: (1) to close the abdomen and treat the gallbladder bed (previously outlined by metal clips) with postoperative radiotherapy; or (2) to close the abdomen and return in three months for a second look on the theoretical grounds that "curable" recurrent disease would still be localized and perhaps resectable, that "incurable" disease would be recognizably out of bounds, and that finding no disease would require no further resection and allow a more favorable prognosis.

My bias is that if there is any chance at cure in the situation presented to us, it is with extended resection at the first procedure. "Bias" is the correct noun to describe a "gut" feeling unsupported by scientific evidence; "naively optimistic" might be appropriate qualifiers of that noun.

BIBLIOGRAPHY

1. Adson MA: Carcinoma of the gallbladder. *Surg Clin North Am* 1973; 53:1202–1216.
2. Foster JH: Carcinoma of the gallbladder, in Way LW, Pellegrini CA (eds): *Surgery of the Gallbladder and Bile Ducts*. Philadelphia, WB Saunders Co, 1987.
3. Glenn F, Hayes DM: The scope of radical surgery in the treatment of malignant tumors of the extrahepatic biliary tract. *Surg Gynecol Obstet* 1954; 99:529.
4. Nevin JE, Moran TJ, Kay S, et al: Carcinoma of the gallbladder. *Cancer* 1976; 37:141–148.
5. Vaittinen E: Carcinoma of the gallbladder: A study of 390 cases diagnosed in Finland 1953–1967. *Ann Chir Gynaecol Fenn* 1970; 168 (suppl):7–81.

26

Alcoholic Pancreatitis With a Chain of Lakes

A 35-year-old male alcohol abuser and cigarette smoker (20 pack-years) was admitted to the Emergency Department for the fourth time in 1 1/2 years due to symptoms of epigastric pain radiating through to the back, as well as nausea and vomiting. The patient had lost his job because of frequent absence from work and his hospitalizations. The patient claimed he had not imbibed alcohol for the past three months after being told his pancreatitis was alcohol-related. The diagnosis of pancreatitis was based on elevated levels of serum amylase and calcifications seen on his flat film. During the past six months his stools had become foul-smelling, greasy, and floated. He had lost 10 lb in weight.

Consultant: Charles F. Frey, M.D.

HOSPITAL COURSE

The patient was admitted and started on intravenous fluids and nasogastric suction. He was given meperidine (Demerol) for his pain. His alkaline phosphatase level was elevated at 150 international units (IU) (normal being 120). His fasting blood glucose level was normal, and there were mild elevations of GTT and amylase. A computed tomography (CT) scan showed an enlarged pancreatic duct in the body and tail of the pancreas. The intrahepatic biliary ducts were somewhat dilated. An upper gastrointestinal (GI) series and endoscopy were unremarkable, and ultrasound of the gallbladder showed no calculi. A surgical consultation was requested by the gastroenterology consult.

While the CT scan and evidence of malabsorption clearly indicated marked structural damage to the pancreas, not all such patients have pain. Therefore, an abnormal CT scan, evidence of pancreatic calcification on flat film of the abdomen (KUB), or malabsorption are not in themselves operative indications. On the other hand, pain in association with structural changes in the pancreas is an indication for operation. The pain in a patient with a history of alcoholism may be of nonpancreatic origin and may be related to gastritis or duodenal ulcer, and these causes should be ruled out before operation on the pancreas is contemplated. Confirmation that the cause of pain is due to pancreatitis should be sought. In patients in whom it is confirmed that chronic pancreatitis is the cause of the pain, every attempt should be made to alleviate it before operatively approaching the pancreas. If the patient has biliary disease or a primary hyperlipidemia as well as a history of alcoholism, the biliary pathology or hyperlipidemia should be corrected and eliminated as a cause of pain; if the pain still persists, then an operative approach to the pancreas should be considered.

After talking with the patient, we decided on the following plan: If the patient recovered from his current episode of pancreatitis, we would treat his steatorrhea. Working with the dietitian, we planned a 25-gm fat content in each meal, at which time he was to take 8 capsules of pancrelipase (Pancrease). He was also placed on Ranitidine 150 mg twice a day. In order for clinically apparent steatorrhea to occur, pancreatic secretion of lipase must be reduced by 90% or more of normal. In chronic pancreatitis, steatorrhea precedes azotorrhea as lipase secretion is adversely affected sooner than secretion of proteolytic enzymes. Thirty percent of patients with chronic pancreatitis coming to operation have, on biochemical examination of the stool, some evidence of abnormal fat loss. The limiting factor in enzyme replacement therapy of pancreatic exocrine insufficiency is the small amount of lipase in the commercial enzyme preparations and the fact that lipase may be destroyed by a low pH in the stomach. In order to be effective, the enzymes (specifically lipase) must reach the duodenum intact. Proteolytic enzymes are more resistant to a low acid pH. DiMagno and Clain have shown that only 5% of the maximal lipase output of the normal pancreas is sufficient to eliminate malabsorption or 28,000 IU of lipase per 25 gm of fat per meal. Of the commercially available pancreatic enzyme preparations, pancrelipase and panenelipase (Viokase) have the highest amounts of lipase per capsule, about 4,000 and 3,500 units, respectively. (A new product, Creon, approved by the FDA for the treatment of cystic fibrosis, is said to contain 8,000 units per capsule.) Therefore, 8 capsules per meal of pancrealipase or Viokase should be taken if malabsorption is to be eliminated. H_2 blockers are necessary to maintain the gastric pH above 4 to allow the enzymes safe passage through the stomach to reach the duodenum intact. While we choose to use the clinical response to our enzyme therapy as a measure of the adequacy of our therapy of pancreatic insufficiency, stool fat measurements (less than 5% of ingested fat should appear in the stool normally) or the triolen breath test can be used to confirm the effect of treatment. The triolen test is not accurate in patients with chronic obstructive pulmonary disease or diabetes.

The patient was interviewed by our psychiatrist and was instructed to be seen in our pain clinic after discharge. The patient also vowed he would seek help for his alcohol dependency. After discussion with his primary physicians, we agreed the patient would not be sent home on a regimen of narcotics. This latter point is one that I believe deserves emphasis. The patient with proved chronic pancreatitis needs to be told that if he cannot function in the absence of narcotics due to the severity of the pain, he needs an operation for pain relief. The practice of providing more and more narcotics for these patients is shameful, but unfortunately it may be resorted to by physicians frustrated by their inability to cope with the patient's complaints. When this regrettable practice is pursued, we end up with a patient already dependent on one drug (alcohol) now dependent on narcotics, an even more difficult problem to manage. Patients addicted to both alcohol and narcotics seldom achieve a satisfactory operative result. In such patients, one never knows whether their complaints of continued pain are due to failure of the operation to provide relief or to their craving for more narcotics.

Although our patient was encouraged to continue his abstinence from alcohol, once major structural changes have occurred in the pancreas (e.g., obstruction of the major pancreatic duct and/or small pseudocysts from fibrosis and intraductal calculi), cessation of alcohol by the patient seldom provides pain relief. However, progression of the structural changes may be slowed by abstinence. Continued ingestion of alcohol often precipitates or exacerbates the patient's pain, and progression of structural changes in the pancreas continues unabated.

Ten days after the patient's admission, he was discharged home with enzyme supplements and H_2 blockers. Before his scheduled return visit, he called to say that his pain had recurred and he would like surgery for pain relief. When seen two days later, the patient wanted to proceed with an operation.

ROLE OF THE SURGEON

It is important for the surgeon to verify that the patient is having significant pain and that the patient fully understands the risks of the operation including the development of diabetes, the results to be expected with regard to pain relief, and the complications associated with the operation. An absolute indication to halt is reluctance or hesitancy on the part of the patient to proceed with an operation after being educated as to its effect on exocrine and endocrine function and informed of the results regarding operative complications and pain relief. Chronic pancreatitis is a disease of many years' duration that may be punctuated by exacerbations and remissions. Only the patient can weigh the severity of pain and balance it against the risks, benefits, and consequences of the operation proposed. Often patients having an initial reluctance may return later for surgery if the pain increases in severity and the patient's resolve to live with the pain is weakened. Patients having pain of unclarified severity should not be sent home with a narcotics regimen.

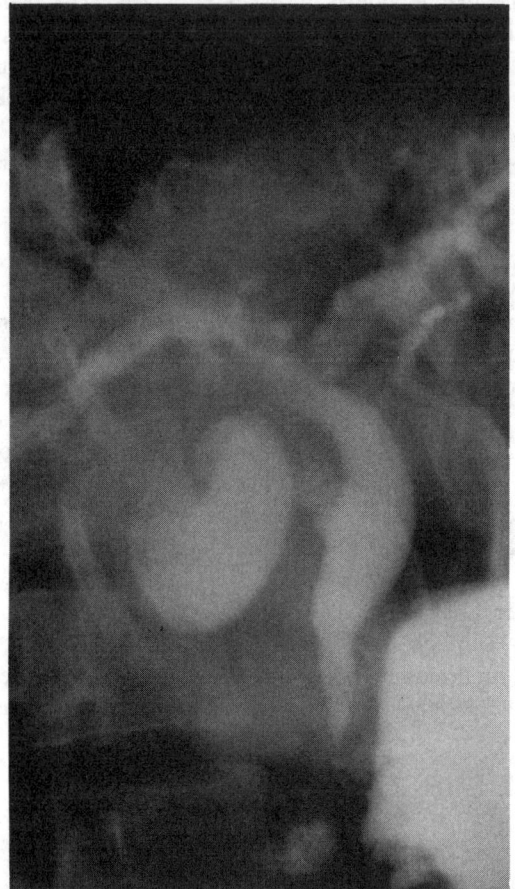

FIG 26–1.
The intrapancreatic portion of the common bile duct is narrowed with mild proximal dilatation.

COMMITMENT OF THE SURGEON

Pancreatic surgery, particularly for chronic pancreatitis, is different from many other types of surgery. The surgeon must be willing to make a major commitment to following up these patients. The patients, particularly the alcoholic patients, need encouragement and close follow-up to maintain abstinence from alcohol, as well as assistance in the management of any exocrine and endocrine insufficiency. The surgeon must also be prepared for patients who fail to achieve pain relief because of the choice of operation or patient selection. The stress of failed relationships and job frustrations more often than not produce recidivism with regard to alcohol abuse. Complications and multiple hospitalizations may result, and the surgeon is usually consulted. These patients are time-consuming and often vexing, a fact that surgeons should consider before becoming involved in their care.

QUALIFICATIONS OF THE SURGEON

The surgeon should be prepared and familiar with the various operative procedures available to deal with the structural abnormalities which may be associated with chronic pancreatitis, such as common bile duct obstruction, small pseudocysts in the head of the pancreas, pseudoaneurysms, an enlarged thickened head of the pancreas, left-sided portal hypertension or vascular anomalies of the hepatic artery, as well as the major complications associated with operations on the pancreas. The surgeon should be certain that he/she has sufficient resources in terms of staff, intensive care facilities and equipment to manage the preoperative, operative and postoperative care of the patient with chronic pancreatitis. Finally, it is the surgeon's ethical and legal responsibility to accurately represent to the patient the qualifications and experience he/she has to perform pancreatic surgery.

SELECTION OF THE MOST APPROPRIATE OPERATION

In selecting an operation for a patient with chronic pancreatitis, I try to judge the appropriateness of the selection by the following criteria:

1. Does the operation correct all structural abnormalities?
2. Does the operation have a low morbidity and mortality?
3. Does the operation relieve the patient's pain for a prolonged period?
4. Does the operation require abstinence from alcohol to be successful?
5. Does the operation minimize postoperative exocrine and endocrine insufficiency?

In order to complete our understanding of the structural abnormalities now that we are committed to the operation, an endoscopic retrograde cholangiopancreatography (ERCP) and angiogram are obtained. Antibiotics should be given before and after the ERCP. I believe it is best to attempt to delineate in advance of the operation the structural abnormalities of the pancreas and biliary tree and the major vessels in order to think through and plan an appropriate operative strategy. In this patient, the ERCP showed a stricture of the major pancreatic duct 2 to 3 cm from the ampulla of Vater (Figs 26–1 and 26–2). The ERCP confirmed the findings of an obstructed major pancreatic duct first noted to be dilated on the CT scan (Fig 26–3) and delineated the site of the stricture in the main pancreatic duct. The ERCP also showed an intrapancreatic stricture of the common bile duct and some dilatation of the common duct. The elevation of alkaline phosphatase level and the dilatation of the common bile duct indicate a need to decompress the common bile duct as well as the major pancreatic duct. Selective angiographic studies of the celiac and superior mesentery artery are useful in delineating the vascular anatomy in the region of the pancreas. Knowing the vascular anatomy is helpful if we find it necessary to core out a portion of the head of the pancreas. This may be done if the head is markedly thickened. The coring-out of the head of the pancreas is done in addition to performing a

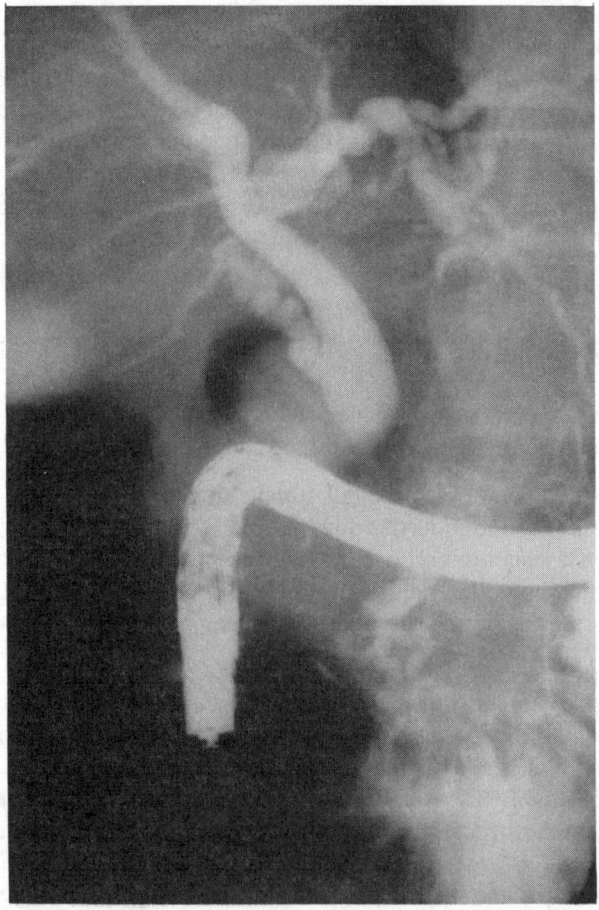

FIG 26–2.
The major pancreatic duct is strictured and does not fill distally.

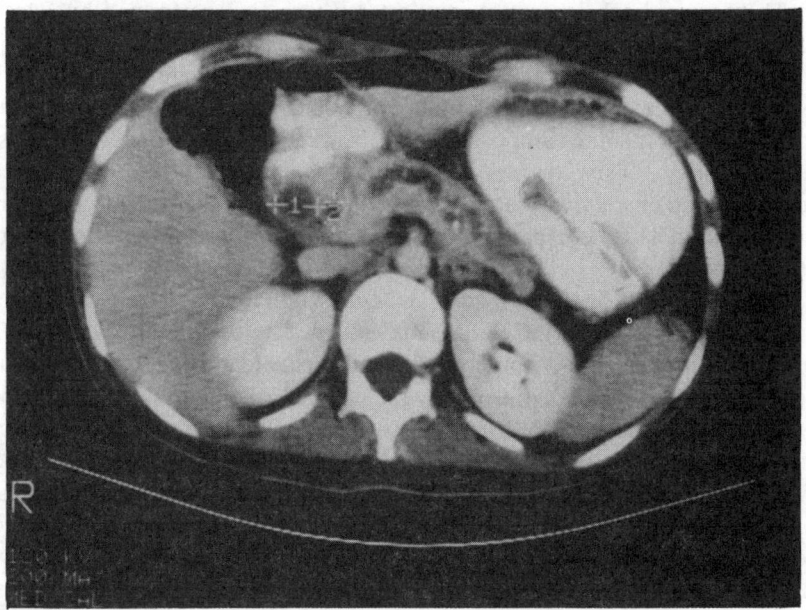

FIG 26–3.
The major pancreatic duct in the body and tail of the pancreas is dilated and has a chain-of-lakes appearance. The common bile duct is enlarged.

longitudinal pancreaticojejunostomy. When the coring-out process is performed, it is important to know, in order to avoid injury to the structures, if there is a replaced right hepatic or common hepatic artery arising from the superior mesentery artery and coursing through the uncinate process pancreas. This common anomaly occurs in 25% of patients. The venous phase of the angiogram may also show us if we will have to deal with left-sided portal hypertension due to thrombosis of the splenic vein or portal hypertension secondary to thrombosis of the portal vein. Splenic vein thrombosis is a common complication of chronic pancreatitis. Evidence of vascular encasement on the angiogram may be the first indication we are dealing with a cancer of the pancreas rather than chronic pancreatitis. In this patient, the angiogram showed normal anatomy.

The longitudinal pancreaticojejunostomy appropriately deals with the structural abnormalities of our patient. The major pancreatic duct is moderately dilated (normal 2 to 3 mm) at about 7 mm. While longitudinal pancreaticojejunostomy does not result in the loss of appreciable amounts of pancreatic tissue, exocrine and endocrine function may be expected to continue to diminish because of the progression of the underlying pancreatitis. In a patient who has lost 90% or more of his exocrine function, as evidenced by steatorrhea, a significant measure of damage to his islets would have to be assumed.

The longitudinal pancreaticojejunostomy was first performed by Puestow and Gilesby (1956) and modified by Partingtan and Rochelle (1960) to make splenectomy unnecessary. It should be considered the operation of choice when the major pancreatic duct is 5 to 6 mm or more and has multiple areas of stricture and/or impacted calcium carbonate calculi. Pain relief results from decompressing the dilated hypertensive duct. We have found pressures in the main pancreatic duct in our patients coming to operation with chronic pancreatitis to range from 18 to 40 cm of H_2O, compared to the normal ductal pressure of 8 to 12 cm of H_2O.

Decompressing the major pancreatic duct will not relieve the stricture in the intrapancreatic portion of the common bile duct. Two options are available. The Roux-en-Y limb used to decompress the major pancreatic duct can also be used to decompress the common bile duct with a choledochojejunostomy, or the head of the pancreas can be cored out, removing the fibrotic pancreas that is constricting the common bile duct (Fig 26–4). The Roux-en-Y limb is then used to cover the defect in the head, and no segmental biliary anastomosis is necessary (Fig 26–5). Another option for decompressing the common bile duct, choledochoduodenostomy, is usually not technically feasible in these patients with markedly enlarged pancreatic heads, as the duodenum is narrowed and edema-

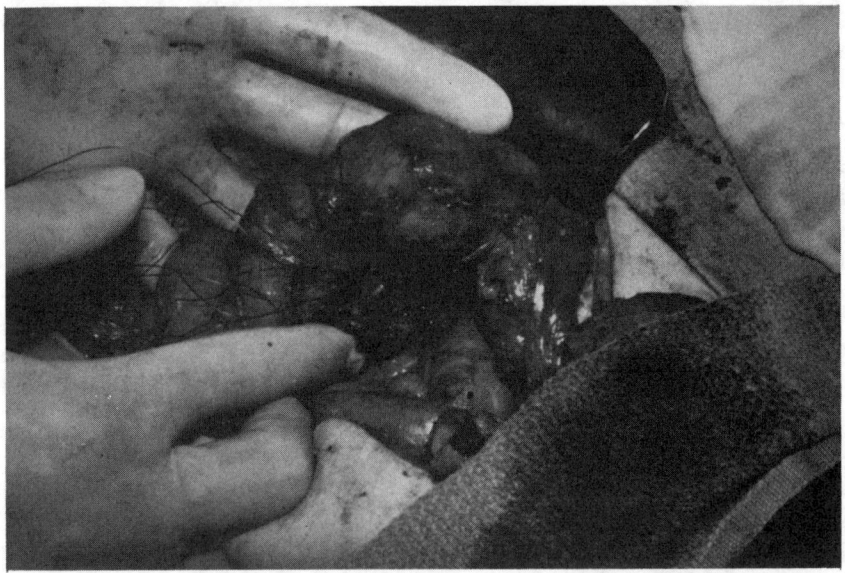

FIG 26–4.
The duodenal head is partially excised, leaving a rim of pancreas along the inner aspect of the duodenum.

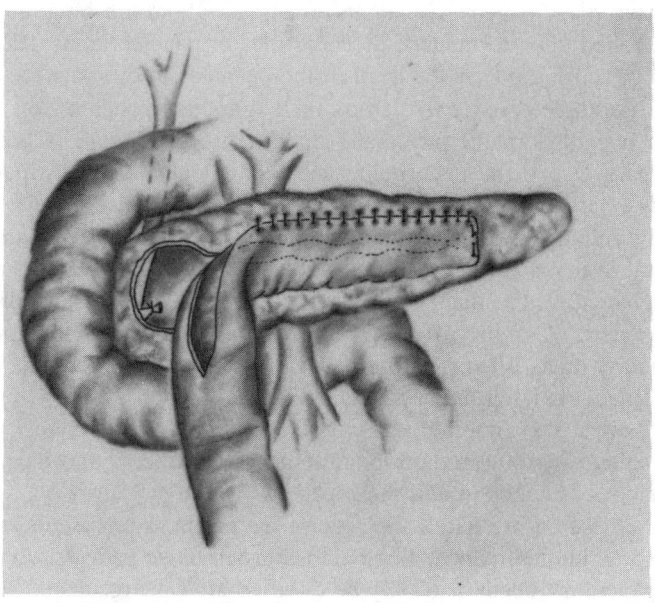

FIG 26–5.
The duodenal-preserving resection of the head of the pancreas is combined with Roux-en-Y longitudinal pancreaticojejunostomy. The cored-out head is drained by the Roux-en-Y limb in continuity with the major pancreatic duct.

tous. We have used both the coring-out procedure and Roux-en-Y choledochojejunostomy for decompressing the common bile duct with some success. We find the coring-out of the head of the pancreas is particularly useful in patients in whom the head of the pancreas is very enlarged, even when the common duct is not obstructed. In such patients it is difficult to decompress the ducts in the head and uncinate process adequately with the conventional longitudinal pancreaticojejunostomy. Small cysts remain undrained, and calculi embedded in tributary ducts may be impossible to dislodge.

Another reason for using this new operation in which the head of the pancreas is cored out is dissatisfaction with the results of operations first developed in the 1940s and 1950s. There is recognition that over time the results of longitudinal pancreaticojejunostomy have not held up as well as after pancreaticoduodenectomy or 95% distal pancreatectomy. Taylor and associates showed a progressive decline in the percentage of good results after longitudinal pancreaticojejunostomy so that by five years only 25% had good pain relief. The pancreaticoduodenectomy is a very long, technically difficult operation with a higher mortality (9%) than either longitudinal pancreaticojejunostomy (4%) or 95% distal pancreatectomy (4.4%). The 95% distal pancreatectomy, while giving excellent pain relief, causes exocrine and endocrine insufficiency that complicates the postoperative management of patients, many of whom are binge drinkers and cannot be relied upon to manage their diabetes or pancreatic insufficiency. We employed the coring-out of the head of the pancreas in our patient.

There are three reasons for failure of longitudinal pancreaticojejunostomy. Failure to open the major pancreatic duct to the duodenum is one cause of recurrent pain in patients undergoing pancreaticojejunostomy. In patients with a markedly enlarged pancreatic head, even carrying the incision to the duodenum may not provide adequate drainage of either the main duct of Wirsung or of the other ductal systems in the head and uncinate process of the pancreas. These other ducts include the duct of Santorini and the ductal system draining the uncinate process. Coming off the main Wirsung ductal system may be small cystic tributary ducts filled with milky calcium deposits or containing impacted, densely adherent calcium carbonate calculi. These small tributary ducts dilated into small cysts may not be decompressed or be accessible for removal of impacted calculi by the standard longitudinal pancreaticojejunostomy when the pancreatic head is enlarged and thickened.

Whether this coring-out of the head of the pancreas represents an improvement over longitudinal pancreaticojejunostomy in those patients with markedly enlarged pancreatic heads will only be clarified after the results of three to five years of follow-up are evaluated, particularly in regard to pain relief.

SUMMARY

In patients with an enlarged major pancreatic duct and a small pancreatic head, we recommend longitudinal pancreaticojejunostomy. If the head of the pancreas is markedly enlarged, a coring-out of the head of the pancreas should be considered in addition to longitudinal pancreaticojejunostomy. If there is an intrapancreatic narrowing of the common duct by fibrosis and inflammation or compression of the bile duct or pseudocysts, the coring-out procedure is an option to consider as an alternative to choledochojejunostomy. For successful results in operative management of patients with chronic pancreatitis, there is no substitute for a committed surgeon, a team approach, careful patient selection, thorough evaluation of the structural abnormalities in the pancreas and biliary ducts, and choice of the most appropriate operation.

BIBLIOGRAPHY

1. DiMagno EP, Clain JE: Chronic pancreatitis, in Go VL, et al (eds): *The Exocrine Pancreas, Biology, Pathology, and Disease.* New York, Raven Press, 1986, pp 541–575.

2. Frey CF, Bodai BI: Surgery in chronic pancreatitis. *Clin Gastroenterol* 1984; 13:913-940.
3. Frey CF: Partial and subtotal pancreatectomy for chronic pancreatitis, in Nyhus L, Baker R (eds): *Mastery of Surgery,* ed 2. Boston, Little Brown & Co, in press.
4. Taylor RH, Bagley FH, Braasch JW, et al: Ductal drainage or resection for chronic pancreatitis. *Am J Surg* 1981; 141:28-33.

27

Gallstone Pancreatitis

A 29-year-old woman is admitted with a sudden onset of severe epigastric pain radiating through to the back. Levels of alkaline phosphatase, amylase, and bilirubin are all mildly elevated. Over the next 24 hours the pain fails to subside; amylase level continues to rise, and white blood cell count increases to 16,000/cu mm. Her requirement for crystalloid increases to approximately 4 L/24 hours. The alkaline phosphatase level rises to 1,260 units/ml (normal, 0 to 240 units/ml), and the patient appears icteric. Bilirubin level rises to 4.5 mg/dl. An emergency ultrasound reveals dilated extrahepatic bile ducts and the suggestion of a stone in the area of the ampulla.

Consultant: John P. Welch, M.D.

Much of the controversy currently associated with gallstone pancreatitis stems from the frustration and sometimes disastrous results following treatment of severe forms of the disease. The operative techniques used in these patients are important, although an individual's outcome depends in large part on the severity of the pancreatitis induced by the migrating gallstone. The majority of patients have a mild form of illness that resolves quite rapidly, and both emergent and semi-emergent operative approaches are successful under most circumstances. When the outcome or the diagnosis is in doubt, however, there is more emphasis on early operative intervention, and the risk of postoperative complications becomes greater.

In this discussion we must concentrate on a small, important subgroup of patients, comprising perhaps 10% to 15% of the entire population with gallstone pancreatitis. These patients develop either: (1) chemical (Ranson's prognostic signs) and clinical evidence of severe or worsening pancreatitis, or (2) symptoms of a potential surgical emergency of unknown etiology, including high intestinal obstruction, mesenteric ischemia, gangrenous cholecystitis, or obstructive cholangitis. The patient under consideration has deteriorated clinically with fever and unabating abdominal pain, and ultrasonography suggests obstruction of the pancreatic and common bile ducts. Based on her requirements for intravenous fluids, there have been significant losses of plasma volume in a short period of time.

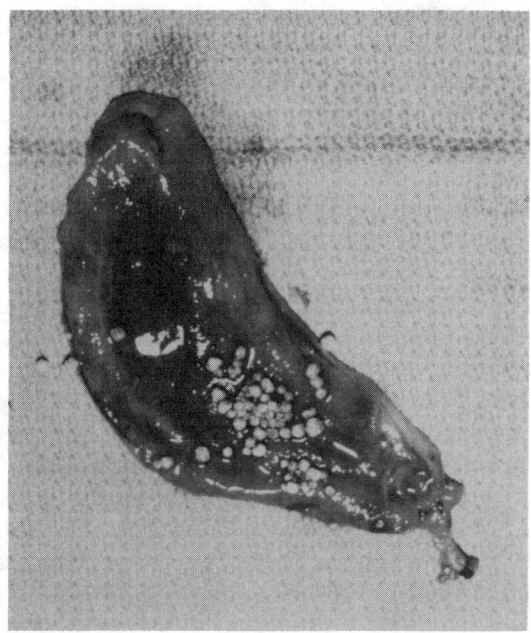

FIG 27–1.
Gallbladder removed from a patient several days after hospital admission for an attack of gallstone pancreatitis. Note the small size of the calculi.

HISTORICAL APPROACH

Opie introduced the common channel theory in 1901 when he discussed the autopsy of a patient who died of pancreatitis. He theorized that an impacted ampullary stone gave rise to a common channel between the common bile duct and the duct of Wirsung. More recent anatomical evidence suggests that a common channel is present in a high proportion of patients with gallstone pancreatitis. Microcalculi (mean size, less than or equal to 3 mm) frequently lie within the gallbladder (Fig 27–1), and ampullary stone impaction is confirmed more often during emergent than during elective procedures, suggesting the transient nature of most impactions. Further insight was gained in the mid-1970s when controlled studies showed that most patients pass calculi in the stools soon after the onset of the attack, while patients with gallstones but no evidence of pancreatitis (e.g., hyperamylasemia) do not pass calculi.

CLINICAL APPROACH

The clinical management of gallstone pancreatitis has undergone some modifications with time. Until two decades ago, most patients were discharged following acute attack, with plans for elective cholecystectomy within a few months. Unfortunately, as many as 30% to 50% of these patients developed recurrent episodes of acute pancreatitis during this "waiting period." In the past decade, controversy about the *acute* management of patients with gallstone pancreatitis has increased, fueled considerably by a report by Acosta et al., who emphasized the advantages of an aggressive surgical approach in *all* patients with gallstone pancreatitis. Their retrospective data and a later controlled trial suggested the safety of early operative intervention, with routine duodenotomy and ampullary stone disimpaction if necessary. Currently, most surgeons believe that the majority of patients can be managed in a more conservative manner, undergoing definitive operation a few days following admission for the acute attack. In fact, only 5% of patients have impacted ampullary stones if they are operated upon following clinical improvement. Thus, the case under discussion is an uncommon example involving clinical deterioration (attributable to pancreatitis, obstructive cholangitis with hyperamylasemia, or both) that *should* be treated on a more urgent basis. In pathophysiologic terms, this patient may have an obstructed common channel together with an elevated pancreatic intraductal pressure and reflux of infected bile into the pancreatic duct.

DIAGNOSTIC AND PREOPERATIVE APPROACH

All basic preparatory steps should be taken for prompt operative intervention. Intravascular volume is evaluated by frequent monitoring of vital signs and urinary output. Central venous pressure readings are less vital in a young, healthy patient without cardiopulmonary risk factors than in an older individual. Values for serum electrolytes (including calcium levels) should be determined sequentially, and pulmonary function is evaluated by arterial blood gas determinations and chest x-rays. A wide-spectrum antibiotic such as mezlocillin is administered because of the risk of cholangitis, given the obstructed biliary system. Since significant duodenal ileus is likely, a nasogastric tube is passed. Meperidine (not morphine) may be required for pain control.

Are any further diagnostic measures recommended? The ultrasonographic findings (dilated extrahepatic ducts, probable distal calculus) strongly suggest an impacted ampullary stone. It is conceivable that this stone will pass into the duodenum within a few more hours. Were this event to occur, the biliary obstruction would be relieved spontaneously and immediate operation might be unnecessary. On the other hand, the patient is at risk of developing progressive pancreatitis or cholangitis.

Two forms of investigation could give expeditious information. A HIDA scan showing early drainage into the duodenum would indicate that obstruction is not complete. Similarly, a transhepatic cholangiogram could provide an accurate anatomical depiction of the common duct, including the presence and position of the offending gallstone and the patency of the cystic and common ducts (Fig 27–2). If either of these studies suggested that the stone had passed or disimpacted, the patient could be observed further in the intensive care unit.

OPERATIVE APPROACH

Given the evidence at hand, it is likely that the calculus will remain impacted. With a young, hemodynamically stable patient, I would proceed to the operating room without further maneuvers (such as peritoneal lavage). The abdomen is opened through a subcostal or upper midline incision. The transverse colon and its mesentery, proximal jejunum, gallbladder, liver, extrahepatic bile ducts, pancreas, and duodenum should be carefully examined. The pancreas may be edematous or, less frequently, hemorrhagic or necrotic. Widespread fat necrosis may be seen in the immediate vicinity. The duodenum is studied for evidence of a penetrating ulcer, and the viability and patency of the small bowel is evaluated, especially if adhesions are present from previous celiotomies.

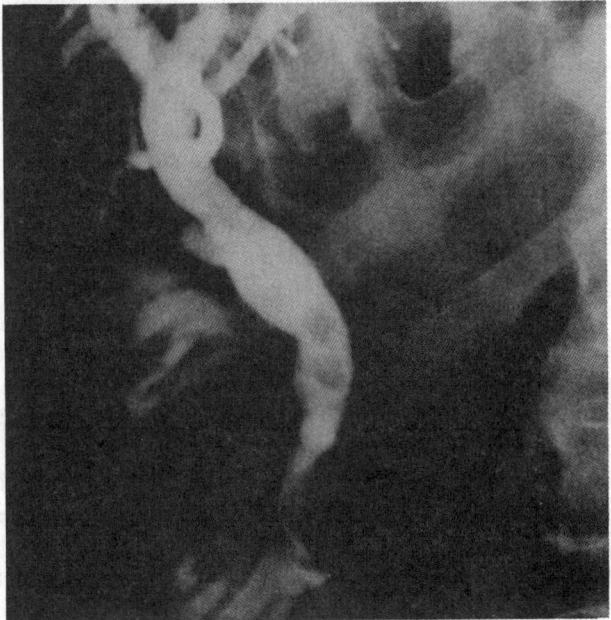

FIG 27–2.
Transhepatic cholangiogram in patient with gallstone pancreatitis. Extrinsic compression of the distal duct is present (*arrow*), together with choledocholithiasis (these stones are larger than the usual microcalculi). Of importance, the distal duct is patent, with flow of contrast into the duodenum. (From Welch JP, White CE: *Am J Surg* 1982; 143:120. Used by permission).

Cholecystectomy is the initial step in most cases. An exception would be in an elderly, unstable patient when a cholecystostomy would be more expeditious. Cholecystectomy eliminates the source of further gallstones and is of obvious benefit if acute cholecystitis is present. A cystic duct cholangiogram is useful (unless a preoperative transhepatic study is already available). Bile is gently aspirated from the catheter to assure that no air bubbles are present in the system. An appropriately positioned patient (with the left side of the abdomen elevated) ensures that the critical common duct anatomy is not distorted by the vertebral column. If the cholangiogram is normal, a common duct exploration is unnecessary. If air bubbles are suspected, another film can be taken after the patient's position is changed (e.g., to the reverse Trendelenburg position) to look for movement of the bubbles. Glucagon (1 mg) is administered intravenously if spasm of the distal duct is suspected, and another cholangiogram is done a few minutes later. If there is suspicion of a stone or a confirmed calculus, the common duct should be explored.

The basic principle underlying common duct exploration is gentle operative technique, involving as little manipulation of the ampullary region as possible. If there is severe pancreatitis, the procedure should be limited to T-tube decompression of the common duct. Frankly necrotic pancreas should be debrided and peripancreatic drainage established. A complete common duct exploration is usually possible, although acute inflammation may obscure the porta hepatis.

After the common duct is opened near the cystic duct entry point, it is gently irrigated with red rubber catheters. Sometimes the offending stone will escape from the duct during this maneuver or following gentle manipulation using stone forceps. If no stone is retrieved, the flexible choledochoscope is inserted through the choledochotomy. Stone extraction is attempted with a basket or Fogarty balloon catheter, or the stone can be fragmented with biopsy forceps. It is usually apparent within 15 to 30 minutes that stone extraction with the choledochoscope will be successful; if it is not, the duodenum should be opened. It is not necessary to insert Bakes dilators blindly, in the hope of forcing the impacted stone into the duodenum or of establishing patency adjacent to the stone; such maneuvers only invite further complications such as exacerbation of the pancreatitis or perforation of the common duct.

The duodenum is kocherized, and an oblique incision is made over the papilla of Vater; if technically possible, passage of a Fogarty catheter into the duodenum simplifies this maneuver. Usually the impacted stone is palpable at the papilla, and it can be freed by means of transduodenal sphincterotomy; a formal sphincteroplasty is time-consuming and unnecessary. The object of sphincterotomy is to relieve the biliary and pancreatic duct obstruction without exacerbating the pancreatitis. The duodenotomy is closed with two layers of sutures.

In the postoperative period, further elevations of the serum amylase level occur frequently and sequelae of pancreatitis may persist or worsen, e.g., gastric outlet obstruction, fever, tachycardia, and further pooling of fluid in the abdomen and retroperitoneum. The duodenotomy may be complicated by an intra-abdominal abscess or a duodenal fistula. (*Editor's note:* Because of the high incidence of technical and other complications following operative intervention and especially duodenotomy, gastrostomy and jejunostomy should be carried out. They are invaluable in the management of a fistula.) If the patient continues to deteriorate, the pancreas should be evaluated serially with ultrasonography and computerized tomography for possible development of a pancreatic abscess or pseudocyst.

An alternative approach in this patient would be early endoscopic papillotomy. This procedure has not been evaluated prospectively in large numbers as yet, and laparotomy is still performed in the good-risk patient. Hemorrhage or worsening of the pancreatitis may follow papillotomy; the mortality is in the range of 1% or less. Papillotomy can establish duct drainage successfully, with relief of clinical symptoms and correction of abnormal laboratory parameters. Unlike a formal laparotomy, it can be done in a short period of time with the patient under sedation rather than general anesthesia. While there are theoretical advantages to papillotomy in the acute setting (especially in older patients), I would not recommend the procedure unless the local endoscopist was very skilled. Just as the surgeon, the endoscopist must use careful technique in these patients in the hope of keeping morbidity at low levels. He/she should have the judgment to cease if the duct cannot be cannulated easily because of distorted anatomy. The pancreatic duct should not be filled with dye, and the common duct stone should be allowed to pass into the duodenum spontaneously rather than following forceful endoscopic extraction.

SUMMARY

Most patients with gallstone pancreatitis can be managed successfully with a "wait-and-see" approach. The patient discussed here is atypical, since she has followed a deteriorating clinical course necessitating early operative intervention. In the future, endoscopic papillotomy may gain a more prominent position in the treatment of this disorder.

BIBLIOGRAPHY

1. Acosta JM, Rossi R, Galli DM, et al: Early surgery for acute gallstone pancreatitis: Evaluation of a systematic approach. *Surgery* 1978; 83:367–371.
2. Coppa G, LeFleur R, Ranson J: The role of chiba-needle cholangiography in the diagnosis of possible acute pancreatitis with cholelithiasis. *Ann Surg* 1981; 193:393–398.

3. Kelly TR: Gallstone pancreatitis: The timing of surgery. *Surgery* 1980; 88:345–350.
4. Neoptolemos JP, London N, Slater N, et al: A prospective study of ERCP and endoscopic sphincterotomy in the diagnosis and treatment of gallstone acute pancreatitis: A rational and safe approach to management. *Arch Surg* 1986; 128:697–702.

28

Pseudocysts

A 45-year-old man, a known alcoholic, is admitted with an acute episode of pancreatitis, his fifth admission. He had been drinking heavily. Amylase level is 600 units/dl; alkaline phosphatase and bilirubin values are normal; serum glutamic oxaloacetic transaminase level (SGOT) is mildly elevated. After an initial period of quiescence, over the next seven to ten days, increased abdominal pain is reported and an attempt to feed the patient results in increased exacerbation of the patient's symptoms. Ultrasound reveals a 5-cm pseudocyst in the area of the body of the pancreas.

Consultant: Edward L. Bradley III, M.D.

OVERVIEW

While pancreatic pseudocysts may occasionally be seen following disruption of the pancreatic duct due to trauma, the overwhelming majority of these lesions are associated with pancreatitis. Although it has been estimated that 10% of patients with pancreatitis will develop a pancreatic pseudocyst, the actual frequency of pseudocyst development may be much higher. If all peripancreatic collections of fluid in patients with the *acute* form of pancreatitis are considered to be pseudocysts, then the incidence of "pseudocyst" might be as high as 40% to 50%. However, if a pancreatic pseudocyst is defined as a collection of pancreatic juice, either within the substance of the pancreas or immediately adjacent to the pancreas, and is enclosed by a fibrous capsule that is devoid of an epithelial lining, then the frequency of development will decline. It is therefore clear that natural history information may vary according to the definition of pancreatic pseudocyst.

PATHOPHYSIOLOGY

Little is known of the pathophysiology of pancreatic pseudocysts. Pancreatic ductal rupture has been assumed to be the underlying defect in pathogenesis for two reasons: (1) the fluid in pancreatic pseudocysts has been demonstrated to be pancreatic juice; and (2) the majority of pancreatic pseudocysts can be demonstrated to be in connection with a branch of the pancreatic ductal system. While these observations seem convincing, the actual dynamics of pseudocyst formation are less clear. Pseudocysts can frequently be demonstrated by endoscopic pancreatography. Since such a pseudocyst is open all the way to the duodenum, it is unclear why the communicating pseudocyst persists in the face of what is apparently adequate drainage. From a physical standpoint it is unlikely that the pressure within the pancreatic pseudocyst can ever exceed the secretory pressure of the pancreas. If pressure were to ever exceed this value, further pancreatic secretion into the pseudocyst would cease. Pressures within pancreatic pseudocysts have been documented to be in the range of 20 to 60 cm H_2O relative to the ampulla. Such a pressure, while not sufficient to result in rupture of tissue per se, might be enough to cause a pseudocyst to persist relative to a duodenal pressure if some as yet unrecognized partial obstruction existed in the ductal system.

Since approximately 50% of pancreatic pseudocysts cannot be demonstrated to be in connection with the pancreatic ductal system, it has been presumed that these pseudocysts have lost the connection at some point during their process of development. Rarely, amylase is not found in noncommunicating pseudocysts. The absence of amylase can be explained by amylase degradation over time. Several groups have found that intracystic deamination of amylase is a constant feature of pancreatic pseudocysts and may, in fact, be related to the "age" of the pseudocyst. Whether such observations will have sufficient discriminative value to enable clinical dating of pseudocyst formation remains to be determined.

ACUTE PSEUDOCYSTS

From a clinical standpoint it is extremely useful to separate pseudocysts into acute and chronic categories. Differentiation between acute and chronic pseudocysts is important since the natural histories are different between the two conditions. In essence, an acute pseudocyst is a pseudocyst that develops in a patient with an acute episode of pancreatitis. Such a fluid collection is the earliest recognizable form of a pancreatic pseudocyst. Under these conditions the collection of pancreatic juice is enclosed by a relatively immature fibrous membrane. Thickening of the enveloping membrane has been shown to be time-dependent. If acute pseudocysts are defined as those pseudocysts that develop within a three-week period following an episode of acute pancreatitis, it has been demonstrated that 30% to 40% of such fluid collections will resolve spontaneously. These observations have important implications for therapy. Clearly, any form of interventional drainage would be contraindicated in uncomplicated pseudocysts within three weeks of formation. Accordingly, acute pseudocysts are best managed expectantly in hopes of spontaneous resolution. Interventional drainage is withheld until: (1) a complication of the acute pseudocyst develops; or (2) the pseudocyst becomes chronic.

CHRONIC PSEUDOCYSTS

In contrast to patients with acute pseudocyst, chronic pseudocysts develop in patients without any recent evidence of an acute episode of pancreatic inflammation. Symptoms in such patients tend to be more related to the space-taking properties of the pseudocyst or those related to the underlying chronic pancreatitis. Since it has been convincingly demonstrated that persistent observation of chronic pancreatic pseudocysts invites development of morbid complications, there is little place for persistent medical therapy. When the diagnosis of chronic pseudocyst has been made, endoscopic retrograde cholangiopancreatography is indicated. This procedure can assist the surgeon in determining whether other forms of chronic pancreatic disease (such as common bile duct stricture or pancreatic duct dilatation) exist concomitantly with the pancreatic pseudocyst. Upon occasion it will be necessary to combine the drainage of the pseudocyst with other procedures designed to relieve other complications of chronic pancreatitis.

ILLUSTRATIVE CASE REPORT

This case typifies the clinical problems that present in the management of pancreatic pseudocysts. Classically, the majority of patients with pancreatic pseudocysts are alcoholics. Since this particular patient has had previous admissions, it is a fair presumption that chronic alcoholic pancreatitis is the underlying cause. The fact that he has acute inflammatory symptoms with an amylase level of 600 units/dl suggests that this is an acute exacerbation of chronic pancreatitis. However, it cannot be stated with certainty whether this case represents an acute pseudocyst in a patient with chronic pancreatitis and an acute exacerbation, or whether the patient had a chronic pseudocyst preceding the acute pancreatitis. Under these circumstances it is best to assume that this is an acute pseudocyst and treat the patient accordingly. The fact that the levels of alkaline phosphatase and bilirubin are normal would suggest that no obstruction of the common bile duct exists. In keeping with the general policies of managing a patient with an acute pseudocyst, expectant supportive treatment is the preferred approach.

One of the more common mistakes in treating patients with acute pancreatitis is resuming enteral feeding too soon. In general, all oral intake should be held until complete clinical recovery has taken place. When the patient is afebrile, the abdominal examination is normal, and the white blood cell count and amylase level have returned within the normal range, only then should oral feeding be instituted. Theoretically, a pseudocyst that is in fact present is prima facie evidence of pancreatic ductal obstruction. Since pancreatic juice volume and enzyme secretion occur in response to enteral feeding, stimulation in the face of obstruction may aggravate the underlying pancreatitis. Distal enteral alimentation as supplied by transnasal long feeding tube has also been shown to result in pancreatic stimulation and should be proscribed along with oral alimentation. Accordingly, management of such a patient should include intravenous hyperalimentation.

Since this patient exhibited no signs of clinical sepsis, continued supportive observation is in order. Our practice is to monitor the size of the pseudocyst on a weekly basis. Should the pseudocyst rapidly increase in size, we would prefer earlier intervention. However, a pseudocyst maintaining its size during this period is permitted to continue maturation of its fibrous capsule in anticipation of surgery. Should the pseudocyst decline in internal diameter, as measured by serial sonography, additional attempts would then be made to prolong the period of nonsurgical observation. Should the pseudocyst cease to decline in size, surgical exploration would be considered. In the absence of specific complications of acute pseudocysts, the patient can be discharged when all evidence of pancreatic inflammation has disappeared. Such patients are then followed up on an outpatient basis for six weeks following onset of the episode of pancreatitis. At this time, consideration is given for a surgical intervention for persistent pseudocysts. By definition, a pseudocyst of this duration would be a chronic pseudocyst and amenable to surgical drainage.

On the other hand, if the pseudocyst is judged to be chronic on admission, no waiting period for "maturation" of the cyst wall is required. Such patients can undergo endoscopic pancreatography and interventional drainage whenever sufficient preoperative data has been obtained.

SURGICAL PROCEDURES

General

In all patients with pancreatic pseudocysts, internal drainage is preferred to external drainage for two primary reasons: (1) internal drainage has a lower mortality than external drainage, and (2) the complication rate following external drainage is higher than that for internal drainage. In general, external drainage is reserved for those patients with complicated pseudocysts in which internal drainage is either not technically possible because of immaturity of the cyst wall or because secondary infection is present that could result in breakdown of a pancreatic suture line.

Transcutaneous drainage of pancreatic pseudocyst via a radiologically guided catheter technique is a recent addition to the therapeutic methods available. While the number of cases so far has been too small to permit definitive recommendations, the early results of this technique would suggest that transcutaneous drainage should not be selected as primary therapy for the following reasons: (1) the rate of pseudocyst recurrence is higher, (2) the incidence of both intracystic hemorrhage and secondary infection is higher, and (3) no opportunity for histologic identification of the cyst wall is possible. Several instances of transcutaneous drainage of malignant pancreatic cysts have been reported. We currently reserve this technique for those patients who evidence signs of sepsis and in whom the pancreatic cyst may be secondarily infected, or for that group of patients with massive pseudocysts whose respiratory function is compromised by the size of the pseudocyst. While it may be logical to presume that the group of pseudocysts that cannot be demonstrated to be in connection with the pancreatic ductal system by endoscopic pancreatography could conceivably have transcutaneous external drainage, the final role of transcutaneous drainage awaits further study.

External Drainage

As previously mentioned, external drainage is reserved for those patients with pancreatic pseudocysts in whom the wall is not sufficiently matured to hold sutures or for those who have suffered secondary complications of a pseudocyst such as intracystic hemorrhage or infection. Under these conditions, external drainage is the preferred technique of surgical management. A large mushroom catheter (28 to 30 F) is introduced into the cyst and passed through the omentum and the abdominal wall. Although some have advocated operative pancreatography through the catheters, it has not been our experience that this has changed the surgical technique. We would, however, obtain a pancreatogram through the catheter seven to ten days after surgery if large volumes of pancreatic juice were recovered from the catheter. In such circumstances, pancreatography often will show communication with the pancreatic duct.

The primary indication for surgical drainage by catheter is the presence of clinical sepsis in a patient with pancreatic pseudocyst in whom the pseudocyst can be demonstrated to be secondarily infected. (*Editor's note:* While I agree with this general approach, one periodically inadvertently performs internal drainage on patients who are not clinically septic, yet whose pseudocyst fluid grows an organism. In my experience, outcome in this situation is not different from those patients whose pseudocyst fluid is sterile. Patients with grossly purulent pseudocyst fluid should, of course, be drained externally.) A Gram stain of the pseudocyst fluid is obtained at surgery in all patients with clinical sepsis, and if this is positive for bacteria and white blood cells, external drainage is chosen over internal drainage in order to reduce the possibility of anastomotic breakdown. Since we have followed a policy of nonintervention in acute pseudocyst, it has been rare to perform external drainage because of immaturity of the pseudocyst wall.

Should a persistent pancreatic fistula develop following external drainage, the large mushroom catheter should be replaced with successively smaller catheters. Only rarely will a surgical procedure be necessary to correct a persistent pancreatic fistula. In those rare instances, the pancreatic fistulogram will show complete obstruction of the pancreatic duct distal to the fistula. We have rarely had to wait over six months for eventual closure.

Resection

While it is tempting to consider resection of a small pseudocyst in the body and tail of the pancreas, the surgeon should resist such an approach for the following reasons: (1) as the majority of patients with chronic pancreatic pseudocyst will have underlying chronic pancreatitis, any further sacrifice of pancreatic tissue will result in an increased incidence of exocrine and endocrine insufficiency; and (2) the morbidity and mortality rates for resection are considerably higher than those for internal drainage (10% vs. 5%). Accordingly, pancreatic resection is reserved for those patients with cysts of the pancreas that could not reasonably be expected to resolve with internal drainage. Example of this would be true cyst of the pancreas (those with an epithelial lining) and malignant cysts. Malignancy in a pancreatic cyst is suggested by one or more of the following observations: (1) a cyst wall exceeding 1 cm in thickness, (2) multiple cystic structures in excess of three or four cysts, (3) hemorrhagic fluid within a pancreatic cyst, or (4) mucoid cystic contents. Since many of the patients with malignant pancreatic cysts have excellent five-year survival rates following aggressive resection, a frozen-section biopsy of all suspected pancreatic pseudocysts is a sine qua non for surgical treatment. It is my opinion that resection therapy for pancreatic cysts should be restricted to those patients with a demonstrated malignant form of pancreatic cystic disease.

Internal Drainage

Internal drainage is indicated in the vast majority of patients with uncomplicated pseudocysts of the pancreas. The specific form of internal drainage—whether cystogastrostomy, cystoduodenostomy, or cystojejunostomy—should be chosen primarily by the anatomical location of the pseudocyst. As mentioned above, at the time of internal drainage, a biopsy of the pseudocyst wall is always obtained for frozen section.

If a pseudocyst is presenting in the body or tail of the pancreas and is closely adherent to the posterior wall of the stomach, cystogastrostomy may be chosen as the preferred procedure. As in all types of internal drainage, needle aspiration of the cystic contents is performed first for two reasons: (1) as an aid to localization of the pseudocyst, and (2) to prevent massive hemorrhage, i.e., a major artery has been eroded by the pseudocyst. If bright red blood should be obtained on aspiration, the possibility of a pseudoaneurysm from arterial erosion from the pseudocyst should be strongly considered and appropriate steps (such as aortic control) taken before the pseudocyst is open. In the specific performance of cystogastrostomy, the anterior stomach wall is opened with electrocautery and aspiration is attemped through the posterior gastric wall into the adherent pseudocyst. If the posterior gastric wall is not adherent to the pseudocyst, another form of drainage such as cystojejunostomy should be performed. In the presence of such adherence, the posterior wall of the stomach is opened with electrocautery into the pseudocyst for approximately 2 in. in length. A biopsy of the pseudocyst wall is taken at this time, and interrupted or continuous sutures of 2-0 Vicryl are placed through the adherent walls in an attempt to maintain hemostasis.

A cystoduodenostomy is chosen when the pancreatic pseudocyst presents primarily in the pancreatic head and transduodenal aspiration determines that the cyst is within 1 cm of some portion of the duodenal wall. This technique is in many ways analogous to cystogastrostomy, in that a longitudinal incision is made over the antimesenteric duodenal border and aspiration is then carried out through the medial duodenal wall into the pseudocyst. When the pseudocyst fluid has been recovered, electrocautery is used to open into the pseudocyst through the medial wall of the duodenum. Care must be taken in this technique to avoid the pancreaticoduodenal arcades as well as the ampulla and the common duct. If any of these structures appears to be in immediate danger, cystoduodenostomy is terminated. When so-called transduodenal cystoduodenostomy is performed in this fashion, it is a safe and effective technique. However, when the adjacent wall of the duodenum is sewn to the side of the pseudocyst (so-called laterolateral cystoduodenostomy), the tension on the suture line from derotation results in a prohibitively high risk of combined duodenal and pancreatic fistula.

Cystojejunostomy is chosen whenever the pseudocyst is not adherent to the posterior gastric wall, those in the pancreatic head not in proximity to the duodenum, or for extremely large pseudocysts in an attempt to obtain dependent drainage. Cystojejunostomy is best performed in a Roux-en-Y fashion in case of an anastomotic dehiscence. The author's preferred approach is through the transverse mesocolon, with care being taken to avoid the middle colic vessels. The end of the Roux-en-Y limb is closed and a side-to-side cystojejunostomy more than or equal to 2 in. in length is constructed with a single suture of interrupted 3-0 Vicryl. The author employs closed drainage for both cystoduodenostomy and cystojejunostomy Roux-en-Y. Such drains are left in place for seven to ten days. It has not been my practice to drain cystogastrostomies.

Failure to recognize the presence of multiple pseudocysts is a known cause of postoperative "recurrence." Since multiple pseudocysts have been estimated to occur in 10% to 15% of cases, a thorough search should be made. Often the presence of multiple pseudocysts is suggested by preoperative sonography or computed tomography. When multiple pseudocysts are present in anatomical approximation, a cystocystostomy may provide for internal drainage of the two cysts, and a subsequent cystojejunostomy Roux-en-Y can be performed for drainage. If multiple cysts are present that are not in anatomical proximity, a double cystojejunostomy to the same Roux-en-Y limb is appropriate.

COMPLICATIONS

Should this patient suffer a complication of his acute pseudocyst while under a six-week period of observation, our proposed management of delayed internal drainage would have to change correspondingly.

Rupture

Rupture of a pancreatic pseudocyst is being recognized with increasing frequency. While originally thought to be a rare catastrophic and fatal event, it is now known that the most common form of pseudocyst rupture is manifested clinically as pancreatic ascites or pancreatic hydrothorax. These conditions are diagnosed by the finding of an elevated amylase level in the ascitic or thoracentesis fluid, as well as an albumin concentration less than 2.5 gm/dl in these aspirated fluids. While the majority of these ruptured pseudocysts will resolve with supportive treatment (hyperalimentation and external drainage of the pancreatic fluids in an effort to bring the peritoneal and pleural surfaces in opposition), occasionally it will be necessary to operate upon such a patient. If after three weeks of supportive treatment the fistula is still present, a pancreatogram is done in an effort to demonstrate the site of the leak. If the leak is in the body or tail, pancreatic resection is undertaken. A leak in the head of the pancreas is best managed by a Roux-en-Y loop placed over the site of the leak.

Hemorrhage

Hemorrhage associated with pancreatic pseudocysts may occur free into the abdominal cavity, into the pseudocyst itself with conversion of the pseudocyst into a pseudoaneurysm, or into the pancreatic duct resulting in a condition known as hemosuccus pancreaticus. Hemorrhage into the free abdominal cavity and hemorrhage into the pancreatic pseudocyst are true surgical emergencies. If time permits, an arteriogram should be performed to determine the vessel involved. Commonly, however, the luxury of time does not exist and the diagnosis must be made as to the source of bleeding in the operating room. It is of some comfort to know that the overwhelming majority of such bleeding episodes occur from the splenic artery. A helpful technique under such circumstances is controlling the abdominal aorta prior to opening the pseudocyst cavity. Operative methods of control have included ligation of the offending vessel prior to entry into the pseudocyst, or direct intracystic suture ligation of the offending vessel. Control of hemosucceus pancreaticus often requires pancreatic resection, an undesirable approach in these severely stressed patients.

Infection

Secondary infection of pancreatic pseudocysts can be a clinically difficult diagnosis. It is frequently uncertain whether a patient with a pseudocyst, spiking fever, and elevated white blood cell count represents secondary infection of the pseudocyst or merely reflects inflammatory pancreatitis. Under such circumstances, guided needle aspiration with bacterial smear and culture can prove useful. If bacteria are found in the pseudocyst, transcutaneous external drainage is a satisfactory therapeutic approach. Should bacteria not be identified, it has been our practice to attribute the inflammatory signs to pancreatitis and to continue to manage the patient in a supportive manner until such time as the pseudocyst converts to chronic.

Obstruction

Obstruction can occur either in the enteric tract as gastric outlet duodenal, jejunal, or colon obstruction, or as common bile duct obstruction with jaundice or cholangitis. When such complications occur with an acute pancreatic pseudocyst, a guided transcutaneous aspiration of the pseudocyst is effective therapy. In patients with chronic pseudocysts, it has been my experience that the pseudocyst is rarely responsible for the obstruction, per se. Accordingly, if one operates upon a chronic pseudocyst associated with an elevated bilirubin level and/or common bile duct obstruction, it will be necessary to obtain a cholangiogram following drainage of the pseudocyst. In most of these patients, it has been the underlying chronic pancreatitis that has caused the obstruction and not the pseudocyst. Accordingly, a secondary procedure other than pseudocyst drainage may be required.

LONG-TERM FOLLOW-UP

Regardless of the type of pseudocyst or the method of therapy employed, it will be necessary to follow up all patients with pancreatic pseudocyst for a prolonged period of time. Mere drainage of a pancreatic pseudocyst can hardly be expected to influence the course of an underlying chronic pancreatitis. Many of these patients will develop other complications of chronic pancreatitis that will require further surgical intervention. Furthermore, it has been estimated that pseudocysts will recur in 10% of patients. However, this figure may reflect multiple pseudocysts unappreciated at the initial exploration.

Combination surgical procedures, such as drainage of an obstructed common duct, pancreatic pseudocyst, and an obstructed pancreatic duct, are occasionally indicated. Simultaneous complications of chronic pancreatitis occur with a low degree of frequency. Therefore, prophylactic bypass of any of these structures in conjunction with pancreatic cystenterostomy is not indicated. Because many patients with pancreatic pseudocyst will have underlying chronic pancreatitis, patients should be aware that preoperative symptomatology cannot be attributed to pancreatic pseudocyst and that persistence of symptoms in the postoperative period may indicate the necessity for further surgical intervention.

BIBLIOGRAPHY

1. Bouman DL: Pancreatic pseudocyst, in Cameron J (ed): *Current Surgical Therapy*, ed 2. St Louis, CV Mosby Co, 1986.
2. Bradley EL III: Pseudocysts in *Complications of Pancreatitis*. Philadelphia, WB Saunders Co, 1982.
3. Frey CF: Pancreatic pseudocyst: Operative strategy. *Ann Surg* 1978; 188:652–662.

29

Acute Pancreatitis

A 63-year-old man, previously healthy and not known to be an alcoholic, was admitted with severe epigastric pain radiating through to the back. Shortly after the onset of pain, he collapsed. On admission to the emergency ward, he was tachycardic and pale, complaining of severe epigastric pain. Temperature was 36.5°C, white blood cell (WBC) count was 18,000/cu mm and amylase level was elevated at 800 units/dl. History revealed a period of fasting due to increased business commitments, followed by a large meal with several alcoholic drinks consumed. Over the next 24 hours, 6 L of crystalloid was administered, and hypoxemia developed (PaO_2 54 mm Hg) requiring intubation and placing the patient on a respirator. The BUN level increased from 15 mg/dl to 28 mg/dl, and the serum calcium value was reported at 6.4 mg/dl. Clinical tetany was not observed nor elicited.

Consultant: John H.C. Ranson, M.D.

The initial phase of management of this patient is directed to three general objectives: (1) establishment of diagnosis and exclusion of life-threatening extrapancreatic disease; (2) prognostic evaluation to determine the possible need for special monitoring or therapy; and (3) management of cardiovascular, respiratory, renal, and other complications.

DIAGNOSTIC ASSESSMENT

The most important part of the diagnostic evaluation is a detailed history and careful physical examination. The features described in this patient are consistent with acute pancreatitis, but they do not exclude other acute illnesses such as perforated peptic ulcer or mesenteric infarction. A calcium level of 6.4 mg/dl is unusual in patients with acute abdominal pain secondary to extrapancreatic disease, but hypocalcemia can occur in patients with perforated peptic ulcer. Plain radiographs of the chest and abdomen reveal findings supportive of a diagnosis of pancreatitis in 79% of patients. The most common findings are a small bowel ileus in the left upper abdominal quadrant (sentinel loop), loss of the psoas margins, and dilatation of the transverse colon. Most of these findings are relatively nonspecific. The most valuable positive finding on plain radiographs is duodenal ileus, with an air-filled duodenum outlining an enlarged pancreatic head; this finding is present in only 11% of patients. The computed tomography (CT) examination may show signs of pancreatitis such as pancreatic enlargement, obliteration of peripancreatic fat planes, and intrapancreatic or peripancreatic fluid collections. While these findings strongly support a diagnosis of acute pancreatitis, they do not exclude the possibility of coexistent duodenal perforation, mesenteric infarction, or other life-threatening extrapancreatic disease in the occasional patient. Furthermore, no evidence of pancreatitis has been recognized on CT studies in 14.5% to 67% of patients with a clinical diagnosis of pancreatitis. A normal scan does not, therefore, exclude the diagnosis of pancreatitis.

When simple clinical, biochemical, and radiologic evaluation leaves doubt about the diagnosis, it is our practice to carry out radiographic evaluation of the upper gastrointestinal tract using water-soluble contrast material. Such studies occasionally show positive evidence of acute pancreatitis, but their main purpose is to reduce the possibility of an overlooked perforation or obstruction of the upper gastrointestinal tract. In patients with known or suspected gallstones and with clinical deterioration, it may become necessary to exclude obstructive cholangitis or gangrenous cholecystitis. In this condition ultrasound may show gallbladder stones, but it rarely provides reliable information concerning common bile duct stones or intrinsic inflammation of the gallbladder. Biliary scanning may demonstrate cystic duct obstruction in approximately 20% of patients with acute pancreatitis, and it is, therefore, an unreliable method for diagnosing acute cholecystitis in this setting. When accurate anatomical information about the biliary tree is essential for patient management, this is best obtained either by endoscopic retrograde cholangiography or percutaneous transhepatic cholangiography. We have generally preferred the latter, because it avoids the risk of exacerbation of pancreatitis that is associated with the endoscopic approach.

In the occasional patient, it is necessary to undertake exploratory celiotomy to exclude or treat life-threatening extrapancreatic disease. In this 63-year-old man who has required large amounts of fluid and mechanical ventilatory assistance during the first 24 hours of treatment, the possibility of an error in diagnosis must be carefully evaluated. The clinical and laboratory data all support a diagnosis of acute pancreatitis, but if serious uncertainty persists, laparotomy should be undertaken. If early operation is required for diagnostic purposes, it should include careful exploration of all abdominal contents to establish the diagnosis beyond question. If gallstones are present in severe acute pancreatitis, but there is no evidence of intrinsic acute cholecystitis or of cholangitis, I would limit biliary operation to cholecystostomy and operative cholangiography. In patients with mild pancreatitis, definitive correction of associated cholelithiasis can usually be safely undertaken at the time of early diagnostic laparotomy to reduce the risk of recurrent pancreatitis. However, in patients with severe pancreatitis, cholecystectomy and common bile duct exploration have, in our experience, been hazardous. There is no evidence that cholecystostomy or any other early biliary surgery ameliorates the course of gallstone-associated pancreatitis. The availability of easy radiographic access to the biliary tree may, however, simplify subsequent management. If uncomplicated acute pancreatitis is found at early diagnostic laparotomy, no pancreatic procedure should be undertaken. In fulminant acute pancreatitis, early formal pancreatic resection has been advocated. However, there is no convincing evidence that this approach results in decreased morbidity or mortality, and it is associated with a higher incidence of diabetes among surviving patients. Early drainage of the lesser omental sac or peripancreatic retroperitoneum has also been advocated. Again, there is no evidence that this reduces the morbidity of the overall disease. In fact, in our experience with patients who underwent laparotomy within the initial 48 hours of treatment, usually because of diagnostic uncertainty, the risk of later pancreatic sepsis was 86% in 14 patients in whom the pancreas was drained. (*Editor's note:* This was also true of the early experience at Massachusetts General Hospital in which triple tubes, gastrostomy, cholecystostomy, and feeding jejunostomy were placed together with drains in the lesser sac. The inflamed, necrotic pancreas is a wonderful culture medium.) Late pancreatic sepsis decreased to 30% in 20 patients in whom no pancreatic drains were placed.

The role of peritoneal lavage in severe acute pancreatitis will be discussed later, but I would place a soft catheter, such as a Jackson-Pratt drain, into the pelvis by a separate stab incision for postoperative lavage if diagnostic laparotomy was required in this patient.

PROGNOSTIC EVALUATION

The clinical course of this patient during the initial 24 hours already indicates that he is severely ill. However, the overall risk of death or life-threatening complications can be estimated objectively by recording the 11 prognostic features listed in Table 29–1. Each of these findings correlates on a statistical basis with overall morbidity, and the relationship between the number of these prognostic signs present and risk is shown in Figure 29–1. Our present patient is 63 years old; his initial WBC count was 18,000/cu mm. He has developed hypoxemia, with a PaO_2 of 54 mm Hg, and his serum calcium level was 6.4 mg/dl. He thus has at least four positive prognostic signs. Blood urea nitrogen has risen from 15 mg/dl to 28 mg/dl, despite administration of 6,000 ml of crystalloid. Estimated fluid sequestration, BUN change, and change in hematocrit reading can, however, only be calculated at the end of the overall initial 48-hour period. A high urine output during the second 24 hours of management or a fall in BUN level may result in these findings being negative for a poor prognosis.

TABLE 29-1.
The 11 Early Objective Signs Used to Classify the Severity of Pancreatitis

At admission or diagnosis
   1. Age over 55 yr
   2. WBC count over 16,000/cu mm
   3. Blood glucose level over 200 mg/dl
   4. Serum lactic dehydrogenase level over 350 international units/L
   5. Serum glutamic oxaloacetic transaminase over 250 Sigma-Frankel units/dl
During initial 48 hr
   6. Fall in hematocrit reading greater than 10%
   7. Rise in blood urea nitrogen level more than 5 mg/dl
   8. Serum calcium level below 8 mg/dl
   9. Arterial PaO_2 below 60 mm Hg
  10. Base deficit greater than 4 mEq/L
  11. Estimated fluid sequestration more than 6,000 ml

TREATMENT

Early measures designed to limit the morbidity of acute pancreatitis fall into two broad categories. The first measures are those that are intended to limit the severity of pancreatic inflammation or to interrupt the pathogenesis of its complications. This category includes: (1) inhibition of pancreatic secretion by nasogastric suction, anticholinergics (*Editor's note:* I share Dr. Ranson's preference for nasogastric suction and anticholinergic drugs despite the fact that numerous controlled trials fail to reveal any advantage to these therapies) and other drugs, or by hypothermia; (2) inhibition of pancreatic enzymes by drugs such as aprotinin or soybean trypsin inhibitors; (3) corticosteroids; (4) antacids; (5) antibiotics; and (6) anticoagulants. Many of these measures have been evaluated by controlled clinical trials over the past 10 to 15 years, and none has yet been demonstrated to be effective in reducing the morbidity of acute pancreatitis. Most of these trials suffer from two major flaws. First, the number of patients studied is small. In a condition in which the natural history is as varied as that of acute pancreatitis, controlled clinical trials tend to show no difference between treatment groups unless very large numbers of patients are studied or the patient population is carefully stratified. Second, many clinical trials include a large proportion of patients with mild alcohol-associated disease. It may be inappropriate to apply the findings from such trials to other patients. Thus, despite controlled clinical trials that fail to show a benefit from nasogastric suction in mild pancreatitis, in this severely ill patient I would recommend this measure to limit abdominal distention and reduce vomiting. It is also important to withhold all oral feedings in patients with acute pancreatitis until all evidence of pancreatic inflammation has resolved. Again, despite clinical trials that fail to show a benefit from antibiotics in mild pancreatitis, I would recommend the administration of a broad-spectrum antibiotic such as cefotxitin to this patient. In patients with severe acute pancreatitis, positive blood cultures have been observed early in their course despite no identifiable focus of established infection. (*Editor's note:* The source of these organisms may be the gut, with breakdown of the normal barrier and translocation of bacteria.) It is possible that antibiotics may benefit such patients.

Early surgical measures intended to ameliorate pancreatic inflammation and its complications include early biliary intervention in gallstone pancreatitis, early pancreatic drainage, early pancreatic resection, and peritoneal lavage. In our studies, no early formal intra-abdominal surgical procedure has been of benefit to any group of patients in terms of limiting the severity of their pancreatitis. We continue to believe, however, that peritoneal lavage by catheters introduced into the peritoneal cavity with the patient under local anesthesia may be beneficial. We have begun lavage in patients with three or more positive prognostic signs within 48 hours of diagnosis. Lavage is continued for two to seven days, depending upon the patient's clinical status. This measure has, in our experience, reduced the early (day 0 to 10) mortality from 10% to 4%. Other controlled

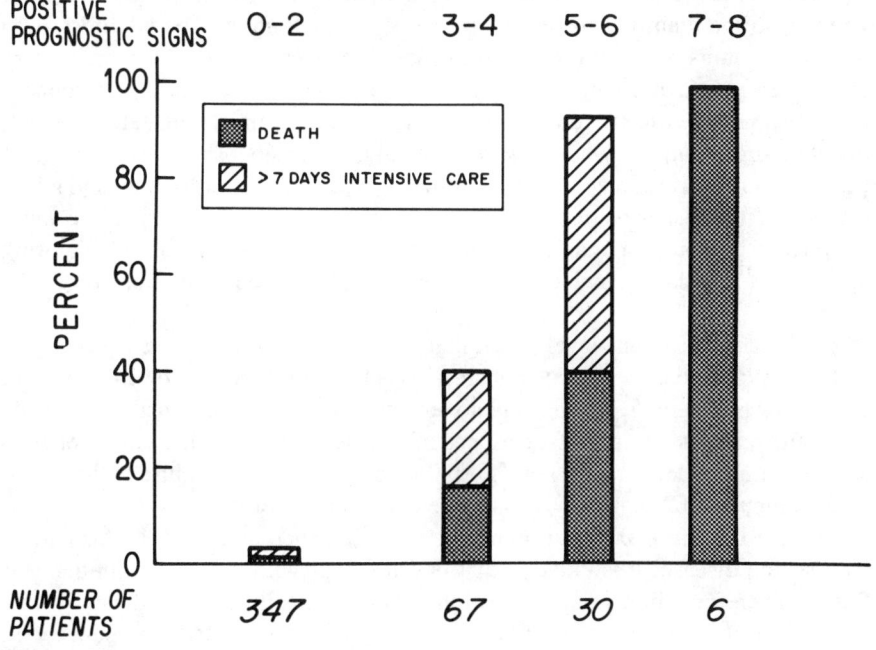

FIG 29–1.
The relationship between the number of positive early prognostic signs recorded and the percent mortality and morbidity, as reflected by the need for more than seven days of treatment in an intensive care unit. (From Ranson JHC, Spencer FC: *Ann Surg* 1978; 187:566. Used by permission.)

clinical trials have not confirmed this finding. However, the dramatic clinical improvement that sometimes occurs with lavage continues to be impressive. (*Editor's note:* One does occasionally see a dramatic response to peritoneal lavage that probably is not coincidental.) Disappointingly, our experience, in keeping with that of others, is that peritoneal lavage, at least as currently used, does not reduce the overall mortality of severe pancreatitis. This is because it does not appear to prevent the occurrence of late infection around the pancreas.

Since there presently is no clear way to reduce pancreatic inflammation, most of the measures that are recommended in acute pancreatitis are designed to support the patient and treat complications. Effective intravascular volume and cardiovascular function must be restored and supported. In this 63-year-old man with large fluid requirements, deteriorating renal function, and respiratory insufficiency, hourly urine output should be monitored and a Swan-Ganz catheter placed to help monitor his volume status and cardiac function. The characteristic hemodynamic picture in severe acute pancreatitis is of a high cardiac output and low peripheral vascular resistance. Appropriate management is greatly assisted by full hemodynamic monitoring. The patient has already received 6,000 ml of crystalloid intravenously. This may have been to try to restore intravascular volume, to maintain perfusion, or to increase urine output. The administration of large amounts of fluid intravenously may, however, be a factor in pulmonary insufficiency in acute pancreatitis. In those who have deteriorating pulmonary function, we have tried to reduce the volume of fluid administered and, if needed, maintain urine output by administration of diuretic drugs. The primary goals of fluid administration and cardiovascular management are the restoration and maintenance of tissue perfusion. There is no evidence that colloid fluids are more effective in this purpose than crystalloid. In this patient with hypoxemia requiring mechanical ventilatory assistance, the use of positive-end respiratory pressures is helpful.

The serum calcium level has fallen to 6.4 mg/dl without tetany. A major factor in hypocalcemia in acute pancreatitis is hypoproteinemia. Ionized calcium levels may be relatively normal and no replacement of calcium is usually needed.

Pain relief is an important aspect of management, and it is traditional to administer meperidine rather than morphine for this purpose because of the spasm of the ampulla of Vater that is associated with the latter drug.

Marked nutritional depletion occurs in acute pancreatitis and, in this patient with severe disease, it is unlikely that oral feedings will be tolerated in the near future. Therefore, intravenous nutrition should be instituted after the early cardiovascular instability has subsided. The safety of intravenous fat preparation in patients with acute pancreatitis is controversial. While uncertainty exists, I believe that lipids should be avoided as a primary calorie source.

With current early supportive treatment, this patient can be expected to survive the early cardiovascular respiratory and renal complications of his pancreatitis. The major cause of morbidity and mortality is the possible occurrence of infection of devitalized pancreatic and peripancreatic tissues. The overall risk of this complication in patients with three or more positive prognostic signs is about 30%. It is higher in those who have extensive changes on early CT studies. The diagnosis of pancreatic infection may be apparent at any time, but it is usually reached during the third or subsequent weeks of treatment. It is marked by fever (100%), abdominal distention (94%), and leukocytosis (78%). The CT scans have been enormously helpful in delineating the anatomy of infection, but two points should be stressed. First, the demonstration of a fluid collection by CT scan is not by itself an indication for drainage. Approximately 50% of fluid collections visualized by CT scans in acute pancreatitis resolve without any specific therapy. Second, infection can be present without a demonstrable fluid collection on CT scans. In 15% of our patients with infected necrosis secondary to severe acute pancreatitis, CT scans showed no fluid collection.

Percutaneous aspiration and bacteriologic examination of peripancreatic fluid have been advocated as a means for the early detection of infection in this setting. We have not used this measure up to now because needle aspiration seems inappropriate in patients who are not suspected of harboring infection, while if infection was strongly suspected on other grounds, a negative aspiration may not accurately reflect the status of the whole peripancreatic area.

In patients with suspected infection, treatment should be by radical debridement and wide drainage. The approach we have favored is illustrated in Figure 29–2. The patient is positioned supine, with the left side elevated approximately 20 degrees. A long bilateral subcostal incision is made, extending from the anterior axillary line on the right to the midaxillary line on the left. The lesser omental sac is opened widely by dividing the gastrocolic omentum, and the entire anterior surface of the pancreas is exposed, including the pancreatic head. The duodenum is mobilized and the area posterior to the pancreatic head is exposed. The area posterior to the tail of the pancreas is examined by exploration carried posteriorly at the inferior margin of the distal one third of the pancreas. The areas posterior to the ascending and descending colon are explored and the root of the small intestinal mesentery is examined closely.

Penrose drains and soft sump catheters are placed anterior and posterior to the head of the pancreas, along the body of the pancreas, and anterior and posterior to the tail of the gland. Additional sump drains are placed into any other large abscess cavities identified. The drains are brought through separate incisions as far posteriorly as possible. A feeding jejunostomy is constructed, and a cholecystostomy is added if gallstones are detected. It is essential that the drains used should be soft in order to minimize visceral injury. We have maintained continuous irrigation and suction to the sump drains and they have been kept in place for an average of 25 days in surviving patients. Mortality with this approach has been 17% in the past 30 patients.

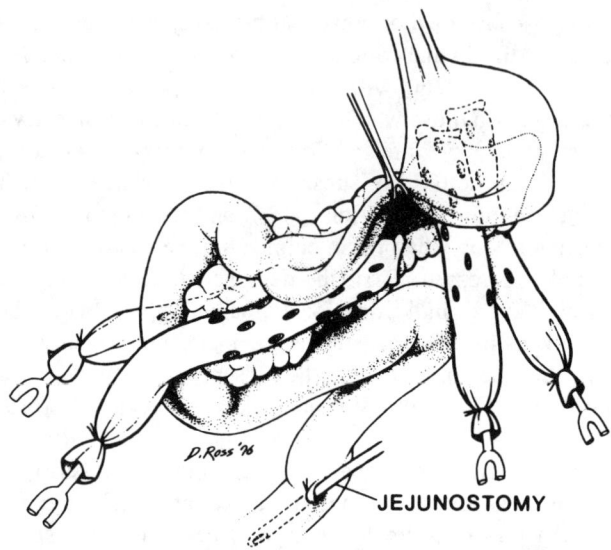

FIG 29–2.
Diagrammatic representation of the technique of wide sump drainage of the peripancreatic retroperitoneum recommended for patients with pancreatic abscesses. (From Ranson JHC: Curr Probl Surg 1979; 16(11):1. Used by permission.)

A different approach has been advocated by Davidson and Bradley. This consists of blunt operative debridement and packing of the retroperitoneum, with the patient returned to the operating room every 48 hours for further debridement and repacking. Davidson and Bradley have recently reported a mortality of 12% in 30 patients treated by this approach. I agree that reoperation and redebridement may often be needed in these patients. However, a large group of patients treated by wide sump drainage recover without further surgery.

SUMMARY

The overall mortality for acute pancreatitis following the general approach outlined above is 6%. The patient presented has at least four positive prognostic signs. In recent years, all patients with three or four positive signs have survived. Appreciable mortality continues to occur in patients with five or more positive signs, and is usually related to the sequelae of pancreatic and peripancreatic necrosis and infection.

BIBLIOGRAPHY

1. Davidson ED, Bradley EL: "Marsupialization" in the treatment of pancreatic abscess. *Surgery* 1981; 89:252–256.
2. Ranson JHC: Acute pancreatitis. *Curr Probl Surg* 1979; 16(11):1–84.
3. Ranson JHC: Acute pancreatitis: Pathogenesis, outcome and treatment, in Creutzfeldt W (ed): *Clinics in Gastroenterology*. London, WB Saunders Co, 1984, pp 843–863.
4. Ranson JHC: The diagnosis and early treatment of acute pancreatitis, in Moody FG, et al (eds): *Surgical Treatment of Digestive Disease*. Chicago, Year Book Medical Publishers Inc, 1986, pp 462–475.

30

Variceal Bleeding

A 45-year-old man, with a known heavy alcohol intake and previous hospitalization for ascites with a known diagnosis of Lacnncc's cirrhosis, presents in the emergency ward with massive hematemesis, hypotension, and syncope. Physical examination reveals a well-nourished man in seemingly good health who is not icteric or comatose. While there is palmar erythema and an early Dupuytren's contracture, as well as increased telangiectasia around the nose, there is no ascites. The liver span is approximately 16 cm and there is no umbilical hernia. Nasogastric intubation reveals large amounts of dark blood, which does not clear on iced-saline lavage. The patient remains tachycardic with a pulse of 120 beats per minute and with postural hypotension.

Consultants: W. Dean Warren, M.D.,
William J. Millikan Jr., M.D.

DISCUSSION

Hemorrhage from gastroesophageal varices remains the most dramatic complication of the portal hypertensive syndrome, and this case represents a typical presentation for many patients. During the last ten years, there have been changes in therapy for variceal bleeding that have improved patient survival and quality of life without impacting adversely on health care expenses. No single therapy represents the best treatment for all patients. The algorithm presented in Figure 30–1, however, presents a flexible approach.

DIAGNOSIS

The first step in both diagnosis and treatment is emergent/urgent upper gastrointestinal endoscopy. Our approach to this patient would be to move him to the intensive care unit and prepare him for endoscopy while acute resuscitation is carried out. After effective plasma volume is restored with 5% albumin (or type-specific blood if the patient has hypotension), the patient's stomach is lavaged

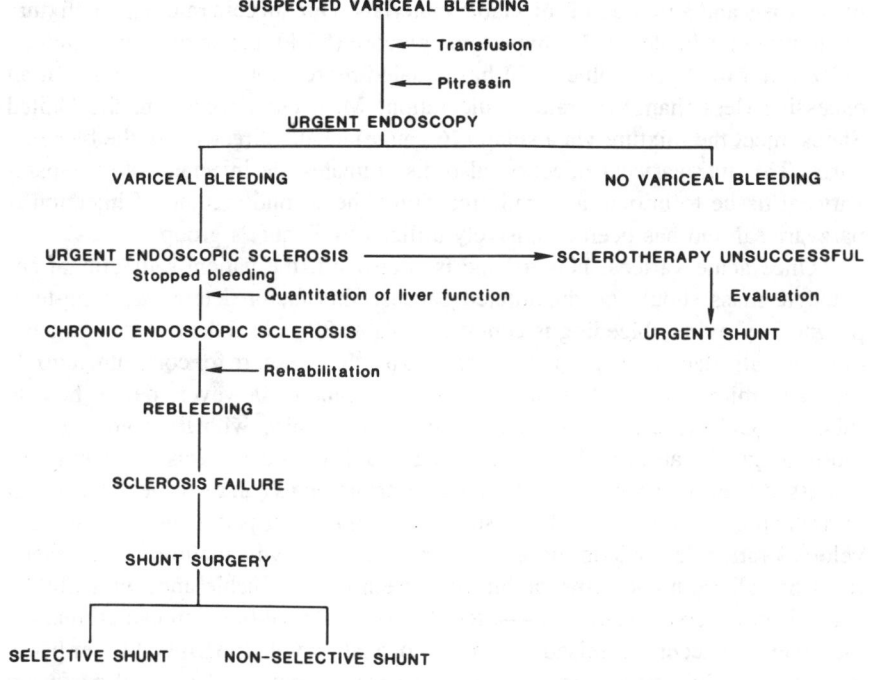

FIG 30–1.
Algorithm for therapy of variceal bleeding.

with saline administered via an Ewald tube to remove blood and clots. If there is any question of encephalopathy, the patient can be endotracheally intubated to minimize the risk of aspiration pneumonia. Intubation with muscle relaxants also facilitates endoscopy and sclerosis in the uncooperative or combative patient. After 6 to 8 L of lavage, the majority of patients' stomachs have been cleared of blood and endoscopy can be carried out. Emergency endoscopy is significantly more challenging than elective procedures, but clearing the stomach of blood usually allows accurate diagnosis of the source of bleeding. The goal of urgent endoscopy is not only to diagnose (and treat) varices, but to exclude other sources of upper gastrointestinal bleeding because 10% to 15% of cirrhotics will bleed from nonportal hypertensive lesions. (*Editor's note:* Some authorities consider gastritic bleeding, or at least some of it, a complication of portal hypertension, and one that should be treated surgically, if necessary, not by gastrectomy but by portal decompression.) For this reason, it is crucial to visualize the duodenum and top of the stomach to exclude peptic ulcers and Mallory-Weiss tears.

In the majority of cases as described above, upper gastrointestinal endoscopy will reveal a varix bleeding at the gastroesophageal junction. In over 95% of cases, injection of this varix will stop bleeding. There are two different methods of sclerosis and a myriad of injectable materials. Our success rate with a mixture of sodium morrhuate (40%), hypertonic glucose (55%), cephalosporin antibiotic (42%), and methylene blue (1%) has equaled more exotic mixtures without an excessive (less than 5%) rate of ulceration. Most endoscopists in the United States inject the mixture via a small (26-gauge) needle directly into the bleeding varix. This intravariceal injection also disseminates the injectate into the paravariceal tissue to initiate a fibrotic reaction. The second method of injection is paravariceal and has been extensively utilized by Paquet's group.

Once acute variceal hemorrhage is controlled, the patient's functional hepatocyte mass should be quantitated because this factor determines long-term prognosis provided bleeding is controlled. Table 30–1 lists the component parts of the hepatic data base. The Child's class is a valuable score for communication's sake and mirrors clinical status over time. It cannot, however, define hepatic function. Galactose elimination capacity does; coupled with liver volume and morphology, it can provide valuable data to aid in clinical decision-making, as discussed later. *(Editor's note:* As much information as can be retrieved is useful in assessing operative risk. Each surgeon dealing with portal hypertension develops a rationale for judging operative risk. In my own situation, the synthetic functions albumin and prothrombin time seem most valuable and, with Child's classification, give a statistical—after all, no predictive function can correct for intraoperative technical misadventures—correlation with mortality.) Liver package angiography documents patency of the portal vein, grades portal perfusion (hepatopedal, hepatofugal), and defines anatomical relationships between the splenic and renal vein in case selective shunt is required in the future.

The studies of the hepatic data base usually require five to seven days to complete. A second elective sclerosis session in which all varices at the gastroesophageal junction are injected is performed one week after the initial acute sclerosis.

If the above patient is like the majority of young alcoholic cirrhotics evaluated at our hospital over the last ten years, his liver biopsy showed Laennec's cirrhosis with some degree of inflammatory response (alcoholic hepatitis). His liver size will be normal (1,200 to 1,400 gm), and his galactose elimination capacity excellent (greater than 300 mg/minute, functional hepatocyte mass =

TABLE 30–1.
Hepatic Data Base

Child's score
Liver biopsy
Liver package angiography
Computed tomography scan for liver volume
Galactose elimination capacity

1 200/300 = 0.25). In addition, this subset of cirrhotics usually demonstrate prograde (hepatopedal) flow of portal blood to the liver.

THERAPY

What is the best therapy for this patient at this time? Data from both controlled trials and uncontrolled experience show that portal perfusion and survival are better preserved in alcoholics when bleeding is controlled without surgery by chronic sclerosis. Therefore, in this patient, a trial of chronic endoscopic sclerosis is indicated. The schedule for chronic sclerosis varies, but we recommend monthly outpatient sclerosis sessions performed using local anesthesia in patients with small- or moderate-size esophageal varices. In patients with very large varices in which rebleeding is more common, a more frequent two- to three-week schedule is utilized. Four to eight sessions will usually obliterate varices at the gastroesophageal junction. Endoscopy is then repeated every three months. (*Editor's note:* This is not the universal experience. See the recent report of Cello and associates in which a significant number (40%) of patients required portal decompression despite an average of 6.1 sclerotherapy sessions.)

There is another therapeutic modality that must be instituted in alcoholic cirrhotics—treatment of their alcoholism. Surgeons are not trained in this field of therapy but must lend encouragement. Psychologists, psychiatrists, social workers, ministers, and organizations like Alcoholics Anonymous are; thus, unless patients are exposed to these support systems, their treatment is inadequate.

What if this patient rebleeds between sclerotherapy sessions? Fifty percent of patients do, but in most patients rebleeding is not life-threatening and is controlled by additional sclerotherapy. However, some patients with variceal bleeding will fail sclerotherapy and require surgical intervention. These patients present the most important unanswered question concerning chronic sclerotherapy: What defines a sclerotherapy failure?

Some information regarding this question can be obtained by reviewing the last 75 sclerotherapy failures shunted at Emory. All had multiple rebleeding episodes requiring transfusion after the institution of sclerotherapy. Twenty-six percent had gastric varices, which most endoscopists agree cannot be permanently eradicated with sclerotherapy. Most, however, rebled from esophageal varices above the gastroesophageal junction or from recurrent varices at the Z line. Two different bleeding patterns were observed: multiple (more than 4) small (1 to 2 units of blood) bleeds or one or more major (more than 4 units of blood) rebleeding episodes requiring hospitalization in an intensive care unit. In the first subset, the decision to shunt the patient was a risk-benefit analysis, e.g., is the risk of hepatitis secondary to multiple blood transfusions greater or less than the operative mortality of elective surgery plus the long-term morbidity associated with changes in hepatic function and hemodynamics after shunt. In the second group of sclerotherapy failures, the decision to operate was more straightforward because these patients frequently required emergent/urgent operation for uncontrolled bleeding. Operative morbidity and mortality was higher, however, because the patients were not in optimal condition. Based on this experience, we believe that sclerotherapy failure can be defined as follows: (1) bleeding from gastric varices or portal hypertensive gastritis; (2) three or more minor rebleeding episodes from esophageal varices in which each rebleed required two or more transfusions; and (3) two or more major rebleeds typified by the need for multiple transfusions (more than 3) and hospitalization in the intensive care unit. (*Editor's note:* It is difficult to know whether the enthusiasm for sclerotherapy will persist over a decade, as few patients will continue to return for any therapy indefinitely.)

CLINICAL DECISION-MAKING

The clinical situation that exists when a patient is declared a sclerotherapy failure often dictates the type of shunt surgery performed. Unfortunately, until there is a clear consensus on the definition of sclerotherapy failure, many cirrhotics will be referred for surgery when the only option is H-graft portosystemic shunt because the patient has uncontrolled active bleeding and massive ascites. The increased mortality and morbidity of this type of surgery that deprives the liver of portal flow is well known. In the ideal situation, the above patient would be defined a sclerotherapy failure before the only surgical option was emergency nonselective shunt. Let us assume that this patient rebled from gastric varices after eight sclerosis sessions had obliterated esophageal veins. Injection therapy temporarily controls the gastric varix, and the patient stabilizes. Because this patient had not rebled in eight months and had abstained from alcohol, his Child's score has improved. Ultrasound reveals that his portal and splenic veins are still patent and hepatopedal flow to the liver persists. Repeat studies of the hepatic data base are performed and confirm that this patient has preservation of functional hepatocyte mass.

The decision to be made at this point is which shunt procedure is best for this patient. Although controlled trials have not shown the superiority of selective shunts in alcoholics, it is intuitively obvious that a surgical procedure that preserves portal flow to the liver (selective shunt) would be better for this patient with hepatopedal flow than a procedure that deprives the liver of hepatotropic factors (nonselective shunt). Our previously published work (1984) has shown that standard selective shunt in alcoholic cirrhotics initially preserves portal flow to the liver, but portal flow is frequently lost as transpancreatic and transgastric collaterals evolve between the high-pressure portal circulation and the low-pressure splenorenal shunt (pancreatic siphon). (*Editor's note:* My own preference is for a central splenorenal shunt, which a randomized prospective trial has shown the equivalent of distal splenorenal shunt. Functionally, it is a small side-to-side shunt, with long-term patency at least equivalent to any prosthetic shunt. A basic issue is where the retained collaterals drain from. An old idea is that following some shunts, particularly central splenorenal shunts, trophic hormones from the pancreas continue to perfuse the liver through the pancreatic branches of the superior mesenteric vein. This concept remains to be established.)

To preclude the development of the pancreatic siphon and improve preservation of hepatopedal flow long-term, Warren and Inokuchi independently developed an extension of selective shunt—splenopancreatic disconnection. This variation of selective shunt has been shown to preserve portal flow and hepatic function in alcoholic cirrhotics better than standard selective shunt. Another surgical option to selective shunt is small-bore (8-mm) interposition H-graft portacaval shunt, originally introduced by Sarfeh. This procedure, which is technically less challenging than selective shunt or splenopancreatic disconnection, portends to achieve adequate decompression of portal pressure to control bleeding while preserving hepatopedal flow to the liver.

Again assuming the best situation, the above patient would undergo elective splenopancreatic disconnection, and because portal perfusion is preserved and abstinence of ethanol is observed, functional hepatocyte mass is maintained. The above patient is an alcoholic cirrhotic. If the patient were a nonalcoholic cirrhotic, the algorithm would change only in that standard selective shunt could be utilized because controlled trials have shown that this operation preserves portal flow and hepatic function for ten years after surgery. If the above patient was a noncirrhotic with hepatic fibrosis or extrahepatic portal vein thrombosis, we would recommend earlier intervention with selective shunt because chronic sclerosis may accelerate splenic vein thrombosis in this subset.

Other Surgical Options

Nonshunt procedures—gastric devascularization with or without splenectomy—have assumed a nontherapeutic role for variceal hemorrhage because rebleeding recurred in at least 50% of patients. The combination of sclerosis plus nonshunt procedure, whose role was projected by Crafoord in his original report of sclerotherapy, now is a viable option for selected patients. This modality should be considered in patients with nonalcoholic cirrhosis or extrahepatic portal vein thrombosis if selective shunt cannot be performed.

Orthotopic liver transplantation is also an option in nonalcoholic cirrhotics and reformed alcoholics with end-stage liver failure. Compared to selective shunt, liver transplantation has a significantly greater operative mortality and expense, and at this time should be recommended only to those patients with severely impaired functional hepatocyte mass.

BIBLIOGRAPHY

1. Cello JP, Grendell JH, Crass RA, et al: Endoscopic sclerotherapy versus portacaval shunt in patients with severe cirrhosis and acute variceal hemorrhage: Long-term follow-up. *N Engl J Med* 1987; 316:11–15.
2. Millikan WJ Jr, Warren WD, Henderson JM, et al: The Emory prospective randomized trial: Selective vs. nonselective shunt to control variceal bleeding: Ten year follow-up. *Ann Surg* 1985; 201:712–722.
3. Paquet K-J, Feussner H: Endoscopic sclerosis and esophageal balloon tamponade in acute hemorrhage from esophagogastric varices: A prospective controlled randomized trial. *Hepatology* 1985; 5:580–589.
4. Warren WD, Henderson JM, Millikan WJ Jr, et al: Distal splenorenal shunt versus endoscopic sclerotherapy for long-term management of variceal bleeding: Preliminary report of a prospective, randomized trial. *Ann Surg* 1986; 203:454–462.
5. Warren WD, Millikan WJ Jr, Henderson JM, et al: Splenopancreatic disconnection: Improved selectivity of distal splenorenal shunt. *Ann Surg* 1986; 204:346–355.
6. Warren WD, Millikan WJ Jr, Henderson JM, et al: Selective variceal decompression after splenectomy or splenic vein thrombosis with a note on splenopancreatic disconnection. *Ann Surg* 1984; 199:694–702.

31

Divided Common Bile Duct

A 23-year-old woman with cholelithiasis undergoes elective cholecystectomy, apparently uneventfully. On the second postoperative day, the patient is noted to be icteric. Acholic stools are noted and the urine turns dark. Bilirubin level increases to 9 mg/dl and alkaline phosphatase level is markedly elevated. The patient becomes febrile to 103°F. A Jackson-Pratt drain in the right upper quadrant begins to drain bile.

Consultant: Rayford Scott Jones, M.D.

PRESENTATION

We will assume that this patient's health was normal except for gallstones and that she had no hepatic abnormalities and no hemolytic disorders. On the second postoperative day she developed jaundice with a bilirubin level of 9 mg/dl. Because of the elevated alkaline phosphatase level, it was probably obstructive jaundice. She developed fever to 103°F and developed bile drainage from her right upper quadrant drain. This combination of jaundice, fever, and abnormal biliary drainage most likely represents an injury to the extrahepatic bile ducts. It is, nonetheless, important to contemplate the differential diagnosis of each of the three components of this syndrome.

The fever, of course, could be due to nonhepatic and nonbiliary causes, such as pneumonia or atelectasis, or perhaps a wound infection. In relation to the biliary disease, it is possible that she could be developing a subphrenic abscess or an intrahepatic abscess, or the fever could represent septicemia from cholangitis due to bile duct obstruction. The jaundice could be due to the postoperative aggravation of some preexisting liver disease, or the patient could have experienced hemolysis. Both of those explanations could probably be excluded on the basis of antecedent clinical knowledge. Jaundice early after cholecystectomy would point primarily to two occurrences. One would be a retained or overlooked common duct stone, and the other possibility, of course, would be an intraoperative bile duct injury. Finally, an analysis of the bile drainage would almost certainly be related directly to the operation, and the differential diagnosis would include bile duct injury, dislodgement of a cystic duct ligature or clip, or perhaps a bile leak from the gallbladder fossa.

The patient could be experiencing some combination of these events. For example, she could have a bile duct injury and a subphrenic abscess, or a retained stone and cholangitis, or a retained stone and a hepatic abscess. Because the symptoms and signs are occurring on the second postoperative day, certain of the diagnoses are less likely. For example, it would be highly unlikely for a subphrenic abscess to develop and to produce these symptoms by the second postoperative day. In addition, a simple bile leak from a cystic duct ligature or from the gallbladder fossa is unlikely to produce the patient's syndrome because the level of bilirubin and the elevation of alkaline phosphatase level are more than one would anticipate from a simple bile leak. A bilirubin level of 9 mg/dl and the elevated alkaline phosphatase level strongly suggest significant obstruction. Therefore, the combination of fever, obstructive jaundice, and significant bile drainage strongly suggests extrahepatic bile duct injury.

The anatomical site of ductal injury during cholecystectomy include, in decreasing order of frequency, the common hepatic duct, the common duct, the lobar duct confluence, the right lobar duct, and the left lobar duct. An isolated lobar duct injury is highly unlikely in this case. Although occlusion of a lobar duct will produce marked elevation of the alkaline phosphatase, it would not produce jaundice if the liver function had otherwise been normal. If there is a ductal injury in this case, it is most likely one involving the common hepatic duct or the common bile duct. There must be an occlusion, at least a high-grade partial occlusion of the duct in association with a defect in ductal integrity on the hepatic side of the lesion.

DIAGNOSIS

In approaching this case, physical examination of the patient would be important in confirming the presence of jaundice. The nasogastric drainage, if present, should be inspected for the presence of bile. In view of the high fever, a specimen should be collected for blood culture. It would also be appropriate to culture the drainage from the right upper quadrant drain site. The most likely organisms to be producing the pyrexia would be either *Escherichia coli, Klebsiella,* enterococcus, or *Bacteroides;* antibiotics effective against those organisms should be administered.

After evaluation of the patient, careful examination of the surgical record, and the institution of antibiotic therapy, an essential goal will be to consider the differential diagnosis as outlined above and to establish an anatomical diagnosis with precise delineation of the biliary anatomy. An ultrasound examination would be a reasonable first test and could reveal information about the following questions: (1) Is there evidence of intrahepatic or extrahepatic ductal dilatation? (2)

Is there evidence of subhepatic fluid collection or other fluid collection within the peritoneal cavity? (3) Is there evidence of a liver abscess? If there was evidence of ductal dilatation, the appropriate next step would be to perform a percutaneous transhepatic cholangiogram. Percutaneous cholangiography (PTC) provides detailed anatomical evaluation of the intrahepatic and extrahepatic bile ducts; it would localize, quantify, and delineate the bile fistula (Figs 31-1 and 31-2). Second, the transhepatic cholangiogram would establish whether a bile duct injury was present and, if so, where it was located; it would also provide information about the integrity of the bile ducts. If there was a partial injury of the ducts, it might be possible with the use of a guidewire to pass the transhepatic catheter through the obstruction into the duodenum. If possible, that would be a very helpful maneuver.

If after ultrasound the bile ducts did not appear dilated, or if an attempted PTC was unsuccessful, then endoscopic retrograde cholangiopancreatography (ERCP) should be performed to obtain anatomical information about the location and nature of the injury. A bile duct injury and an external biliary fistula can be localized accurately using ERCP. (*Editor's note:* A skilled endoscopist may be able to pass a stent retrograde if the injury is partial.) Another diagnostic test to consider in this circumstance would be a HIDA scan. Our experience with that technique is not great, because we rely heavily upon PTC or ERCP in cases such as this.

TREATMENT

Having obtained an accurate anatomical diagnosis, one must decide how to correct the anatomical abnormalities and when to do so. The timing of the treatment will generally depend upon the condition of the patient. Generally, a 23-year-old woman on the second day following an elective cholecystectomy would be in good nutritional status and would probably be in a state of normal fluid and electrolyte balance. The presence of infection clearly deserves attention, because one would generally refrain from performing biliary reconstructive surgery in the presence of infection; thus, the presence of subhepatic infection especially must be considered and preferably controlled before treating the duct injury. Similarly, if the fever was due to cholangitis, one should endeavor to correct that before taking other measures. The administration of antibiotics and the placement of the percutaneous transhepatic tube in most cases would correct sepsis due to cholangitis.

If at this point the transhepatic catheter can satisfactorily be placed, it might allow alleviation of the jaundice and perhaps even the quantity of drainage through the biliary fistula. If both of those can be controlled, one would have to decide whether to perform early reconstruction or to wait until all infection and edema has resolved. This can be a difficult question; if one cannot alleviate

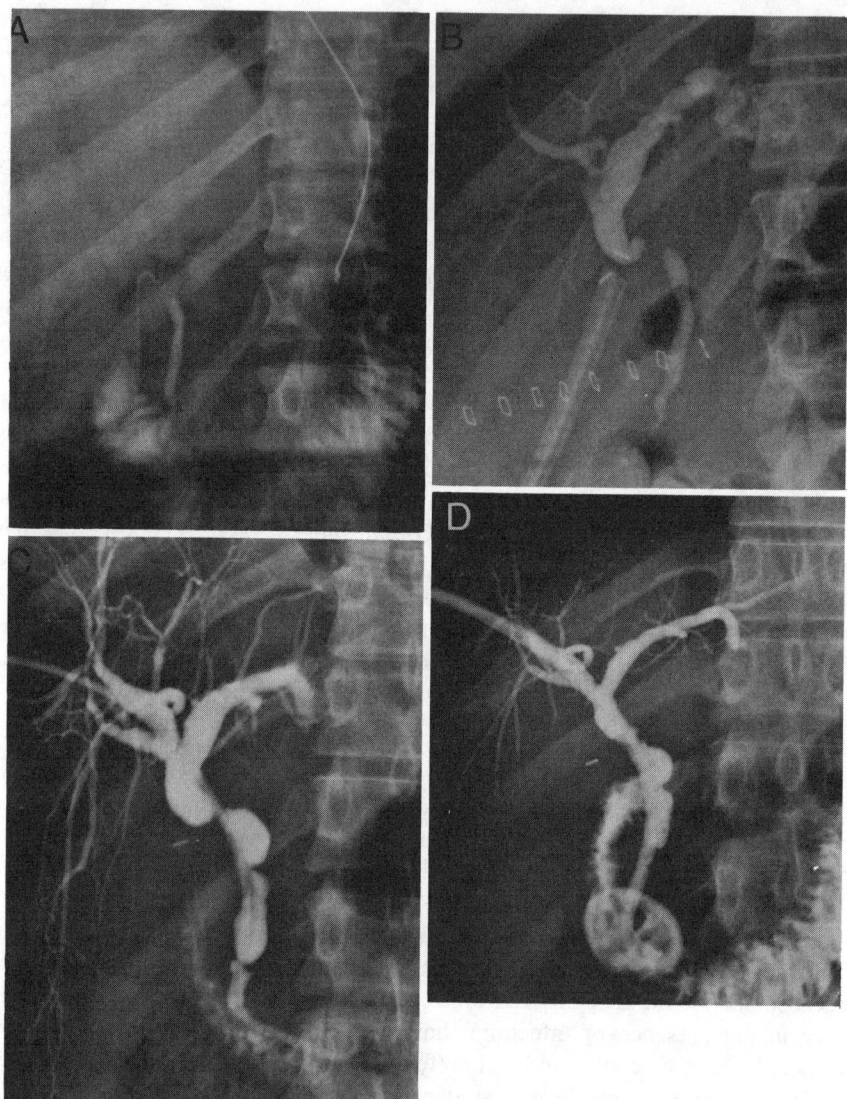

FIG 31-1.
A, during a routine cholecystectomy in a 25-year-old woman, this cholangiogram was obtained revealing that the surgeon had mistaken the common duct for the cystic duct. He removed the ligature, repaired the duct, and completed the cholecystectomy. **B,** postoperatively the patient became jaundiced; percutaneous transhepatic cholangiogram performed on the seventh postoperative day revealed stricture. **C,** a percutaneous transhepatic tube was passed through the stricture into the duodenum. Following placement of this transhepatic stent, the stricture was treated by balloon dilatation. **D,** balloon dilatation effectively relieved the stricture. The stent remained in place several months before removal. The patient has remained asymptomatic for two years. This case illustrates the utility of percutaneous transhepatic techniques in certain bile duct injuries.

the obstruction, then operation should be carried out as soon as sepsis can be controlled. Generally speaking, attempts at extrahepatic biliary reconstruction should not be attempted in an infected operative field. This particular case will likely resolve into an extrahepatic bile duct stricture with or without external biliary fistula. It is possible that the fistula could close as the stricture forms, or it is possible that the patient could be left with a persistent fistula proximal to the stricture. After infection has been controlled, the patient should undergo repair of the bile duct stricture. In most cases, that will be accomplished by a hepaticojejunostomy Roux-en-Y. Although resection of a stricture with end-to-end, duct-to-duct anastomosis is attractive theoretically, practically speaking it is usually impossible to perform because either the distal duct cannot be found, or sufficient length of duct has been damaged so that end-to-end anastomosis is impossible without excessive tension.

Another possible therapy for extrahepatic bile duct stricture, especially for a short stricture, would be transhepatic balloon dilatation. The question about stenting following repair of a stricture often arises, and there is surprisingly little data upon which to base recommendations. If one is repairing a bile duct stricture with a dilated bile duct that is otherwise normal, so that normal, healthy dilated bile duct is sutured to normal, healthy Roux-en-Y jejunum, then stenting is not truly necessary. If, on the other hand, a stricture is treated by balloon dilatation

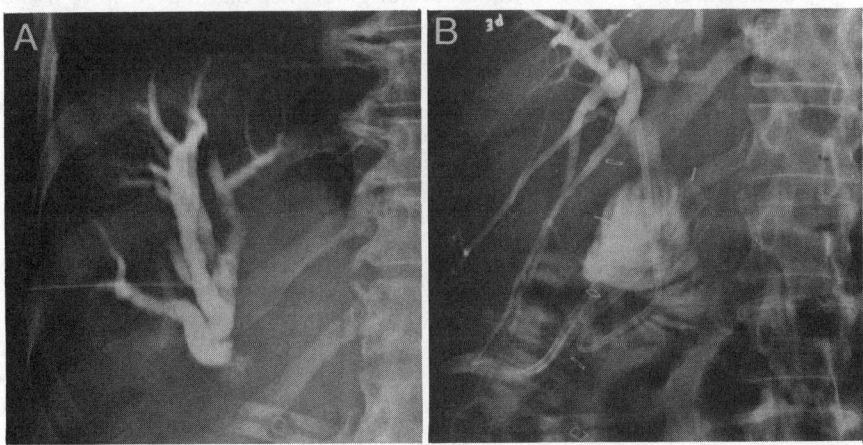

FIG 31–2.
A, a 52-year-old woman became jaundiced in the early postoperative period following a routine cholecystectomy. Percutaneous transhepatic cholangiogram showed complete biliary obstruction at the hilum of the liver. **B,** the patient underwent reoperation following the cholangiogram. The surgeon found that the common hepatic duct had been ligated and divided. He treated this injury by hepatic jejunostomy Roux-en-Y. The patient is asymptomatic. This case illustrates the usual therapy for bile duct injury.

and the scar is left in place, then stenting should be carried out for several months until the scar can stabilize in the open position.

The first attempt at repair of a bile duct injury has the best chance for success. For that reason, the timing and the technique for the first repair should be the best possible. The possibility for long-term satisfactory results following repair of bile duct injury approximates 80%. Of bile duct injuries occurring during cholecystectomy 85% to 90% are not recognized during that cholecystectomy. Such injuries may occur in a routine or an easy procedure performed on a thin patient. Reflection upon the operation or review of operative notes often provides no helpful information in such cases. If the surgeon recognizes the bile duct injury at the time, repair at that time, of course, has the best possibility of good long-term results. If a common duct is simply partially or completely cut during cholecystectomy, immediate repair should be carried out, and generally a T-tube should be left in for follow-up care and for stenting. If a segment of duct is resected during cholecystectomy, then hepaticojejunostomy Roux-en-Y should be the immediate treatment of choice. The frequency of bile duct injury during cholecystectomy is almost impossible to determine. If we accept that about 0.2% of patients undergoing cholecystectomy have a bile duct injury, and if 500,000 cholecystectomies are performed in the United States annually, then approximately 1,000 iatrogenic bile duct injuries occur each year in this country.

We should always bear in mind several guidelines that may help to avoid injuring bile ducts: (1) Always strive for excellent exposure and lighting. (2) Do not clamp bleeders in the porta hepatis in an uncontrolled manner (remember the Pringle maneuver). (3) Do not clamp, tie, clip, or divide structures without simultaneous definitive identification of the cystic duct, the common duct, the common hepatic duct, and the cystic artery. (4) Think of cholangiography during difficult dissections. (5) In difficult cholecystectomies, a cholecystostomy or partial cholecystectomy may be better than risking common duct injury. (6) Do not encroach upon the common bile duct while tying the cystic duct. (7) During routine "easy" cholecystectomies, watch the bile ducts and not the clock.

BIBLIOGRAPHY

1. Blumgart LH: Bile duct strictures, in Fromm D (ed): *Gastrointestinal Surgery*. New York, Churchill Livingstone Inc, 1985.
2. Blumgart LH: Benign biliary strictures, in *Surgery of the Liver and Biliary Tract*. London, Churchill Livingstone Inc, 1988.
3. Nahrwold DC: Benign stricture of the bile duct, in Moody FG, Carey LC, Jones RS, et al (eds): *Surgical Treatment of Digestive Diseases*. Chicago, Year Book Medical Publishers Inc, 1986.
4. Warren, KW, William CI, Tan EGC: Bile duct injuries and strictures, in Schiff L, Schiff ER (eds): *Diseases of the Liver*. Philadelphia, JB Lippincott Co, 1987.

32

Hepatic Transplant

A 45-year-old woman is known to have biliary cirrhosis, first diagnosed at age 25. Cholesterol level was elevated, as was the level of alkaline phosphatase, but she was not icteric. Over the past three years, she has gradually become more icteric, with persistent elevation of the level of alkaline phosphatase and with anorexia. Episodes of hepatic encephalopathy become more frequent, responding to protein restriction and finally to catharsis, lactulose, and neomycin. For the past six months, she has noticed a gradually increased protuberance of her abdomen and an umbilical hernia. Two weeks ago, she was hospitalized with increased lethargy, increasing abdominal distention, and failure to eat. She is barely arousable; bilirubin level is 12 mg/dl; alkaline phosphatase, 1600 units/L. Serum albumin value is approximately 1.8 gm/dl and there is peripheral edema.

Consultants: Leonard Makowka, M.D., Ph.D.
Thomas E. Starzl, M.D., Ph.D.

GENERAL COMMENTS

Primary biliary cirrhosis (PBC) or chronic nonsuppurative obstructive cholangitis represents one entity in a spectrum of hepatic disorders termed "chronic cholestatic liver disease" that also includes sclerosing cholangitis in adults and biliary atresia and intrahepatic cholestasis in children. The progressive loss of bile ducts is the feature common to all of these hepatic disorders. (*Editor's note:* This is an unusual but, at least to me, very attractive concept. Evidence as to common etiology is as yet not abundant.) The etiology of PBC is unknown, although it is thought to be an autoimmune disorder, with antimitochondrial antibodies (AMA) being positive in over 90% of the patients. The disease overwhelmingly afflicts middle-aged women (female:male ratio of approximately 10:1), as illustrated by the present case.

The disease is characterized clinically by jaundice, pruritus, hepatosplenomegaly, early fatigability, and malabsorption, with vitamin deficiencies, malnutrition, and bone disease and fractures of varying severity. Once the end-stage of this disease develops, the patient can present with the complications of cirrhosis and hepatic failure, including ascites, encephalopathy, and variceal hemorrhage that often represent the terminal events. The diagnosis of PBC is based on these clinical findings, accompanied by abnormal biochemical parameters reflecting a cholestatic pattern of liver injury, the presence of circulating autoantibodies, particularly AMA, increased immunoglobulins (IgM), and an increased complement turnover.

The exact histologic characterization of PBC is critical, especially when one considers orthotopic liver transplantation (OLTx) for this entity and as it relates to the differential diagnosis of posttransplant liver dysfunction, as will be described below. The pathologic characteristics have been described to represent the stages and progression of the disease, ranging from the early findings of a chronic inflammatory process, with lymphocytic infiltration of the portal tracts and interlobular bile ducts and granulomata, and finally leading to the end-stage findings of an absolute paucity of bile ducts, fibrosis, and frank cirrhosis.

Previously, medical management has been directed at the prevention, early recognition, and treatment of the symptoms and systemic complications of PBC. The results of therapy with such agents as penicillamine, chlorambucil, colchicine, and cyclosporine have been disappointing. These approaches have had little influence on survival; the progression of the disease is inevitable, and patients succumb to liver failure and its complications such as variceal bleeding.

Orthotopic liver transplantation has revolutionized the approach to and management of patients with end-stage liver disease. The survival results of this procedure have advanced dramatically over the past seven years as a result of improved immunosuppression with cyclosporine and improved methods of multiple organ harvesting and preservation, and with technical refinements in the recipient procedure. Now OLTx should be considered the treatment of choice for patients with PBC. The survival is excellent, with a projected five-year actuarial survival of at least 70% in our group of PBC patients, which represents the largest single series of such patients undergoing OLTx (165 out of the first 1,000 transplant patients during the cyclosporine era). These results are even more striking when one considers the survival of those patients treated by alternate methods or not at all, and the fact that successful transplantation represents a cure allowing the patient to resume, in the majority of cases, a normal life and not one of a chronic and relentless disease. In fact, PBC is currently the second most common indication for OLTx in adults at our institution, being exceeded only by posthepatic cirrhosis, and represents a primary indication for OLTx at most other transplant centers.

The patient described here in many respects typifies the ideal candidate for OLTx. With the current state of the art, one might argue that liver replacement should have been considered at an earlier stage of her disease, prior to the most recent marked deterioration in her condition. The preoperative evaluation, operative approach, and important postoperative considerations pertaining to this case will be outlined.

PREOPERATIVE EVALUATION AND CONSIDERATIONS

Once referred to the transplant center for evaluation as a candidate for OLTx, the patient undergoes a thorough and extensive evaluation to determine the suitability and fitness for the procedure. A careful history and physical examination are carried out. Alcohol and/or drug abuse, prior blood transfusions, concomitant illnesses, prior surgical procedures, medications, and exposure to toxins are important details. Physical examination will offer an estimate of how advanced the liver disease is (i.e., the presence of the stigmata of end-stage liver disease and cirrhosis), and may also offer clues as to the etiology of the liver disease that at times may be very difficult to diagnose (i.e., the presence of xanthomata and Kayser-Fleischer rings in PBC and Wilson's disease, respectively).

The presence and degree of encephalopathy should be documented and graded. The presence of hepatic encephalopathy should initiate a search for precipitating factors such as dehydration, infection, or gastrointestinal bleeding that should all be treated. Spontaneous bacterial peritonitis (SBP) is a very important associated finding and must always be considered and ruled out by appropriate cultures. The SBP can usually be easily managed with appropriate antibiotics. When all other circumstances are appropriate, and the patient is a candidate for OLTx, and a suitable donor organ is available, the presence of a recent SBP should not be considered a contraindication to OLTx since SBP represents a manifestation of end-stage liver disease. Severe cases of encephalopathy should be managed in an intensive care setting, with consideration being given to endotracheal intubation to prevent aspiration. All patients should also receive neomycin and lactulose.

A full battery of blood tests are performed that include blood cell count, full coagulation profile, electrolyte studies, liver function tests, glucose level, and renal function tests, along with more specialized determinations for specific disease entities (i.e., autoantibodies, copper and iron studies, etc.). Any evidence of coagulopathy should be corrected insofar as possible prior to undertaking any invasive procedures. Abnormalities in renal function must be further investigated to distinguish the hepatorenal syndrome from both simple dehydration due to chronic diuretic therapy and ascites, and intrinsic renal disease. This differentiation is extremely important, since renal failure during the posttransplant period increases morbidity and mortality. Hepatorenal syndrome is completely reversible after successful OLTx. However, OLTx candidates with significant preoperative intrinsic renal disease are best managed by combined liver and kidney transplants during the same operative procedure. This combined approach to end-stage liver and kidney disease has now been carried out in 18 patients at our institution with excellent results.

The functional reserve of the liver can be determined further using an indocyanine green clearance study, particularly in patients who are not deeply jaundiced. Endoscopy of the gastrointestinal tract can be performed to detect esophageal varices and other pathology such as inflammatory bowel disease in patients with primary sclerosing cholangitis. Patients with a history of bleeding esophageal varices undergo injection sclerotherapy.

Doppler ultrasonography is used to determine the patency of the portal vein, hepatic artery, hepatic veins, and vena cava. Selective angiography is reserved for patients whose portal vein cannot be visualized by noninvasive means or for patients with previous portasystemic venous shunts in whom the status of both the shunt and portal vein are very important technical considerations. A general evaluation of pulmonary, cardiac, and renal status is carried out to asssess the surgical risk and to prepare the patient for major surgery.

The patient's weight, height, ABO blood group, and ultrasound and/or computed tomography (CT) scan determination of the liver volume are the most important variables in the selection of a suitable donor. The ultrasound and CT scan are also useful to detect the presence of liver tumors and to exclude extrahepatic extension. Donor-recipient matching is mainly based on blood type and organ size. Although ABO blood group barriers have been violated in emergent situations (i.e., fulminant hepatic failure, retransplantation, or in pediatric patients for whom the supply of donor organs is critical), we recommend that for the elective or semielective OLTx, donors of the same ABO blood group be selected. Knowledge of the recipient liver volume as assessed by ultrasound and/or CT scan has proved to be very helpful in the size matching of the donor organ. The liver volume may be very small in relation to the body weight in certain hepatic disorders such as postnecrotic cirrhosis, and therefore an organ harvested from a donor of similar body weight as the recipient could prove to be too large for that recipient, who would better accept a liver from a smaller weight donor. Conversely, the liver in diseases such as PBC and sclerosing cholangitis is quite large or oversized, and thus such recipients are able to accept organs from much higher weight donors. It is important to remember that whatever the liver size, it can always be easily accommodated by a much larger recipient; however, the opposite situation can result in disaster.

It is important to consider certain "risk factors" and discuss how the approach to these have changed. These risk factors have included age, previous abdominal surgery, previous portasystemic shunt procedures, and the presence of active infection. The presence of extrahepatic acute infection should preclude OLTx at the time of the active infection. However, the presence of intrahepatic sepsis such as cholangitis and hepatic abscesses, as may occur with hepatic artery thrombosis in a transplanted liver, should not be contraindications for liver transplantation. Similarly, as already mentioned, the presence of treated spontaneous bacterial peritonitis, a manifestation of chronic liver disease, should not preclude successful OLTx.

In the past, an age of 55 years or greater was considered a relative contraindication to OLTx. The concept of age has undergone a dramatic reevaluation at our institution over the last two to three years. With careful selection criteria and individualization of patient management, and by establishing accurate criteria for adequate cardiovascular, pulmonary, and neurologic function, the survival results in patients older than 50 years, and even in patients older than 60 years, have approached the results in the younger age groups. In fact, in a recent review of the first 1,000 liver transplants at our institution, who were immunosuppressed with cyclosporine, there were 121 patients between the ages of 50 to 60 years old, 47 patients between 60 to 70 years old, and one patient who was 76 years old at the time of OLTx.

The case of the 76-year-old patient who underwent OLTx illustrates clearly the impact that liver transplantation can have on the delivery of health care to and the management of geriatric patients; it also highlights the importance of considering and evaluating each candidate as an individual. This patient was a 76-year-old woman with primary biliary cirrhosis who was bedridden because of incapacitating bone disease. Jaundice was moderate and the main indication for OLTx was her debilitating bone disease. She was carefully evaluated, both medically and psychosocially, and there was unanimous agreement at the candidate selection committee that she should undergo OLTx. She underwent an uneventful transplant procedure, with an uncomplicated postoperative course, and was discharged at three weeks after transplantation. She is now about 18 months posttransplant, doing extremely well at home, with normal liver function, and has required no readmissions into the hospital.

There is no doubt that previous abdominal surgery can increase the difficulty, morbidity, and mortality of OLTx. Even simple procedures such as an open liver biopsy or a cholecystectomy can influence the blood loss and operative time. However, it is the mutilating procedures in the hilum of the liver, such as bile duct reconstructions for sclerosing cholangitis and portacaval shunt for bleeding esophageal varices, that can convert an otherwise routine and straightforward liver transplant procedure into a nightmare. In fact, any portasystemic shunt procedure will add tremendously to the complexity and morbidity of OLTx, not only because of the consequences of previous abdominal surgery and adhesions, but also because of marked changes in the quality of the portal vein that can occur with any of these shunt procedures. All of these procedures can at best be considered palliative; the progression of the underlying liver disease is not altered, and rarely do the patients become free from the ravages of a chronic and relentless disease state. Liver transplantation is curative, and with the markedly improved results that have been realized over the last few years, many, if not all, of the procedures such as portoenterostomy, bile duct reconstruction, and portasystemic shunts should become obsolete. The results of OLTx will undoubtedly even improve further as candidates are selected at an earlier stage of their disease and as OLTx is offered to younger patients and prior to undergoing palliative upper abdominal surgical procedures.

The indications for OLTx include a major gastrointestinal (GI) bleed, a history of repeated bouts of encephalopathy, progressive neuropathy, refractory ascites, a recent precipitous deterioration in liver function and jaundice, severe fatigue and pruritus, the rapid progression of incapacitating bone disease, and severe wasting.

Considerations regarding the proper timing of OLTx are also constantly changing and, as already mentioned, OLTx continues to be offered at earlier stages of the disease. It has been somewhat easier to time and offer liver transplantation to patients with PBC than for some of the other indications since a set of prognostic indices have been developed and accepted at most centers; these indices employ the common clinical and pathologic criteria of this entity (i.e., age, total bilirubin level, albumin level, encephalopathy, ascites, GI bleed). In our own large series of PBC patients that underwent OLTx, virtually all met the criteria for advanced disease that would predict that death would have been likely in a year or less without the transplant procedure.

The patient described in the present case report represents an ideal candidate for OLTx. This patient exemplifies most of the common features and characteristics of PBC that have already been outlined above. Moreover, the signs and symptoms that she presents will illustrate many common findings in end-stage liver disease of any etiology that require hepatic replacement. This patient has experienced a rather rapid deterioration of her liver function and exhibits the sequelae from it. This type of patient should immediately undergo an evaluation as outlined above and immediately be considered for OLTx once a suitable donor liver is available. One can easily argue that this patient should have been referred for evaluation of liver transplantation at a much earlier stage in her disease. The importance of knowing a patient well, and of being able to follow the course of a patient's liver disease prior to transplantation, cannot be overemphasized.

OPERATIVE CONSIDERATIONS

Liver transplantation for PBC, as for any disease indication, involves the donor hepatectomy (organ procurement), recipient hepatectomy, and implantation of the new liver into the recipient.

Donor Procedure

The techniques for multiple organ retrieval that are currently used are based on the rapid core cooling of solid organs by the aortic infusion of cold electrolyte-containing or colloid-containing solutions, and for the liver, the additional infusion of cold solution through the portal venous system. These techniques, along with careful donor monitoring and management, and synchronous collaboration with other transplant teams, have allowed the successful harvesting of the liver and/or pancreas, kidneys, and heart or heart and lungs from a single brain-dead, heart-beating cadaveric donor. The suitability of a potential liver donor has been customarily based on traditional indicators of ischemic injury, including liver function tests, parameters of coagulation, oxygenation, blood pressure, level of pressor agent support, the number and duration of cardiac arrests, and the cause of death. We have found that these parameters of donor assessment can be applied too rigorously and, in fact, may be much less reliable in predicting the quality of the liver than has been assumed, thus resulting in a potentially high degree of organ wastage. We have liberalized these conservative criteria for donor acceptance considerably, and have not suffered a discernible penalty.

The conventional method of liver preservation in recent clinical practice has been static, hypothermic (4°C) storage of the liver in Euro-Collins solution. This has necessitated the implantation of the liver within a six- to eight-hour period after aortic crossclamping in the donor. A major advance in liver preservation that has impacted our own clinical practice of liver transplantation has been the development of the University of Wisconsin-Lactobionate solution by Dr. Belzer and his group. (*Editor's note:* A very logical approach to increasing donor organ survival, this is hopefully but the first in a series of metabolic approaches in improving substrate supply to donor organs.) Cold preservation in this new solution has resulted in improved quality of organs after revascularization, after any duration of preservation; however, more importantly, it has allowed us to successfully preserve and transplant livers after more than 20 hours of simple cold preservation.

Recipient Procedure

The recipient hepatectomy in patients with PBC is usually easier to perform than it is in most other instances of adult chronic liver disease. This is especially true in the absence of previous upper abdominal surgery. Specific operative findings include livers that are considerably larger than normal, marked hilar lymphadenopathy, and a minimal-to-moderate degree of portal hypertension. These findings, along with the usual absence of major collaterals in the hepatic suspensory ligaments and the bare areas of the liver, the usually normal consistency and configuration of the suprahepatic and infrahepatic vena cava and the portal vein, and the usual presence of a normal recipient common bile duct, are all features that render the procedure in PBC technically easier than it is for many of the other indications for OLTx.

Veno-venous bypass (without systemic heparinization) was developed for the anhepatic phase of OLTx as a method of decompressing the temporarily obstructed systemic venous (vena caval) and splanchnic venous (portal) systems. The anhepatic phase of OLTx is the most physiologically turbulent period of the entire procedure. Without veno-venous bypass, there is a massive sequestration of blood volume in the peripheral venous circulation of the lower torso and in the mesenteric venous circulation, resulting in diffuse edema of the gastrointestinal tract, high renal vein pressure with deterioration of renal function, increased bleeding from high pressure in the thin-walled venous collaterals found throughout the abdomen in patients with portal hypertension, and marked hemodynamic instability.

Veno-venous bypass is now routinely employed in most adults undergoing OLTx in order to reduce these risks and to maintain physiologic stability during the anhepatic phase. Blood from the inferior vena cava is drained via a cannula placed through the saphenofemoral junction into the cava near the bifurcation of the common iliac veins. A second cannula to drain the splanchnic venous system is placed end-on into the transected portal vein. These two cannulas are joined by a Y-type connector, and the blood is returned to the heart through a cannula placed in the ipsilateral axillary vein using a nontraumatic, centrifugal pump (Biomedicus Inc.). Using such a bypass, it is possible to maintain stable hemodynamic parameters similar to prehepatectomy levels, to reduce postoperative problems of the bowel and ileus by relieving congestion of the intestinal tract, to avoid renal venous hypertension (thus markedly decreasing the incidence of renal failure requiring postoperative dialysis), and to reduce the blood loss by preventing the development of high pressure in venous collaterals.

The technique of veno-venous bypass allows the surgeon to control the length of the anhepatic phase and, in this way, the recipient hepatectomy can be individualized; certain problems can be addressed such as previous surgery or significant portal hypertension. The bypass is established prior to the completion of the recipient hepatectomy and facilitates the final steps of this procedure, particularly the dissection of the vena cava. Once the liver is removed, the large bare areas created by the hepatectomy are carefully inspected and hemostasis is achieved by oversewing them if necessary. The cuffs of the suprahepatic and infrahepatic vena cava are then carefully fashioned and tailored for anastomosis. The donor liver, appropriately prepared at the back table in cold fluid, is then brought up for implantation. The suprahepatic and infrahepatic vena caval cuffs are anastomosed. Prior to the completion of the infrahepatic caval anastomosis, the liver is flushed free of potassium and air with cold solution infused through a cannula in the portal vein. The portal bypass cannula is then removed, and the splanchnic venous system is clamped for the next 10 to 15 minutes while the portal vein cuffs are appropriately fashioned and anastomosed. The liver is usually revascularized on portal flow, and the bypass is then completely stopped and the cannulas are removed. Once the liver is revascularized on portal blood and initial rapid hemostasis is achieved, we then proceed with the hepatic arterial reconstruction. We prefer an end-to-end anastomosis between the recipient hepatic artery and the donor celiac axis, whenever possible.

Our preferred method of vascular anastomoses for the vena cava, portal vein, and hepatic artery is an end-to-end anastomosis with continuous nonabsorbable monofilament propylene suture. A "growth or expansion factor" is employed to prevent suture line stenoses. The running suture is tied several millimeters or more from the vessel wall such that when the vessel distends under pressure or when vasospasm resolves, the suture can easily be soaked up into the vessel, thus preventing deformity at the site of the anastomosis.

Portal vein thrombosis at one time was considered an absolute or at least a relative contraindication to OLTx. However, as the surgical techniques of OLTx have been refined over the last few years, our approach to abnormalities and thrombosis of the portal vein has become much more aggressive, and these situations no longer preclude successful OLTx. We have used vascular grafts of donor iliac vein, harvested at the same time as the liver, to reconstruct recipient portal vein segments of varying length that are either hypoplastic or thrombosed. We have been able to reconstruct the portal vein as far back as the level of the confluence of the superior mesenteric and splenic veins under the neck of the pancreas, in order to achieve satisfactory splanchnic flow to the liver.

One technical problem that is unique to patients with PBC undergoing OLTx is the fragility and friability of the recipient hepatic artery. The media and subintima have a tendency to separate from the rest of the artery, even with the slightest amount of trauma, including the application of vascular clamps in the preparation for anastomosis and/or the ligation of the gastroduodenal artery or other branches. This can result in fragmentation and intramural dissection of the injured vessel proximal to or beyond the level of the left gastric and splenic arterial branches, resulting in a suboptimal arterial supply that is unacceptable for successful OLTx. In this situation, as in any situation in which the hepatic arterial inflow is poor, we use a conduit usually consisting of a free-standing graft of donor iliac artery that is anastomosed to the recipient infrarenal aorta and is passed through a tunnel posterior to the pancreas and duodenum and entering the hilum so that it can be anastomosed to the donor iliac artery. It should be noted that intimal dissection occurred in about 20% of the cases in our large series of PBC patients and required the use of an iliac graft to prevent subsequent thrombosis.

After completing the four vascular anastomoses and achieving adequate hemostasis, the recipient procedure is completed with the biliary tract reconstruction. In PBC patients, the biliary reconstruction of choice, and one that is usually possible, is a duct-to-duct choledochocholedochostomy over an external T-tube stent. The advantages of this method include the preservation of the sphincter of Oddi and the availability of the T-tube to monitor bile production and to perform cholangiography. In certain situations, a direct duct-to-duct repair should not be performed, and in these cases an end-to-side Roux-en-Y choledochojejunostomy over an internal stent should be performed. This technique should be the primary method of biliary reconstruction in patients with preexisting extrahepatic biliary tract disease such as sclerosing cholangitis, when there is significant size discrepancy between the donor and recipient bile ducts, when there is significant bleeding around the bile duct, and for most cases of liver transplantation for hepatic tumors in which the recipient dissection includes the entire supraduodenal lymph node and bile duct areas. Failures of duct-to-duct repair are usually best managed by conversion to this method of reconstruction.

POSTOPERATIVE CONSIDERATIONS

Postoperative immunosuppression in adults usually consists of a rapid steroid taper, beginning with methylprednisolone at 200 mg intravenously the day after surgery; this is reduced by 40 mg each succeeding day until a maintenance dose of 20 mg per day is reached. Cyclosporine is administered intravenously at a dose of 6 mg/kg/day in three divided doses. As gastrointestinal function normalizes, the therapy is gradually switched from intravenous to oral cyclosporine at 17.5 mg/kg/day. The cyclosporine dose is judged on a day-to-day basis by assaying the blood concentration of the drug. Acute rejection episodes are treated with either steroid boluses and recycles, with monoclonal antibody (OKT_3, Orthoclone, Ortho Pharmaceutical Corporation, Raritan, NJ), or with increased doses of cyclosporine when indicated.

The survival in liver transplant patients treated with cyclosporine has improved dramatically. The overall survival rates of the first 1,000 liver transplant patients treated with cyclosporine-steroid therapy at our institution were three times higher than those of the 170 patients treated with azathioprine and steroids before 1980. The five-year actuarial survival for this overall group of 1,000 patients was 64%. The projected five-year actuarial survival of the group of PBC patients who underwent transplantation at our institution is approximately 70%.

An aggressive attitude toward and the frequent use of retransplantation has had a favorable influence on the overall survival results of liver transplantation at our institution, in particular in the group of patients with PBC. In addition to hepatic dysfunction, important factors determining the feasibility of retransplantation include cardiopulmonary status, renal function, and the presence or absence of infection. Since the overall general condition of PBC patients prior to the initial transplant procedure is usually better than that of patients undergoing transplantation for other indications, retransplantation can often be carried out more readily and with better results in the PBC group. In our own series of PBC patients undergoing OLTx, the incidence of retransplantation was less than 1 in 5, and the survival rate in this particular group was almost 50%.

Most of the mortality after OLTx for PBC occurs within the first six months following transplantation. The causes of death are the same as for OLTx for any disease indication. In the group of PBC patients who underwent transplantation at our institution, rejection was the single most important cause of death, either because retransplantation was not possible or because retransplantation was not successful. Other causes of death included primary graft nonfunction, hepatic artery thrombosis, and pneumonia due to bacteria or *Pneumocystis carinii*. Although the morbidity after OLTx has decreased considerably over the last few years, numerous postoperative complications are experienced by patients after this procedure, many of which require surgical intervention. Our review of PBC patients undergoing OLTx revealed that wound infection was the most common problem, followed closely by the need for biliary tract revision for anastomotic stricture or leak. Gastrointestinal hemorrhage and hemoperitoneum were also significant postoperative complications in this group of patients.

The only potential controversy regarding the application of OLTx for patients with PBC has arisen from another group's experience with liver transplantation for PBC in 11 patients who were immunosuppressed with azathioprine and prednisone. Clinical and histopathologic evidence for recurrent PBC was reported in 3 of these 11 patients. However, in our own experience in 165 patients, and with follow-up periods ranging from six months to almost 9 1/2 years, we have not been able to document recurrent PBC in any of the patients who underwent transplantation. Furthermore, we could demonstrate no correlation between the presence of AMA titers before and after transplantation and the function of the graft. Many histologic similarities exist between PBC and rejection, as well as graft vs. host liver disease, and this may therefore account for some confusion when diagnosing recurrent disease after transplantation.

The quality of life after OLTx for PBC has been excellent, with 90% of the long-term survivors achieving full rehabilitation. A significant incapacitating problem in patients with PBC is osteoporosis, which is thought to be caused by a low bone turnover state. Significant bone disease was present in about 40% of the PBC patients who underwent liver transplantation at our institution, and approximately 20% of these patients were totally incapacitated. There was marked improvement in either bone pain or fractures following OLTx in these patients, even though some patients required prolonged postoperative rehabilitative programs. A large number of the long-term survivors have returned to either full-time or part-time work, and there are patients who have become pregnant and have given birth to normal children.

There is no doubt that the survival, and particularly the quality of life, of patients with primary biliary cirrhosis who undergo orthotopic liver transplantation is markedly enhanced when compared to that in patients managed with standard medical therapy. It is expected that these results will even improve further in the future with better and earlier preoperative selection of candidates, as immunosuppression improves or becomes more selective, and as the surgical technique and the postoperative management of these patients becomes more refined.

BIBLIOGRAPHY

1. Esquivel CO, Van Thiel D, Demetris AJ, et al: Transplantation for primary biliary cirrhosis. *Gastroenterology* 1988; 94:1207–1216.
2. Gordon R, Iwatsuki S, Esquivel CO, et al: Progress in liver transplantation. *Adv Surg* 1987; 21:49–64.
3. Iwatsuki S, Starzl TE, Todo S, et al: Experience in one thousand liver transplantations. *Transplant Proc* 1988; 20(Suppl 1):498–504.
4. Starzl TE, Iwatsuki S, Van Thiel D, et al: Evolution of liver transplantation. *Hepatology,* 1982; 2:614–636.
5. Starzl TE: Hepatic transplantation. *Semin Liver Dis* 1985; 5:309–419.

PART IV

Endocrine

33

Medullary Carcinoma of the Thyroid

A 23-year-old man presents with explosive diarrhea of three months' duration. On physical examination a mass that is 3 × 3 cm is palpable in the right thyroid lobe and there is associated ipsilateral lymphadenopathy. Evaluation of the gastrointestinal tract shows no intrinsic lesion, and microbial cultures are negative. The fasting plasma calcitonin level is 25,400 pg/ml (normal, less than 200 pg/ml), and the plasma carcinoembryonic antigen level is 23 ng/ml (normal, less than 5.0 ng/ml).

Consultants: Stanley W. Ashley, M.D.
Samuel A. Wells, Jr., M.D.

DISCUSSION

This patient's presentation with severe diarrhea, a thyroid mass, and increased plasma concentrations of calcitonin (CTN) and carcinoembryonic antigen (CEA) is virtually diagnostic of medullary thyroid carcinoma (MTC). Although among the least often considered diagnoses in patients presenting with chronic diarrhea, a variety of endocrine neoplasms—gastrinomas, carcinoids, vasoactive intestinal polypeptidomas (VIPomas), and medullary thyroid carcinomas—can produce dramatic alterations in bowel habits. Approximately one third of patients with MTC develop some degree of diarrhea during the course of their disease, and this symptom is especially severe in patients with plasma CTN levels in excess of 20,000 pg/ml. Another consideration in a patient presenting with diarrhea of recent onset and a neck mass is hyperthyroidism.

Medullary thyroid carcinoma, which accounts for 5% to 10% of thyroid malignancies, was first identified as a distinct clinical entity by Hazard and associates in 1959. These tumors arise from the parafollicular or C-cells that are derived from the neural crest. During embryonic life, these neural cells migrate to several parts of the body including the pituitary gland, the adrenal medulla, the enterochromaffin system of the gut, and the upper portions of the thyroid lobes. These cells have the common pharmacologic property of *a*mine *p*recursor *u*ptake and *d*ecarboxylation and tumors originating from these cells are called APUDomas. The primary secretory product of the thyroid C-cells is the hormone calcitonin. In some species this 32-amino-acid polypeptide plays an important role in the regulation of calcium metabolism by inhibiting osteoclastic bone resorption. However, in man the specific biologic effect is unclear. Even patients with MTC and high concentrations of plasma CTN have normal concentrations of serum calcium. This hormone does seem to have an effect during embryogenesis and in infancy, when it appears to increase bone formation from the miscible calcium pool. Clinically, plasma levels of CTN are useful for establishing the diagnosis of MTC, especially in patients or kindred members suspected of having the familial syndromes of multiple endocrine neoplasia (MEN), types IIa and IIb. Modest elevations of plasma CTN have been reported in patients with chronic renal failure, in patients who are pregnant and in patients with a variety of other malignancies.

CLINICAL SETTING

It has become evident that MTC may occur in four different clinical settings: MEN-IIa, MEN-IIb, non-MEN MTC, and sporadic MTC. The MEN-IIa is characterized by the concurrence of MTC, pheochromocytomas, and hyperparathyroidism, while MEN-IIb is typified by MTC, pheochromocytomas, multiple mucosal neuromas, and ganglioneuromatosis. Patients with MEN-IIb also have a characteristic physical appearance. In patients with familial non-MEN MTC, there are no associated endocrinopathies. The familial MTC syndromes are characterized by a Mendelian autosomal dominant pattern of inheritance. There is complete penetrance but variable expressivity, such that 100% of affected patients with MEN-IIa develop MTC, while approximately 50% develop pheochromocytomas and 50% develop hyperparathyroidism.

Medullary thyroid carcinoma is most aggressive in patients with MEN-IIb and least aggressive in patients with familial non-MEN MTC. The MTC in patients with MEN-IIa is quite variable. In some patients it progresses rapidly, while in most it grows slowly, and even patients with metastases may enjoy a normal life expectancy.

Medullary thyroid carcinoma presenting in a young adult such as the present case suggests the possibility of familial MTC and should prompt screening to detect MTC in family members at risk. Also, the present patient and affected kindred members should be screened for the presence of associated endocrinopathies. The apparent sporadic MTC may actually represent the index case to a kindred with familial MTC. In such a patient, the presence of a pheochromocytoma and hyperparathyroidism should be searched for and, if found, the pheochromocytoma should be resected before thyroidectomy for MTC. Any surgical therapy in the presence of an undiagnosed pheochromocytoma is associated with a high mortality. We routinely measure 24-hour urinary excretion rates of catecholamines, vanillylmandelic acid, and metanephrines in all patients with confirmed MTC. If the urinary values are elevated or if the patient is to undergo thyroidectomy, an abdominal computed tomography (CT) scan is performed. Measurements of serum concentrations of calcium and parathormone are usually adequate to diagnose hyperparathyroidism. The presence of MEN-IIb can usually be detected by the patient's characteristic physical appearance.

Of critical significance in the screening of family members for MTC has been the recognition that calcium (Ca^{++}) and pentagastrin (Pg) administered intravenously are potent CTN secretagogues. Pathologically, familial tumors are usually preceded by C-cell hyperplasia (CCH) which, with time, progresses to microscopic foci of carcinoma and then to frankly invasive MTC. In contrast with normal subjects, patients with CCH or early MTC may have normal basal plasma CTN levels that significantly increase within minutes after the intravenous administration of Ca^{++} and Pg. We have found that the infusion of calcium gluconate (2 mg/kg/minute) followed immediately by the infusion of Pg (0.5 µg/kg/5 seconds) is the best provocative screening test. Patients at risk for MTC who have minimally elevated plasma CTN levels (250 to 1,000 pg/ml) following provocative testing with Ca^{++} and Pg should either be retested in six months or should have provocative testing repeated immediately with selective venous catheterization of the inferior thyroid veins (ITV). Plasma CTN levels are often strikingly increased in ITV plasma samples (compared to those in peripheral plasma samples) in patients with CCH or microinvasive MTC. Using such methods, it is possible to detect MTC in a preclinical stage when thyroidectomy is associated with a cure rate approaching 100%.

Clinically, MTC usually presents as a firm, rounded painless nodule in the substance of the thyroid. As in the present case, approximately 40% of patients with a palpable nodule will have cervical lymph node involvement. Advanced local disease may produce symptoms of cough, hoarseness, or dysphagia as a result of tracheal, laryngeal, or esophageal involvement. There is usually evidence of capsular invasion and blood vessel involvement. After the cervical lymph nodes, the most common sites of metastatic disease are mediastinum, lungs, liver, bone, brain, adrenals, pleura, and heart, in decreasing order of frequency. A metastatic workup should include a chest x-ray film, liver function tests, and a skeletal survey. As shown in Figure 33–1, the extent of tumor burden seems to correlate directly with the preoperative basal levels of plasma CTN. Patients with palpable tumors often have plasma CTN levels exceeding 1,000 pg/ml, whereas those with extensive metastases may have levels of 50,000 pg/ml or greater. The patient in the present case has an intermediate level suggesting the probability of extrathyroid spread. We have also found that the preoperative stimulated plasma CTN level has prognostic significance, in that patients whose

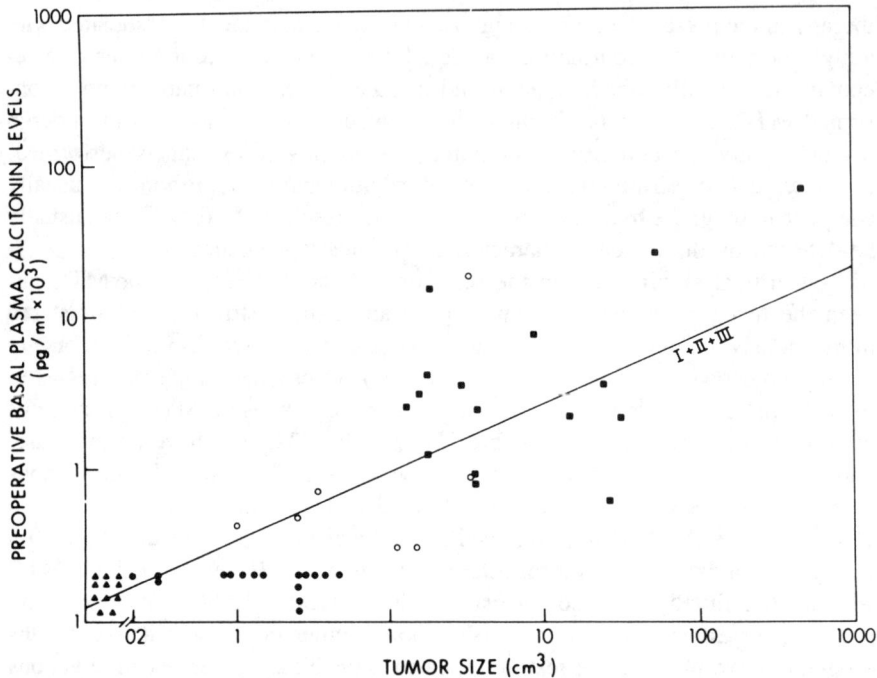

FIG 33–1.
Correlation of tumor size with preoperative basal plasma CTN levels. *Closed circles* and *closed triangles* represent patients with no clinical evidence of MTC whose normal basal plasma CTN levels become elevated after provocative stimulation (I). *Closed triangles* denote patients with C-cell hyperplasia. *Open circles* represent patients who had no clinical evidence of MTC but did have elevated basal plasma CTN levels (II). *Closed squares* represent patients with clinically evident MTC (III). *Diagonal line* represents the least-squares linear regression of data. (From Wells SA Jr, Baylin SB, Gann DS, et al: *Ann Surg* 1978; 188:377. Used by permission.)

preoperative stimulated plasma CTN levels were less than 1,000 pg/ml rarely had lymph node involvement at surgery or residual postoperative MTC as indicated by an elevated stimulated plasma CTN level. Conversely, 60% of patients with preoperative stimulated plasma CTN levels in excess of 10,000 pg/ml had either spread of MTC to regional lymph nodes or residual MTC postoperatively.

As in our patient, the level of carcinoembryonic antigen (CEA) is another plasma marker that is frequently elevated in patients with clinically evident MTC and may serve as a useful prognostic indicator. Some investigators have reported a rise in the level of plasma CEA without a rise in the level of plasma CTN in patients with progressive disease, and others have found that patients with elevated levels of plasma CEA are more likely to develop metastases than are patients with normal levels. It has been suggested that significant CEA production by these tumors is a marker for dedifferentiation, a characteristic that often correlates with more aggressive growth. As shown in Figure 33–2, our group evaluated 37 patients with suspected or clinically established MTC. Plasma CEA levels were elevated in all patients with clinically evident MTC, but they were much less often increased in those with occult disease.

Systemic manifestations of MTC are actually quite uncommon. Diarrhea is the only secondary symptom of any frequency and, in most large series, it develops in 30% to 40% of patients with clinically evident disease. In contrast with the presented patient's explosive history, the diarrhea is typically mild, although over one half of patients will complain of more than five bowel movements per 24-hour period. Stools are usually loose and watery. Urgency is reported in one third of patients, but steatorrhea and significant malabsorption are uncommon. Incapacitating diarrhea typically develops only in patients with a large tumor burden (CTN levels more than 20,000 pg/ml) and metastatic disease. The diarrhea may improve by removing the primary tumor or debulking the metastases, but its persistence is indicative of substantial metastatic disease.

The pathogenesis of the diarrhea is not clear. Disorders of gastrointestinal absorption, secretion, and motility have all been proposed. Most clinical studies suggest that this diarrhea is secretory in nature, with increased water and chloride secretion and decreased sodium absorption in the jejunum and ileum. Medullary thyroid carcinomas have been demonstrated to secrete a variety of substances known to alter gastrointestinal function, including prostaglandins, vasoactive intestinal polypeptide (VIP), substance P, and serotonin. In addition, CTN itself may alter circulating levels of gastrin, motilin, pancreatic polypeptide, and glucose-dependent insulinotrophic peptide (GIP). However, none of these substances is found to be consistently elevated in all patients with MTC and diarrhea. Prostaglandins have been strongly implicated by some investigators, although their role has been questioned by the failure of indomethacin to alleviate symptoms in these patients. At present, the most likely causative agent for the diarrhea is increased plasma concentration of CTN. In both clinical studies and in a variety of experimental animal studies, increased plasma CTN levels are associated with inhibition of fluid absorption and stimulation of fluid and electrolyte secretion in the distal small bowel. It is generally agreed that this is a direct effect of CTN on the intestine, although a mechanism mediated by the central nervous system has also been proposed. In contrast with most secretory diarrheas, changes in mucosal cyclic adenosine monophosphate (AMP) do not appear to be involved. However, it is still not clear how directly circulating plasma CTN levels correlate with the incidence and magnitude of diarrhea. Further studies are needed to determine if some other factor or factors secreted by the MTC is responsible for the symptoms.

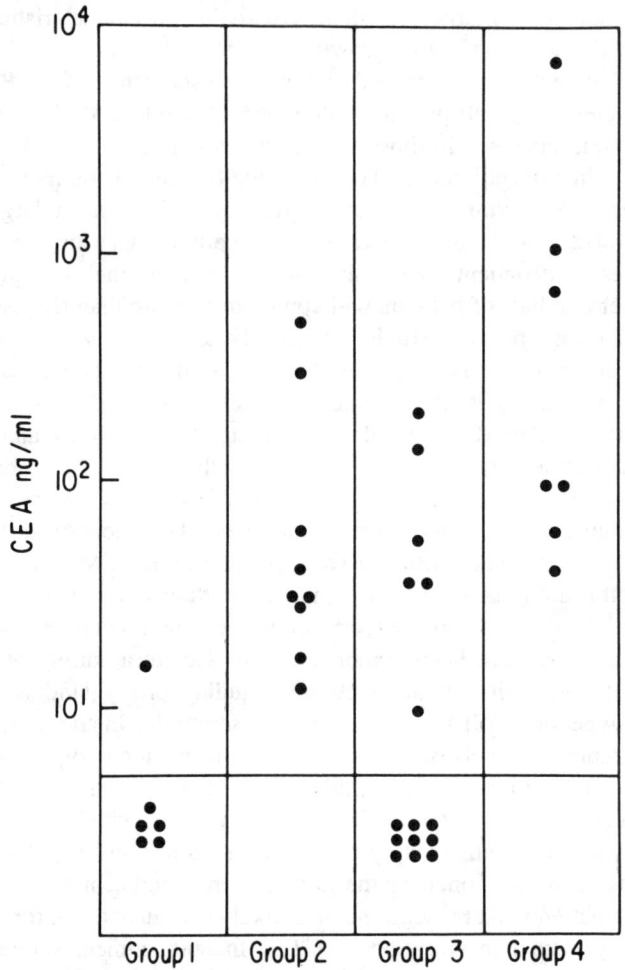

FIG 33–2.
Plasma concentrations of CEA in 37 patients with known or suspected MTC. Patients in groups 1 and 2 were previously unevaluated members of a MEN-IIa kindred at risk for MTC. The patients in group 1 had no clinical evidence of thyroid disease, whereas the patients in group 2 had one or more palpable thyroid nodules. The patients in groups 3 and 4 had previously undergone thyroidectomy for MTC. The patients in group 3 had no clinical evidence of MTC, whereas the patients in group 4 had objective clinical evidence of recurrent local or metastatic MTC. The horizontal line at the bottom of the graph represents the normal plasma level of 5 ng/ml of CEA. (From Wells SA Jr, Haagensen DE, Linehan WM, et al: *Cancer* 1978; 42:1498. Used by permission.)

TREATMENT

Treatment in the presented patient should include total thyroidectomy and resection of enlarged regional lymph nodes in the neck. Because of the high incidence of multicentricity in patients with familial disease and the possibility that even the patient with a presumed sporadic tumor may have affected family members, total thyroidectomy is considered the treatment of choice for all patients presenting with MTC. To avoid recurrence, meticulous removal of all thyroid tissue is essential. Because of the association with hyperparathyroidism, care must be taken to examine all four parathyroid glands. We remove any grossly enlarged glands, even if discovered incidentally. In patients with documented MEN-IIa who have hypercalcemia and four-gland enlargement, total parathyroidectomy with parathyroid autotransplantation to the forearm muscle is performed. Because of the high incidence (approximately 50%) of nodal metastases in the central zone of the neck, lymph nodes from the hyoid bone superiorly to the innominate vessels inferiorly and to the internal jugular veins laterally are routinely removed. Sampling of midjugular nodes on either side is also recommended. If disease is evident, such as in the present case, a modified neck dissection is required.

With lymph node involvement, ten-year survival for affected patients approaches 25%. However, depending on the setting, these tumors may be more or less aggressive. Recent studies by Lippman et al. have suggested that immunohistochemical staining techniques may provide useful information regarding prognosis. Patients whose primary MTC stains homogenously for CTN have a better prognosis than do patients whose tumors stain heterogenously.

It has become our practice to perform provocative testing in all patients within a month of thyroidectomy to determine if residual tumor is present. Patients with normal stimulated plasma CTN levels are then followed up at yearly intervals. The appropriate management for patients with elevated postoperative plasma CTN levels is less well established. Some patients with clear evidence of residual disease may survive for long periods without symptoms. It has generally been our policy not to reexplore patients who have elevated plasma CTN levels following thyroidectomy. Tissel and associates, however, recently reported cases of 11 patients with increased plasma CTN levels postoperatively who had extensive dissection of the mediastinal and cervical lymph nodes at subsequent reexploration. Three of the patients were apparently cured by this technique, since plasma CTN levels were normal following provocation postoperatively.

The use of conventional chemotherapy and x-ray therapy in patients with metastatic MTC has been disappointing. Although regression and prolonged survival have been reported in some cases, MTC is relatively radioresistant. The potential benefits of such therapy must be weighed against the risk of cervical fibrosis, radiation tracheitis, and other radiation-related complications. Neither single- nor multiple-agent chemotherapy has proved to be effective. Our group has treated patients with streptozocin, carmustine (BCNU), doxorubicin, cisplatin, cyclophosphamide (Cytoxan), methotrexate, and fluorouracil (5-FU), but objective responses have been infrequent. Some investigators have reported favorable results with ^{131}I therapy, presumably as a result of radioiodine trapping in remaining follicular cells adjacent to the C-cells. However, we have not found this therapy useful.

The recurrence of diarrhea in the present patient after thyroidectomy should influence therapeutic decisions. Even in the absence of any potential for cure, debulking of recurrent disease can reduce the tumor burden and the plasma CTN levels or other possible diarrheogenic factors in the patient with metastatic disease. In the majority of patients with widely metastatic MTC, opiates and a high-fiber diet may provide significant symptomatic relief. Isolated reports have suggested that somatostatin and bromocriptine may be helpful.

SUMMARY

This patient's presentation with diarrhea and a thyroid mass suggests the presence of MTC. This diagnosis is confirmed by the elevated plasma CTN level, although patients with this magnitude of diarrhea typically present with even higher basal levels of this hormone. Particularly because of his young age, he should be evaluated for the presence of a pheochromocytoma and hyperparathyroidism before thyroidectomy. In addition, family members should undergo provocative testing for MTC. The elevated CEA and ipsilateral adenopathy increase the likelihood that he already has distant metastatic disease. Total thyroidectomy and central and ipsilateral neck dissection are indicated. Postoperatively, provocative testing should be performed and plasma CTN levels determined. The return of diarrhea almost certainly indicates recurrent disease. In the event of a recurrence, aggressive intervention including reoperation may be indicated.

BIBLIOGRAPHY

1. Hazard JB, Hawk WA, Crile G Jr: Medullary (solid) carcinoma of the thyroid: A clinicopathologic entity. *J Clin Endocrinol Metab* 1959; 19:152–161.
2. Lippman SM, Mendelsohn G, Trump DL, et al: The prognostic and biological significance of cellular heterogeneity in medullary thyroid carcinoma: A study of calcitonin, L-dopa decarboxylase, and histaminase. *J Clin Endocrinol Metab* 1982; 54:233–240.
3. Tissel LE, Hansson G, Janson S, et al: Reoperation in the treatment of asymptomatic metastasizing medullary thyroid carcinoma. *Surgery* 1986; 99:60–66.
4. Wells SA Jr, Baylin SB, Leight GS, et al: The importance of early diagnosis in patients with hereditary medullary thyroid carcinoma. *Ann Surg* 1982; 195:595–599.

34

Asymptomatic Hyperparathyroidism

A 34-year-old, asymptomatic male junior executive undergoes a physical examination. An SMA-12 reveals a calcium level of 11.2 mg/dl and a phosphorus level of 2.3 mg/dl. The patient is basically asymptomatic, is not fatigued, and has no history of renal stones, peptic ulcer, or joint pain. Repeat calcium and phosphorus tests reveal consistently elevated values for serum calcium and ionized calcium and a consistently low phosphorus level.

Consultant: Chiu-an Wang, M.D.

DISCUSSION

The patient is a 34-year-old executive who was found to have persistent hypercalcemia (11 to 12 mg/dl) and hypophosphatemia on routine physical examination. He was otherwise totally free of symptoms and in good health. While the plasma parathyroid hormone (PTH) level is not available in the protocol, the differential diagnosis of hypercalcemia has been fully discussed and a diagnosis of hyperparathyroidism is reasonably certain. The patient, however, is totally asymptomatic.

Many questions are raised as to the best way to care for patients who have asymptomatic hyperparathyroidism. Should they undergo neck exploration or should they be treated expectantly? What criteria should be applied in the selection of patients with asymptomatic hyperparathyroidism for surgery? Is there a therapeutic alternative to surgery?

CLINICAL ASSESSMENT

The first step in the care of these patients is to assess the severity of the disease. A mild degree of hypercalcemia seldom constitutes a threat to the patient, and experience has shown that the diseased glands are often very small and can be extremely difficult to find in an asymptomatic but mildly hypercalcemic patient.

Thus, if the disease is mild, it may be well to defer surgery. If it is severe, however, surgery should be performed without undue delay. Furthermore, it is difficult to make a definitive pathologic diagnosis because in these patients the diseased gland is often indistinguishable from the normal glands. Thus, it is definitely advantageous to postpone the explorations until the anatomical as well as pathologic diagnosis is more conclusive.

Generally speaking, the disease is considered severe if the serum calcium level is persistently elevated to 11 to 12 mg/dl and the PTH is double or triple the normal level. When the 24-hour urinary calcium excretion exceeds 200 mg and the formation of renal stones becomes a serious threat to the patient, disease itself must be viewed as grave and exploration is mandatory. We have found that biochemical derangements seldom regress spontaneously. In fact, should the disease follow its usual course, ultimately kidney function is impaired, bone masses are lost, and the patient's general well-being is threatened. At this point, the damage has been done, and it may be too late for surgery to be beneficial.

In the present case, the patient was asymptomatic with a relatively severe biochemical parameter, but without metabolic complications. On the basis of the biochemical derangement alone, this patient is a candidate for surgery and an exploration should be seriously considered.

In addition to the biochemical parameters, factors such as the sex or age of the patient must be considered in deciding whether the patient would benefit by surgical intervention. Osteoporosis in a premenopausal or menopausal woman is inevitably aggravated by hyperparathyroidism. Even if the disease is asymptomatic and mild in degree, surgery should be performed. In a young, healthy, and productive man, as in the present case, the disease should be corrected even if hyperparathyroidism is mild and asymptomatic.

We reported a series of 242 patients with asymptomatic hyperparathyroidism who were operated on between January 1971 and December 1982 at the Massachusetts General Hospital. All were classified as having hyperparathyroidism as defined by a persistently high serum calcium level in the range of 10.5 to 11 mg/dl on serial measurements and an inappropriately high normal or clearly elevated parathyroid hormone level. With the patients on a low-calcium diet, the 24-hour urinary calcium excretion was 150 mg or more in most patients. Other causes of hypercalcemia were excluded in all patients, and none had metabolic complications such as renal function impairment, nephrolithiasis or ureterolithiasis, bone pain, peptic ulcer disease, pancreatitis, or psychiatric disorders.

The decision to proceed with parathyroid exploration was based on the following criteria: (1) sufficient evidence of the deterioration of renal function; (2) loss of bone mass; (3) increase in the serum calcium level to a level greater than 11 mg/dl; (4) elevation of the PTH level; and (5) particularly in women, augmentation of 24-hour calcium excretion to more than 150 mg. Because a female may be at risk for long-term disabling complications or threatened by osteoporosis, we believe it would be appropriate to correct the disease. The interval between the initial detection of hypercalcemia and the diagnosis of asymptomatic hyperparathyroidism requiring operative intervention varied from 6 months to 15 years, with a mean of 3.4 years. The age of the patients at the time of operative intervention ranged from 15 to 82 years, with a mean of 52 years. In this series, there were 187 female (77%) and 55 male (23%) patients. During the 12-year study period, there appeared to be a marked increase in the number of female patients in the sixth decade; there now seems to be an increased awareness of the relationship between osteoporosis and hyperparathyroidism.

In this series, 201 of the patients had an adenoma (83.1%); 39 had primary hyperplasia (16.1%), and 2 had incipient hyperplastic glands that appeared to be early cases of primary hyperplasia (0.8%). We have not encountered any patients with parathyroid carcinoma or so-called multiple adenomas. Interestingly enough, four of the patients in this series had a supernumerary gland; ten patients had multiple endocrine neoplasia type I, and one patient had familial hyperparathyroidism.

The weight and size of the diseased parathyroid tissue generally correlated well with the severity of the disease as reflected by the degree of hypercalcemia and the level of parathyroid hormone. Patients in whom there is mild or borderline elevation of serum calcium and PTH levels had a smaller diseased parathyroid gland, whereas those in whom there was marked elevation of these levels had larger and heavier glands.

The anatomical distribution of the diseased glands in these patients was not very different from that of the symptomatic cases. Of the 201 adenomas removed from the neck, 59% were on the right and 41% were on the left side; 23% were located posterior to the upper thyroid pole; 40% were near the cricothyroid junction; 20% were adjacent to the lower thyroid; 14% were in the thymic tongue, and 2% were in the mediastinum; rarely, one may be found within the thyroid parenchyma.

In 238 (98.3%) of the patients, hypercalcemia reverted to normocalcemia immediately following surgery. The mean serum calcium level fell from 11.1 to 8.9 mg/dl, and the mean serum phosphorus level rose from 2.8 to 3.9 mg/dl. Follow-up study from 9 months to 12 years postoperatively documented maintenance of normal calcium values in these patients. Postoperative persistent hypercalcemia occurred in four patients (1.7%); all of whom required reoperation. There were no deaths or permanent hypocalcemia in this series and there was no recurrent laryngeal nerve palsy. There were six minor complications—a corneal abrasion, a superficial bleeding wound controlled with a subcutaneous suture, one stitch abscess, one postoperative gouty attack, an episode of superficial thrombophlebitis, and one prolonged attack of hypocalcemia lasting four months.

From this study, we have found that not all patients with asymptomatic hyperparathyroidism require surgical correction. If the disease is mild and remains stable, we elect to defer surgery. We believe that mild hypercalcemia will pose little or no risk for them. When the symptoms are mild, certain inherent features of the disease may make surgical treatment difficult at this stage. These are: (1) the characteristic smallness of the glands in the early stage that makes them hard to find; (2) the fact that the pathologic diagnosis is not always clearcut and may be impossible to interpret; and (3) the fact that it is difficult to distinguish a moderately hypercellular parathyroid from a normal gland. For these reasons, surgical exploration should be postponed.

SUMMARY

Our current policy in the management of patients with asymptomatic hyperparathyroidism is to follow expectantly those asymptomatic patients with mild hypercalcemia. We recommend surgery when there is evidence of progression of the disease, when there are relatively more severe biochemical abnormalities, and in a young patient or a menopausal woman. The patient under discussion has a relatively severe hyperparathyroidism and, although asymptomatic, by our criteria should be a surgical candidate.

BIBLIOGRAPHY

1. Bileziuian JP: The medical management of primary hyperparathyroidism. *Ann Intern Med* 1982; 97:142–143.
2. Gaz R, Wang C: Management of asymptomatic hyperparathyroidism. *Am J Surg* 1984; 147:498–502.
3. Graham JJ, Harding PE, Hoare L, et al: Asymptomatic hyperparathyroidism: An assessment of operative intervention. *Br J Surg* 1980; 67:115–118.
4. Russel CF, Edis AJ: Surgery for primary hyperparathyroidism: Experience with 500 consecutive cases and evaluation of the role of surgery in the asymptomatic patient. *Br J Surg* 1982; 69:244–247.

35

Zollinger-Ellison Syndrome

A 43-year-old woman complains of severe epigastric pain occasionally relieved by antacid and partially responsive to histamine H_2 blockers. Six years ago she underwent parathyroidectomy, with the return of an elevated calcium level to normal. Upper gastrointestinal (GI) series reveals not only an ulceration in the first portion of the duodenum but also an ulceration in the third portion of the duodenum and perhaps in the proximal jejunum as well. The gastric mucosa is "wet" and does not coat well with barium.

Consultant: Robert M. Zollinger, M.D.

The clinical symptoms of this patient, the partial response to intense antacid therapy, a history of hyperparathyroidism, and the classic findings of a gastrinoma by upper GI series strongly support the diagnosis of the syndrome of multiple endocrine neoplasia (MEN), type I. I would inquire whether any member of her family had had similar complaints and findings.

DIAGNOSTIC APPROACH

The patient must be made comfortable while various diagnostic tests are performed. Constant gastric suction would undoubtedly provide that comfort as well as document the fact that she is probably making more than the diagnostic 10 mEq of hydrochloric acid every hour. The presence of free acid is essential to establishing a diagnosis of gastrinoma since there are multiple causes of hypochlorhydria, including failing kidneys, that can be associated with hypergastrinemia. The gastric intubation should remain in place several days to determine the frequency and amount of medication required to maintain the gastric acid output below 10 mEq/hour. During this period, determination of serum gastrin levels should be repeated for several days.

If the gastrin level is only marginally elevated, the secretin "push" test should be performed. This consists of the intravenous administration of 2 clinical units of Swedish secretin per kilogram of body weight within 30 seconds. Blood for determination of gastrin levels is taken within 5, 10, 15, 20, 25, and 30 minutes. If the gastrin level rises 200 pg or more, the diagnosis of gastrinoma is strongly supported.

In addition, serum calcium and parathormone levels should be measured since recurrent hyperparathyroidism is not unusual in a patient with the MEN-I syndrome. It has been proposed by Brandi et al. that a mitogenic factor may be responsible for this clinical occurrence. In addition, a more complete endocrine survey can be initiated that should include tests for a prolactinoma and a pheochromocytoma. While the tests are being carried out, the patient should be given sufficient antacid or H_2-receptor antagonist therapy with drugs such as famotidine or omeprazole, if available, to remain comfortable. The patient should be informed concerning the importance of taking the medication as prescribed without fail.

Unless there is evidence of a second endocrine tumor that requires surgical intervention, the best interests of this patient will be served if immediate steps are taken by scans and angiography to locate a gastrinoma in the pancreas and metastases in adjacent lymph nodes or liver. Even when these increasingly accurate tests are negative, a gastrinoma may be found in approximately 25% of these patients.

MANAGEMENT OF GASTRINOMAS

Unfortunately, the gastrinoma remains the only pancreatic islet cell tumor about which there has been consistent debate concerning management. Our medical colleagues tend to be satisfied indefinitely with control of the hormonal effects of these tumors while surgeons are concerned about the malignant potential of the gastrinoma that, according to Thompson et al., has functioning metastases in two thirds of the patients.

When the gastrinoma syndrome was first described in 1955, there were no effective medications available to control the marked gastric hypersecretion. The traditional ulcer operations failed, leaving the removal of all acid-secreting surface by total gastrectomy, a lifesaving procedure. As new drugs became available, it became obvious that patients with gastrinoma could be made comfortable for varying periods of time, which might well exceed ten years. Unfortunately, the tumor continues to grow and the metastases often become more extensive, producing increasing amounts of hormone, and thus ever increasing amounts of medication are required. It must be admitted that the new drugs are very effective in controlling symptoms, but disagreeable side effects can occur. Furthermore, a rigid medication routine is not only difficult to adhere to for many years but also very expensive. Palliation may be accomplished, but the patient with a malignancy should be given every chance for cure.

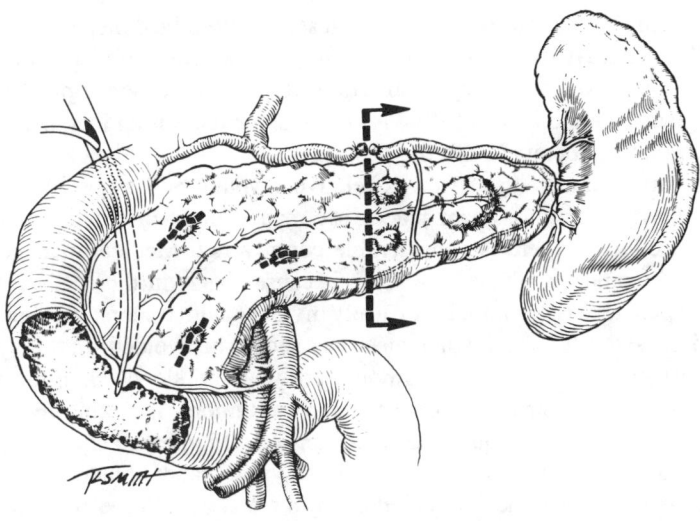

FIG 35–1.
Location of incisions for tumors in head and neck of the pancreas. Multiple tumors in the body and tail are removed by hemipancreatectomy. (Modified from Zollinger RM: Gastrinoma: The Zollinger-Ellison Syndrome, in Scott HW Jr, Sawyer JL (eds): *Surgery of the Stomach and Duodenum.* Boston, Blackwell Scientific Publications, 1988, p 740. Used by permission.)

SURGICAL APPROACH

Early diagnosis and localization of the gastrinoma by scans and angiography have greatly increased the chance of surgical removal of the tumor. Certainly the incidence of complete surgical excision of one or more gastrinomas has increased, with an increasing rate of cure that may approach 20%. The surgical treatment is best managed by a surgeon who is familiar with pancreatic and gastric surgery. Left hemipancreatectomy for tumor in the left half of the pancreas has long been performed, but surgeons have been too hesitant to remove tumor from the head and neck of the pancreas aggressively. It may be helpful to make the incision over the tumor and parallel to the estimated course of the major pancreatic duct in the region of the head and neck of the pancreas. Tumors in the left half of the pancreas are removed by hemipancreatectomy (Fig 35–1). The current trend is to be quite aggressive in searching for, finding, and removing the gastrinoma, regardless of where it is located, even though more than one tumor is found.

If we believe that all gastrinoma has been resected and no metastatic lymph nodes or metastases to the liver are present, we would not hestitate to perform a truncal vagotomy and pyloroplasty. In addition, we have ligated and divided the left gastric artery to decrease gastric vascularity. In poor-risk or elderly patients, or when a gastrinoma cannot be found, a conservative gastric procedure should be considered. However, in the presence of retained metastases or tumor within the pancreas that cannot be resected, we would perform a total gastric resection with a Roux-en-Y reconstruction. At the time of the exploration, both adrenal glands should be carefully visualized since there is an increase in tumors of the adrenals associated with the gastrinoma.

The patient under discussion is relatively young and a good risk, but the history of hyperparathyroidism places her management in another category in which, once again, there is considerable controversy. Medical management of this patient would be advised by some because she is in the MEN-I group in which the pancreas is commonly diffusely involved with tumors, making surgical cure an impossibility. Total pancreatectomy should be avoided. In this syndrome there is a consensus that the gastrinoma grows more slowly than the solitary, so-called sporadic gastrinoma. Other endocrine tumors, including recurrent hyperparathyroidism, may require surgical excision. If hyperparathyroidism should recur in this patient, the removal of $3^1/_2$ parathyroid glands should be performed, marking the location of the residual gland by a metal clip. Some prefer to implant very small fragments of the removed parathyroid glands into the muscle of the nondominant forearm.

Over the years, we have been impressed that these patients are more comfortable during long-term survival when they have had a total gastrectomy. We have not been impressed that there is a significant difference in the more than 10- to 15-year survival after total gastrectomy in the MEN-I patients and those with gastrinoma only.

It can be hoped that in this patient a localized tumor would be suggested by either the scans or angiograms. If it appeared reasonably certain that all gastrinoma had been excised from the pancreas, frozen sections of any enlarged lymph nodes were negative for tumor, and angiography failed to show metastases, I would favor truncal vagotomy, pyloroplasty, and ligation of the left gastric artery. If there was clear-cut evidence that tumor had been left behind, I would perform a total gastrectomy with Roux-en-Y anastomosis. Prolonged survivals have been observed when large metastatic lymph nodes have been resected. Survival with metastases to the liver is limited, but some patients survive for ten years or more.

POSTOPERATIVE COURSE

Regardless of the decisions concerning treatment for this patient's gastrinoma, she is a candidate for recurrent hyperparathyroidism, and there is an increased possibility that she may develop a prolactinoma or adrenal tumor.

Nutrition is surprisingly good in patients with gastrinomas after total gastrectomy. In addition to routinely receiving cyanocobalamin, the caloric intake must be monitored and body weight recorded. The onset of digestive symptoms may be related to stenosis of the esophageal anastomosis, gallstones, or may signal the continued growth of tumor.

The postoperative course extends indefinitely and is unpredictable. Low postoperative gastrin levels may be gradually replaced by rising levels. Our first patient showed an increasing gastrin level that began to rise 25 years after total gastrectomy and excision of a local pancreatic tumor as well as metastasis in a small lymph node (Fig 35–2). Tests for pheochromocytoma, prolactinoma, or recurrent hyperparathyroidism should be repeated every few years in each patient.

The gastrinoma tends to defy an accurate prognosis or yield to the microscope its degree of malignancy for the present or the future. Chemotherapy of various types has been reported, with varying degrees of success. Chlorozotrocin is the only drug that we have observed to have an obvious beneficial effect after varying periods of time.

SUMMARY

The gastrinoma is being recognized earlier and probably more frequently every year. It is time to accept the fact that ridding the patient of this malignant tumor should be the major concern of all physicians. Early surgical intervention will give this patient the best chance for cure or at least effective palliation from the hormonal effects of the tumor. Despite the fact that this patient probably has two endocrine tumors, there is a reasonable chance of prolonged survival over 10 to 15 years.

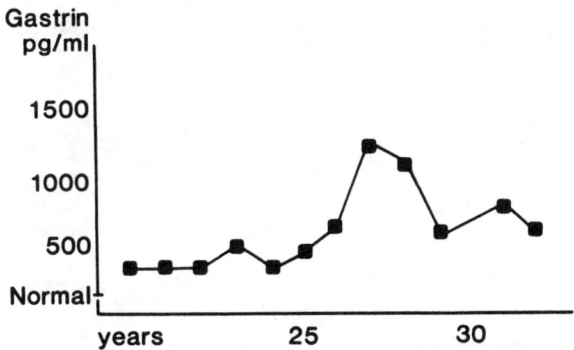

FIG 35–2.
Postoperative gastrin levels in one patient over a period of 32 years.

BIBLIOGRAPHY

1. Brandi ML, Aurbach GD, Fitzpatrick LA, et al: Parathyroid mitogenic activity in plasma from patients with familial multiple endocrine neoplasia type I. *N Engl J Med* 1986; 314:1287–1292.
2. Thompson JC, Greeley GH, Rayford PL, et al (eds): *Gastrointestinal Endocrinology.* New York, McGraw Hill Book Co, 1987.
3. Zollinger RM, Ellison EC, O'Dorisio TM, et al: Thirty years' experience with gastrinoma. *World J Surg* 1984; 8:427–435.

36

Adrenal Cortical Tumor

A 38-year-old woman presents with pain and heaviness in the right upper quadrant. Physical examination reveals a question of a mass that does not descend with respiration. An adrenal mass is present on the right on computed tomography (CT) scan. Level of urinary catecholamines is reported as normal.

Consultant: Donald S. Gann, M.D.

In the management of this case, two critical questions arise. First, is the adrenal mass functioning? Second, is there a malignancy of the adrenal, and, if so, is this a primary adrenal tumor or is it metastatic?

CLINICAL PRESENTATION

The suspicion of adrenal hyperfunction can frequently be aroused by elements in the history. In the case of pheochromocytoma, there may be a history of paroxysmal headache, sweating, light-headedness, or flushing. Similarly, in the case of Cushing's syndrome, the patient may reveal hirsutism, uncontrollable weight gain, and menstrual irregularities. The symptoms associated with primary aldosteronism are more subtle; however, in the full-blown case, polydypsia, polyuria, and weakness are all related to potassium depletion and are frequently present. Although none of these historical features is diagnostic, the presence of any one or more should raise the suspicion of the investigating physician and lead him/her to do definitive laboratory workup.

Except in the case of Cushing's syndrome, the physical examination may be relatively nonrevealing. Occasionally, however, the physical examination may reveal paroxysmal hypertension or orthostatic hypotension, both suggestive of pheochromocytoma. The stigmata of Cushing's syndrome include truncal obesity, moon facies, buffalo hump, and purple striae. Patients with full-blown cases are unmistakable; however, when the stigmata are expressed only partially, they may be confused with subjects with mild hirsutism, weight gain with noncolored striations, and generalized obesity. Again, laboratory tests are required to distinguish such patients from those with true Cushing's syndrome. Besides muscle weakness, there is nothing to be noted on the physical examination of a patient with primary aldosteronism except hypertension.

DIAGNOSIS

Laboratory tests are the primary means of excluding or diagnosing the three primary causes of adrenal hyperfunction in the adult. In the present case, the level of urinary catecholamines has been reported as normal. The finding of an elevated level of urinary catecholamines may be diagnostic of pheochromocytoma, and false-positives are rare; however, false-negatives are not uncommon. The measurement of urinary metanephrines (with an upper limit of excretion of 1 ng/day) probably represents the most sensitive and specific urinary test for pheochromocytoma. However, it is notoriously difficult to collect a complete 24-hour urine sample, even in the hospital setting, so that the validity of a negative test must be questioned. Bravo and colleagues have noted in a large series from the Cleveland Clinic that tests measuring plasma catecholamines are more sensitive and more specific, and in their view measurement of these catecholamines represent the ultimate test for this disease. I prefer to measure plasma catecholamines after the patient has been resting 20 minutes in the supine position, and after the patient has been standing 15 minutes subsequently. In the absence of pheochromocytoma, plasma values fall in the normal range when the patient is supine, and essentially double when the erect posture is assumed. Patients with pheochromocytoma may have a paradoxical fall from an elevated value or may have an exaggerated rise in the standing position. In the latter case, the baroceptor reflex has acted as a provocative test.

Cushing's syndrome is best diagnosed or excluded by the overnight dexamethasone suppression test. In this test, plasma cortisol is measured at 8:00 a.m. on one day. Dexamethasone, 1 mg, is administered orally between 10:00 p.m. and midnight that evening, and the level of plasma cortisol is measured again the following morning. Normal subjects suppress more than 50%, and generally to less than 5 µg/dl after the single dose of dexamethasone. This test is to be preferred to urinary measurements or to attempts at detecting a loss of circadian rhythm, because of the difficulty of urinary collection and because episodic secretion of cortisol, which may be maintained in Cushing's syndrome and is uniformly present in normal subjects, may lead to false conclusions concerning circadian evaluation.

The diagnosis of primary aldosteronism or its exclusion requires the measurement of renin activity when the patient is on a low-salt diet and standing, and the measurement of plasma aldosterone when the patient is on a normal sodium intake and in the resting supine position. The diagnosis is made by the findings of suppressed renin activity despite sodium restriction in the erect posture of an elevated level of plasma aldosterone despite normal sodium intake and the supine posture. The failure to find this combination excludes primary aldosteronism.

The CT scan may also be helpful in the diagnosis of benign adrenal lesions. The benign tumor tends to have regular margins, and these are uniformly distinguishable from surrounding strictures such as kidneys, cava, aorta, and liver. Size alone is not a good index of malignancy in the functioning adrenal tumor, although it is true that small tumors tend to be benign. However, even in the case of aldosterone-producing adenomas, which tend to be quite small, one may occasionally see a mass as large as 8 cm in a perfectly benign adenoma.

The diagnosis of malignancy metastatic to the adrenal depends upon the identification of these malignancies. Since the most common tumor metastatic to the adrenal is cancer of the lung, one should note carefully the presence of cough, hemoptysis, or prolonged smoking history. The presence of risk factors for breast cancer should also be noted, since this tumor is the second most common that metastases to the adrenal in women. Physical examination should similarly address areas of altered ventilation or density in the lungs, or suspicious lesions in the breast. The presence of a palpable abdominal mass in the absence of adrenal hyperfunction should make one suspicious of a malignancy, and this may be the situation in the present case. However, even if there is a palpable mass, there is a substantial likelihood that it will prove to be not a malignant tumor but rather a myelolipoma of the adrenal. These may grow to an extremely large size, and pain and pressure are frequently the only presenting symptoms.

The CT scans will be extremely helpful in the diagnosis of malignancy without hyperfunction. The metastatic adrenal tumor tends to be eccentric and irregular, whereas the primary adrenal tumor tends to have regular borders, except where the tumor may invade surrounding structures. The absence of distinct margins, and especially invasion of the vena cava, the renal vein, or direct extension into the liver, kidney, or pancreas, will establish the diagnosis of a malignancy. The presence of enlarged nodes in the region of the adrenal will also increase suspicion of a malignant lesion. Myelolipoma can be identified by the low density of much of the tissue, although these tumors regularly contain significant amounts of dense vascular stroma as well. It should be noted parenthetically that they should be removed because of the risk of hemorrhage that may occur and be massive in the absence of any warning signs. If the tumor is of primary origin, as determined by the absence of other primary malignancies and by the shape of the mass, then size may be an important determinant of the need for surgery. There is general agreement that adrenal masses larger than 6 cm should be removed because of the suspicion of malignancy, and that those 3 cm or smaller may be followed up without surgery unless there is evidence of hyperfunction. Various workers have different criteria in the 3- to 6-cm range, and general rules may be swayed by features in the history or examination of the patient. Not surprisingly, most surgeons appear to have a lower threshold than many of their internist colleagues. There are also a few laboratory tests that may be useful in the diagnosis of functioning adrenal malignancies. The identification of 3-methoxytyramine in the plasma may be suggestive of a malignant pheochromocytoma. Similarly, the finding of a grossly elevated level of 17-ketosteroids in the urine or of an elevated level of DHEA (dehydroepiandrostenedione) or DHEA-sulfate in the plasma should lead to the suspicion of a functioning adrenocortical malignancy.

SURGICAL APPROACH

The surgical approach will be guided by the studies cited above. If the tumor is thought to be benign, hyperfunctioning, and adrenocortical in origin, it should be approached posteriorly. I use the approach described first by Hugh Young and popularized by Reginald Smithwick. The skin is opened through a hockey stick incision extending from 3 cm lateral to the spine at the level of the ninth rib to approximately 5 cm lateral to the spinus process at the iliac crest. The 12th rib is resected up to its junction with the transverse process of the vertebra dividing the intercostal vessels, but preserving the intercostal nerve. The pleura is swept off the posterior surface of the diaphragm and the latter is then incised between a series of metal clips, carrying this incision superiorly and medially. Access to the vessels is easy through this approach. Respiratory complications are minimal, and gastrointestinal complications are virtually absent. Characteristically, the patient can eat within 24 hours of surgery and may be discharged from the hospital quickly. If the tumor is thought to be benign and is nonfunctioning, it should be followed up. Subsequent removal should be mandated by growth or the appearance of evidence of hyperfunction. If such removal is ultimately carried out for hyperfunction, the above approach is indicated. If it is carried out for suspicion of malignancy, however, the posterior approach is unsatisfactory.

If a malignant tumor of the adrenal is thought to be metastatic, CT guided needle biopsy is indicated. Confirmation of cancer of the lung or breast metastatic to the adrenal obviates the need for further surgery and stages the disease at the same time. The classic approach to primary adrenal malignancies is through a thoracoabdominal incision that is extended through the ninth inner space. The diaphragm is divided to allow retraction of the liver and exposure of the adrenal. Flank incisions have also been used, especially when the procedure has been carried out by a urologist. I personally prefer to explore the patient through a vertical midline incision to determine the need for extension and to ensure that resection is possible. Frequently, a mass can be removed on the left side without further extension of the incision. If the mass is clearly malignant, the adrenal should be removed with the fat of Gerota's fascia, possibly including the kidney

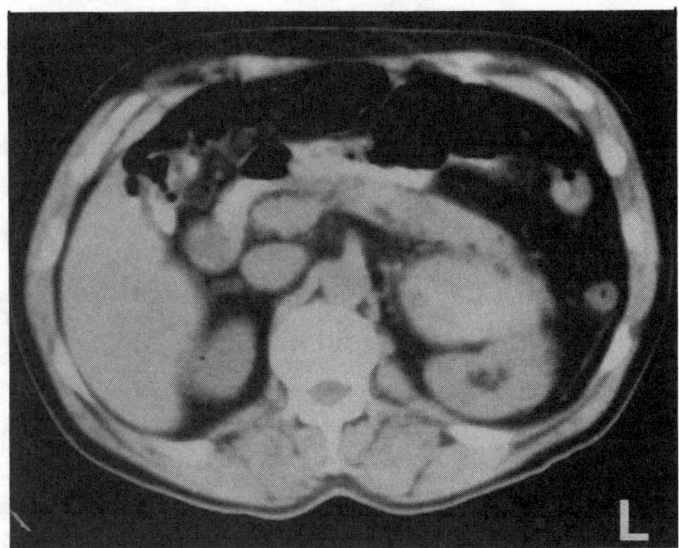

FIG 36–1.
Adrenal carcinoma with extension into liver and vena cava.

(assuming that renal function is normal on the opposite side). Such a resection is mandated by direct extension into the kidney on the left side. The tumor may extend into the tail of the pancreas, requiring distal pancreatectomy as well. A typical case is shown in Figure 36–1. For right-sided adrenal tumors, I have come to prefer medium sternotomy to extension into the right side of the chest. The exposure is just as good, and the subsequent morbidity is less. (*Editor's note:* I agree. As a general rule, sternotomy is preferable to extending the incision into the right side of the chest. The same is true for hepatic resections.) The central tendon of the diaphragm is incised; the right triangular ligament is taken down, and the liver is easily retracted.

Occasionally, the tumor extends directly from the adrenal into the vena cava. Rarely, this extension may be down the adrenal vein into the cava without involvement of the wall of the vena cava, as is seen in renal cell carcinoma. However, it is not uncommon to see direct extension through the wall of the cava. If this is small, the cava may be resected and patched. However, it is not uncommon to see the combination of direct involvement of the cava, and much of its circumference associated with direct extension to the liver. One such case is shown in Figure 36–2. The combination of spread into the liver and into the cava, when massive as in the case shown, may prevent satisfactory resection. Even when the tumor is resectable, adrenocortical carcinoma is associated with dismal postsurgical results. Accordingly, most workers choose to use orthopara DDD as adjuvant therapy since this DDT analog will destroy adrenal tissue. If

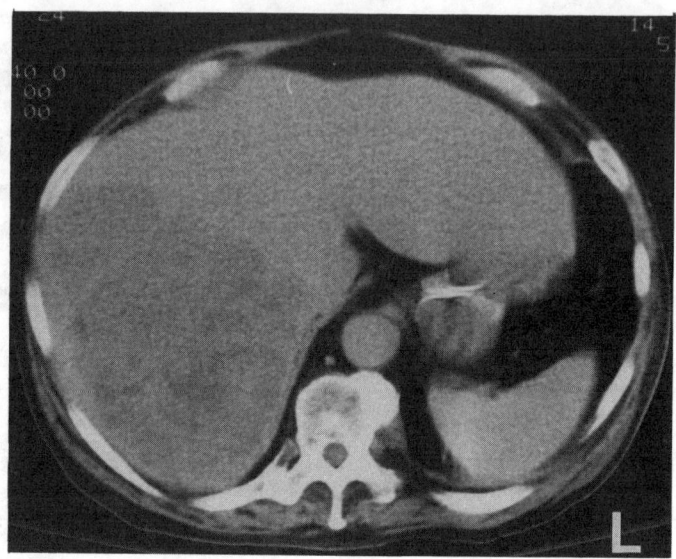

FIG 36–2.
Adrenal carcinoma with extension into left kidney and attached to pancreas.

this is used, it will inevitably produce adrenal insufficiency, and the patient will need replacement steroids. On a few occasions, I have seen previously unresectable tumors regress to the point of being resectable. However, this sort of gratifying response is rare, and one cannot depend upon it.

In the present case, assuming that there is no adrenocortical hyperfunction, I would opt for removal of the tumor. I would use an anterior approach because of the suspicion of malignancy, and I would take a portion of Gerota's fascia without the kidney if there was no evidence of extension of the tumor or metastases to regional nodes. It should be noted that the pathologist can make the diagnosis of adrenocortical malignancy only by identification of the tissue outside of the adrenal gland in the surrounding fat nodes or in adjacent organs. The presence of mitoses in normal adrenal tissue obviates the use of this criterion. If there were signs of extension, I would do a radical nephrectomy as the procedure of choice, extending this only as guided by local invasion. I would emphasize to the patient and to her family that the prognosis is guarded.

BIBLIOGRAPHY

1. Bravo EI, Tarzi RC, Gifford RW, et al: Circulating and primary catecholamine in pheochromocytoma: Diagnostic and pathophysiologic implications. *N Engl J Med* 1979; 301:682–686.

2. Gann DS, DeMaria EJ, Campbell RW: Adrenal gland, in Davis JG (ed): *Clinical Surgery*. St Louis, CV Mosby Co, 1987.
3. Gann DS, DeMaria EJ: The adrenals, in Schwartz SI, Shires GT, Spencer FC, et al (eds): *Principles of Surgery*, ed 5. New York, McGraw-Hill Book Co, in press.

PART V

Small and Large Intestine

- SMA emboli Rx: embolectomy
- SMA Thromby Rx: Ao-mesenteric bypass c̄ autogenous vein
- Aortography is the most specific diagnostic test.
- mortality 80-100%
- Prophylactic revascularization of pts c̄ chronic intestinal ischemia is to be encouraged.

37

Acute Mesenteric Artery Thrombosis

A 70-year-old woman presented with the gradual onset of abdominal pain and distention. Approximately five years earlier, she had suffered a severe myocardial infarction and had been in mild congestive heart failure ever since that time. Her present illness began approximately 72 hours prior to admission, with the gradual onset of crampy abdominal pain, vomiting, and diarrhea. On examination, her abdomen was distended and she had hypoactive bowel sounds, but there was no focal tenderness or peritoneal signs. Her nasogastric aspirate was guaiac negative, and stool obtained on rectal examination was trace positive for blood. The white blood cell count, on admission, was 16,000/cu mm but increased to 22,000/cu mm over the next six hours. A flat plate of the abdomen was nondiagnostic, showing only some distended small bowel loops with scattered air fluid levels. Because of the rising white blood cell count and abdominal findings, the patient was taken to the operating room. At laparotomy, the entire small bowel and right part of the colon were dusky and cyanotic, and no pulse was palpable in the superior mesenteric artery at the base of the transverse mesocolon.

Consultant: Richard F. Kempczinski, M.D.

Although acute mesenteric arterial occlusion is infrequently encountered by most general surgeons, its management remains particularly frustrating because of a persistently high operative mortality and the difficulty in establishing an accurate preoperative diagnosis. A majority of the patients with acute mesenteric arterial insufficiency have embolic occlusion of the superior mesenteric artery (SMA) and present with the classic triad—heart disease, with or without arrhythmia; severe, acute abdominal pain with relatively insignificant physical findings in comparison to their symptoms; and vomiting, with or without diarrhea. Given this presentation, the diagnosis is usually obvious and such patients will be taken to the operating room promptly. If the bowel is not extensively gangrenous at the time of exploration, the mesenteric vascular insufficiency can usually be reversed by embolectomy alone, and 40% to 50% of such patients will survive.

Unfortunately, the onset of symptoms in patients with acute SMA thrombosis is much more insidious; diagnosis is accordingly more difficult; surgical therapy is often delayed, and the results of treatment are predictably dismal. Clearly, if these results are to be improved, clinical suspicion for this condition must be high if patients fall into certain recognized high-risk groups, and diagnosis and treatment must be prompt and appropriate.

CLINICAL FEATURES

The presentation described above is quite typical for patients with this condition. They are often elderly, usually in the seventh or eighth decade of life. Women outnumber men and frequently there will be an antecedent history of other manifestations of their atherosclerosis, especially in the form of coronary artery disease. Patients often suffer from congestive heart failure, with or without cardiac arrhythmias. Because the onset of their symptoms is insidious, there is frequently a delay of one to several days before seeking medical assistance.

Abdominal pain is invariably present. Initially, it may be colicky and periumbilical, but it soon becomes severe, poorly localized, and continuous. Unlike the pain experienced by patients with mesenteric artery embolus, thrombosis of the SMA usually results in a gradual, more insidious onset of pain and abdominal distention, thus mimicking bowel obstruction rather than mesenteric infarction. Although associated symptoms, such as vomiting, nausea, diarrhea, melena, and hematemesis may occur, they are rarely the predominant complaint and are seldom helpful in narrowing the differential diagnosis.

Although abdominal tenderness is present in most patients, it is not usually localized. Early in the course of the disease, the abdominal findings may be relatively insignificant compared to the patient's restlessness, apprehension, and hyperactivity, but hypotension is rarely present. An important physical finding, as reported by Williams, is abdominal distention, despite audible peristalsis. This finding may not be present early in the course of the disease, but it invariably develops after 12 to 24 hours. Evidence of gastrointestinal bleeding can be found in most patients, but it is seldom gross except when colon ischemia is present. If there is a delay in seeking medical attention, the patient may present with significant dehydration, hemoconcentration, and hypotension. Acidosis and leukocytosis are usually prominent findings late in the course of illness. The white blood cell count on presentation usually ranges between 10,000 to 20,000/cu mm but within 12 to 24 hours it almost invariably rises above 20,000/cu mm.

In many patients with SMA thrombosis, an antecedent history of intestinal angina and weight loss can be elicited. Characteristically, this pain occurs 15 to 20 minutes after eating, and it is of such severity that the patients voluntarily refrain from eating once they recognize the association between meals and the onset of their symptoms. This self-imposed starvation results in weight loss that may be quite significant and should further reinforce the suspicion of mesenteric vascular disease.

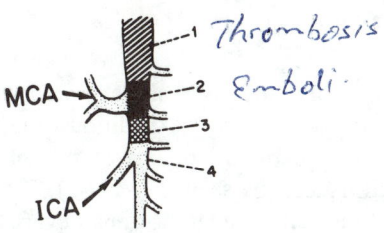

FIG 37–1.
The superior mesenteric artery (SMA) can be divided into four zones based on the origins of the middle colic (MCA) and ileocolic (ICA) arteries. The SMA thrombosis invariably involves zone 1, while emboli usually lodge in zone 2 or beyond. (From Ottinger LW: *Ann Surg* 1978; 188:722. Used by permission.)

DIAGNOSIS

Traditional abdominal plain films are generally of little value, since their findings are typically nonspecific. The presence of intramural gas within the bowel wall or gas in the portal system are unusual findings that occur only in the most advanced cases of mesenteric infarction when it is already too late for effective surgical management. Another nonspecific finding is diffuse small bowel distention with air fluid levels, as was seen in this patient. Typically, the distention involves the entire small bowel and colon up to the splenic flexure (the so-called colon cutoff sign). Perhaps the greatest value of abdominal plain films is in helping to exclude other potential causes for abdominal pain.

The most specific diagnostic test in these patients is adequate *aortography*. It should be considered promptly in all high-risk patients in whom other causes of abdominal pain can be excluded. In order to visualize the origin of both superior mesenteric and celiac arteries, a lateral aortogram must be obtained. Typically, the SMA will be occluded at its origin and collateral vessels will be poorly developed. (*Editor's note:* Patients must be adequately hydrated before this and other angiographic studies in order to minimize the nephrotoxicity of the angiography contrast material.)

In patients with SMA embolus, the clot rarely lodges at the origin of the artery and is more typically found immediately distal to the ileocolic artery (Fig 37–1). It is this sparing of the middle colic artery and the usual absence of disease in the celiac artery that is responsible for the more limited bowel necrosis seen in patients with SMA embolus. Unfortunately, SMA thrombosis usually occurs in patients with severe atherosclerotic stenosis of both superior mesenteric and celiac arteries. When thrombosis occurs, it often propagates distally, and collateral development is impaired because of the associated stenosis in the celiac artery. Accordingly, the extent of bowel involvement is characteristically more extensive.

SURGICAL TREATMENT

Once the diagnosis of acute visceral ischemia is established, the patient should be aggressively resuscitated and expeditiously taken to the operating room for revascularization. At exploration, one of two characteristic patterns of bowel involvement will usually be seen (Fig 37–2). Patients with SMA embolus will have ischemia of the central small bowel and variable portions of the colon, with sparing of the proximal jejunum. By contrast, thrombotic occlusion of the SMA produces a variable pattern of ischemia, but it usually involves the entire small bowel and varying amounts of the large bowel. Specifically, the proximal portion of the jejunum is involved as well as the central small bowel. When the celiac artery is also involved, the duodenum may be ischemic as well.

The diagnosis of mesenteric arterial occlusion can be confirmed by palpating the SMA at the base of the transverse mesocolon. In patients with embolic occlusion, the proximal portion of the SMA will usually be soft and have a strong pulse that ends abruptly at the site of embolus. In patients with thrombotic occlusion, pulsations will be absent in the proximal portion of the artery, and the atherosclerotic involvement of the adjacent aorta and its visceral branches

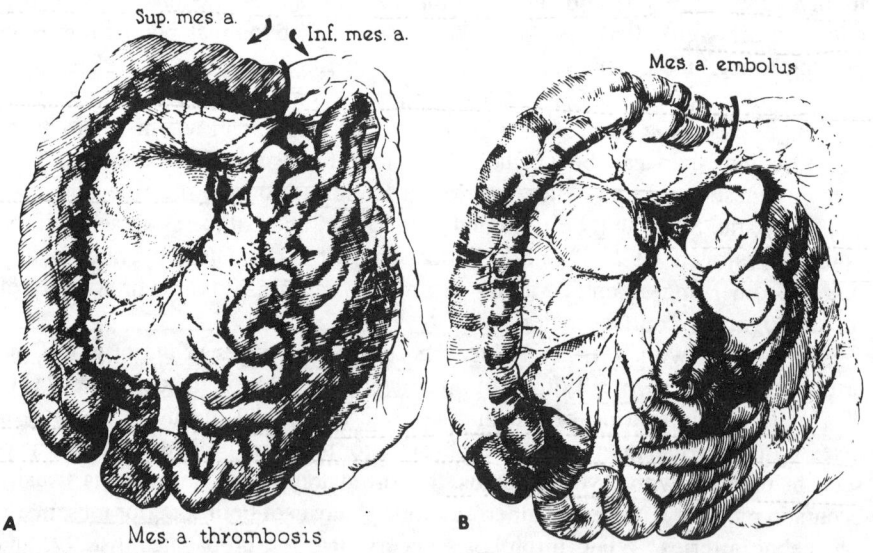

FIG 37–2.
The SMA thrombosis usually results in cyanosis/gangrene of the entire small bowel and right colon **(A)**, while embolus generally spares proximal jejunum **(B)**. (From Bergan JJ: *Surg Clin North Am* 1967; 47:109. Used by permission.)

may often be apparent. If the celiac artery is also diseased, it or its branches will have an absence of pulsations.

Once SMA occlusion is recognized, the surgeon must decide whether to revascularize the artery prior to bowel resection. Resection without revascularization is invariably doomed to failure, as reported by Bergan and colleagues. In patients in whom there is a significant delay between the onset of symptoms and surgical intervention, the entire small bowel and colon may be irreversibly gangrenous at the time of celiotomy. In such patients, revascularization with or without bowel resection will be futile, since the outcome is inevitably fatal. (*Editor's note:* With the currently available techniques of home parenteral nutrition, even if only 6 in. of proximal jejunum are viable and can be anastomosed to a viable portion of the left colon, patients may survive for years provided they can be sustained through a stormy postoperative period.) However, in most patients, even in those with some frankly gangrenous portions of bowel, there will often be significant intestine that is cyanotic but potentially viable. Since it is usually impossible to predict which bowel loops will recover, revascularization should almost always be performed prior to bowel resection. Unlike patients with SMA embolus, in whom revascularization can usually be accomplished simply by removal of the embolus and closure of the arteriotomy with a vein patch, patients with SMA thrombosis usually present a much more challenging technical problem. Simple thrombectomy rarely results in durable revascularization, since the proximal stenosis that resulted in the thrombosis cannot be removed through a distal arteriotomy.

Since the origin of the SMA and adjacent aorta is not easily accessible, most surgeons favor a distal aortomesenteric bypass for visceral revascularization. If there has been distal propagation of the thrombus prior to surgical exploration, it may be necessary to perform an initial balloon catheter thromboembolectomy prior to insertion of the bypass graft. This must be performed with great care, since the artery and its distal branches are quite small and delicate and can be easily traumatized by excessively vigorous thrombectomy. Once a patent distal vessel has been assured, a bypass should be constructed using a segment of autogenous saphenous vein. Although prosthetic grafts have been successfully used for elective revascularization of chronically occluded mesenteric arteries, they are generally inappropriate in acute SMA thrombosis, since the presence of infarcted bowel will result in bacterial contamination of these prosthetic grafts and may result in the dreaded complication of intraabdominal prosthetic vascular graft infection. Once a satisfactory vein graft has been harvested, the distal anastomosis to the SMA can be performed first, followed by the proximal anastomosis to a soft segment of the aorta or iliac artery. The graft should be kept as short as possible to avoid kinking when the intestines are replaced within the abdomen.

Following completion of the anastomoses and restoration of flow, a sterile

Doppler velocity meter probe can be used to document the adequacy of the revascularization. Restoration of a pulsatile arterial signal on the antimesenteric border of the bowel wall is usually a good sign of viability. Some authors have been dissatisfied with the use of the Doppler velocity meter to predict bowel viability; instead they recommend the use of intravenous fluorescein as a more discriminate technique.

If the patient is stable, the surgeon will have to decide whether to proceed with adjunctive revascularization of the occluded celiac artery. Although most vascular surgeons now favor multiple bypasses in patients with chronic visceral artery occlusion, this approach is more controversial in these critically ill patients in whom bowel resection will be required, since the additional dissection and time required to perform such bypasses will often be poorly tolerated. In most patients, single vessel revascularization of the SMA will be adequate to reverse the ischemic changes without exposing the patient to the risk of additional operating time and blood loss. However, if the patient is stable and the bowel ischemia appears to be entirely reversible without need for resection, consideration should be given to performing revascularization of the celiac artery if it is occluded or highly stenotic. This can be performed by entering the lesser sac and performing an additional vein bypass from the suprarenal aorta to the celiac artery or one of its major branches. The anesthesiologist should be alerted prior to release of the vascular clamps and restoration of blood flow, since this maneuver may result in acidosis and hypotension as toxic by-products of intestinal ischemia are returned to the venous circulation.

Following revascularization, the bowel wall may remain cyanotic for a variable period of time. In order to speed reversal of this condition, we replace the intestines in the abdominal cavity that is then irrigated copiously with several liters of warm, normal saline or Ringer's lactate solution. The intestines are covered with warm, moist laparotomy pads and the anesthesiologist is given time to resuscitate the patient. After a period of 20 to 30 minutes, the entire bowel should be carefully reexamined and any sections that are clearly nonviable should be resected. Primary anastomoses of the remaining viable segments can be performed, using whatever technique the surgeon prefers.

Following resection of all nonviable bowel segments and restoration of intestinal continuity, the remaining intestine should be replaced within the peritoneal cavity, which is again liberally irrigated with large quantities of warmed normal saline containing an antibiotic of the surgeon's choice. The abdominal incision is then closed in the usual manner and the patient is returned to the intensive care unit where resuscitation and monitoring can be carefully maintained over the next several days.

Second-Look Operation

The decision to perform a repeat laparotomy 24 hours after revascularization of ischemic intestines should be based on the final appearance of the bowel at the original operation, since there is no combination of clinical or laboratory findings in the postoperative period that will infallibly predict the necessity for reexploration, as reported by Ottinger and Austen. At the completion of the original procedure, if the surgeon has serious concerns regarding potential viability of the remaining bowel segments, a planned elective reexploration within 24 hours is preferable to primary resection of marginally viable intestine.

The interval between operations is usually 24 hours, although this may be modified depending on the patient's condition and availability of operating time. Between the first and second operations, the patient should be vigorously resuscitated with correction of any residual acidosis, hypovolemia, and anemia. At the time of reexploration, further resection of ischemic intestine may be performed or the abdominal cavity may be irrigated and closed if all the remaining intestine is clearly viable and the vascular reconstruction is patent.

RESULTS

Despite early and aggressive therapeutic intervention, the surgical results with SMA thrombosis remain dismal. In most reported series, perioperative mortality ranges from 80% to 100%. This is, in part, due to the advanced age and underlying cardiovascular disease that is frequently present. Furthermore, because of the delay in seeking medical attention that is common in these patients, they must often be taken to the operating room while still critically ill and must undergo a major arterial reconstruction followed by extensive bowel resection.

Since approximately 50% of patients who develop acute thrombosis of the SMA will have an antecedent history of chronic intestinal angina, perhaps the most effective means of lowering the mortality from SMA occlusion is by preventing it. If patients with intestinal angina can be identified early and undergo appropriate *elective* revascularization, we may be successful in improving our results in the management of this otherwise lethal condition.

CONCLUSIONS

Superior mesenteric artery thrombosis is a condition that continues to frustrate the best efforts of surgeons. Elderly patients with known coronary artery atherosclerosis and congestive heart failure who present with the insidious onset of vague, generalized abdominal pain and distention should be suspected of having SMA thrombosis when other more common causes of abdominal pain can be excluded. If arteriography confirms the diagnosis, they should undergo revascularization of the superior mesenteric artery, using an autogenous bypass from the aorta or adjacent iliac artery, followed by resection of clearly nonviable bowel. Even with such an aggressive surgical approach, continuing high mortality is to be expected. Accordingly, the most effective management of this condition must include early identification of patients with chronic intestinal angina and referral for prompt prophylactic revascularization of the intestines before thrombosis and infarction occurs.

BIBLIOGRAPHY

1. Bergan JJ, Dean RH, Conn J Jr, et al: Revascularization in treatment of mesenteric infarction. *Ann Surg* 1975; 182:430–438.
2. Ottinger LW: The surgical management of acute occlusion of the superior mesenteric artery. *Ann Surg* 1978; 188:721–731.
3. Ottinger LW, Austen WG: A study of 136 patients with mesenteric infarction. *Surg Gynecol Obstet* 1967; 124:251–261.
4. Williams LF Jr: Vascular insufficiency of the intestines. *Gastroenterology* 1971; 61:757–777.

38

Ileal Fistula

A patient is admitted with intestinal obstruction several years following a cholecystectomy. At the time of laparotomy, there are dense adhesions and great difficulty is experienced in freeing up the small bowel. A point of obstruction in the distal ileum is noted, with a tight band. After lysis of the band, the bowel is initially compromised but finally appears viable. Following operation the patient does not do well, with a fever of 101°F to 102°F and a prolonged ileus. On the fifth postoperative day, induration and fluctuance of the midpoint of the abdominal wound is noted. Wound drainage obtains pus and the patient's fever subsides. On the sixth postoperative day, intestinal contents are noted emanating from the wound.

Consultant: Josef E. Fischer, M.D.

OVERVIEW

The history described is fairly typical of the development of a postoperative fistula. In recent years, a leading cause of gastrointestinal cutaneous fistula has been abdominal surgery for cancer or inflammatory bowel disease. Neoplasm figures prominently in the etiology of fistulas in other ways, with the fistula either developing secondary to spontaneous perforation of malignancy, following postoperative radiation as treatment for malignancy, or following operation.

With the discovery of the fistula or the presentation of a patient transferred from another institution in whom a postoperative fistula has been discovered, the patient has usually suffered five to six days of septic starvation and is often depleted both from the preoperative preparation (e.g., elective colonic resection) or from the effects of chronic disease such as cancer or inflammatory bowel disease. Anemia, hypoalbuminemia, and contraction of both extracellular and intravascular volume are often present. Breakdown of 300 to 500 gm of protein per 24 hours has created a significant deficit in lean body mass.

APPROACH TO THE PATIENT

As with any complicated clinical situation, it is helpful to divide the approach

Sometimes it is useful to obtain a fistulogram before the abscess is drained.

to the patient into a series of phases so that given problems can be dealt with in a temporally logical and efficient manner. However, it is my belief that surgery has lately tended to rely too heavily on protocols and algorithms; despite the fact that these are often useful, they are not etched in stone, nor are they meant to be rigid. As a matter of convenience in the care of patients with fistulas, the five phases are (1) stabilization, (2) investigation, (3) decision, (4) definitive therapy, and (5) healing phase. It should be emphasized that as complicated as these patients are (and even currently prone to a high mortality), with sophisticated monitoring; perioperative support; and respiratory, antibiotic, and nutritional care, a high success rate with respect to closure and survival can be achieved. The care of the patient with fistulas requires excellent surgical judgment and a knowledge of surgical pathophysiology in yielding a successful outcome.

Stabilization

When a patient such as described here presents or is recognized, he/she generally has deficits in plasma volume and extravascular fluid and is anemic. Resuscitation with red blood cells, crystalloid, and colloid sufficient to bring the serum albumin level to 3 to 3.5 gm/dl is appropriate. It is also necessary to refill intravascular volume to make cannulation of the large veins easier for parenteral nutrition. Parenteral nutrition should be instituted as quickly as possible and delayed only for the drainage of obvious abscesses that are pointing toward the abdominal wall, since hematogenous bacterial catheter implantation, while rare, is possible as a source of catheter sepsis. If an abscess pointing toward the abdominal wall is obvious, the patient should be taken to the radiology department; a needle or a small intracath is placed in the abscess; pus is aspirated for appropriate cultures and bacteriologic studies, and a water-soluble dye injected by the surgeon with a radiologist doing the fluoroscopy. Such examinations yield information concerning the extent and anatomy of abscesses and the source of the fistula that are difficult to achieve otherwise. The abscess is then drained.

Some estimates of caloric and protein requirements are appropriate. For those units in which such monitoring is possible, indirect calorimetry, nitrogen balance studies, and measurement of plasma short-turnover proteins are carried out. When protein and caloric equilibrium are achieved, the patient will be in nitrogen balance, and hepatic synthesis of short-turnover proteins (as evidenced by an increase in serum levels) will be detected, with retinol-binding protein increasing earliest; thyroxin-binding prealbumin, second; and transferrin, third. Albumin will not increase, even with increased hepatic protein synthesis of albumin, for at least 10 to 14 days, owing to its long half-life. Caloric and protein requirements may be estimated by various modifications of the Harris-Benedict equation or by indirect calorimetry. In each situation, some adjustment is required. In my experience, either method is equally accurate provided that

Care of wound: ① *Involve enterostomal therapist.*
② *Stomadhesive & Karaya powder*
③ *Sump c̄ Robinson tubes.*

one bears in mind that in indirect calorimetry determinations, some upward adjustment (e.g., 15% to 20%) for activity must be applied.

Nutritional support should not be delayed except for cardiovascular instability during resuscitation. The breakdown of lean body mass is relentless and sufficiently rapid that after five or six days of starvation, particularly septic starvation, significant deficits occur every 24 hours. Patients with fistulas can be treated with chemically defined diets with reasonable success, as reported by Voitk et al. However, since protein and caloric equivalence takes at least three to five days to achieve, parenteral nutrition should be initiated promptly and discontinued only when intake via the gastrointestinal tract is sufficient to meet the patient's estimated caloric and nitrogen needs. ✓

If the gastrointestinal route is elected for nutritional support, a 4 ft segment of small bowel (either above or below the fistula) is required for adequate absorption. One may administer chemically defined diets into the stomach and have them drain out the fistula. Alternatively, it is possible to place a feeding tube in the fistula and administer the diet distally, with the effluent coming out another fistula or water being absorbed in the colon. If the gastrointestinal route is utilized, patients generally tolerate diets better if their serum albumin level is kept above 3.0 gm/dl. Salt-poor albumin is administered to achieve this level.

If a chemically defined diet is chosen for nutritional support, the mode of administration varies with available gut access. The gastrointestinal tract's defense against osmolality is the stomach, which secretes sufficient material to bring the hypertonic chemically defined diet into isosmolar equilibrium prior to transfer across the pylorus. Gastrointestinal tract feeding is best done as a continuous infusion, starting with a hypo-osmolar concentration (e.g., 200 to 300 milliosmol/L at a rate of 50 cc/hour). If the diet is given intragastrically, osmolality should be increased prior to volume. If the diet is given into the jejunum, which cannot "defend itself" against osmolality, volume is increased before osmolality. Remember that a full-strength hyperosmolar diet may not be tolerated by the jejunum, and it may be necessary to give large volumes of relatively dilute chemically defined diets in order to achieve protein and calorie equilibrium.

Finally, as soon as the patient is diagnosed as having a fistula, wound care assumes a high priority since, if reoperation is necessary, one should not operate through a septic, indurated, cellulitic, and denuded abdominal wall. Each surgeon will develop his/her own method of skin care around fistulas. I prefer to apply Stomadhesive or some other protective agent to the wound edges; once adherent, it may be left in place for six to seven days. A sump is essential, and I generally prefer a variable-size Robinson nephrostomy catheter with a No. 14 angiocath, threaded to the tip to break the suction; it is soft and will not erode at room temperature, can be used to aspirate the fistula contents, and its size may be varied depending on the size of the fistula and the character of the effluent. If it is not possible to protect the wound using Stomadhesive, one may use other materials such as karaya powder, ion-exchange paste (the principle of which is to maintain the pH of the surrounding tissues at an acidic level so that the pancreatic enzymes cannot be activated), or other local favorites. I have found it very useful to involve enterostomal therapists in the care of patients with fistulas, since they have the technical expertise to address difficult wound situations and to keep the wound dry and free of fistula contents.

Investigation

After seven to ten days, when the patient is feeling better and the fistula tract is somewhat matured with sump suction, it is time to define what one is dealing with. Radiographic investigations, in my opinion, are the single most important part of the decision-making process as to whether the patient will require operation; as such, these investigations should be carried out by the senior most responsible surgeon caring for the patient, in conjunction with a senior radiologist. A senior radiologist is very helpful because it is necessary to be expert with both equipment and positioning for best definition of the fistula. If adequate fistulograms are obtained using No. 5 pediatric feeding tubes and a water-soluble dye such as Conray or Hypaque, standard barium gastrointestinal tract examinations such as upper GI series and small bowel follow-throughs and barium enemas are unnecessary, and rarely yield as much information.

What is one looking for? What I look for under fluoroscopy are the characteristics that will tell me whether or not this fistula is likely to close spontaneously. Characteristics associated with nonhealing of fistulas include a large adjacent abscess, intestinal discontinuity, distal obstruction, and poor adjacent bowel (Figure 38–1). Location is also important. The highest rate of closure has been consistently reported for esophageal, lateral duodenal, biliary, pancreatic, and jejunal fistulas. The volume of output does not seem to matter. Small bowel fistulas heal whether output is 300 or 1,000 ml/day. Fistulas of ileum, stomach, and the ligament of Treitz are resistant to spontaneous closure; even in the most optimistic series, that of MacFayden and associates, only 40% of ileal fistulas closed. Etiology is important as well. As Soeters et al. reported in 1979, patients with inflammatory bowel disease, radiation, and recurrent carcinoma are not likely to heal or, in the case of inflammatory bowel disease, tend to close the fistula and then reopen as soon as oral intake is resumed.

If the radiographic situation is anatomically favorable and the patient is not septic, nutritional support should continue. Most authorities, including myself, accept a cutoff point of four to five weeks of adequate parenteral nutrition in a sepsis-free patient for spontaneous closure to occur. It is usually preceded by a decrease in fistula drainage. Nor will fistula closure occur all at once. The fistula will likely close and then, several days later, open and drain a small amount. It is important not to get discouraged as this occurs.

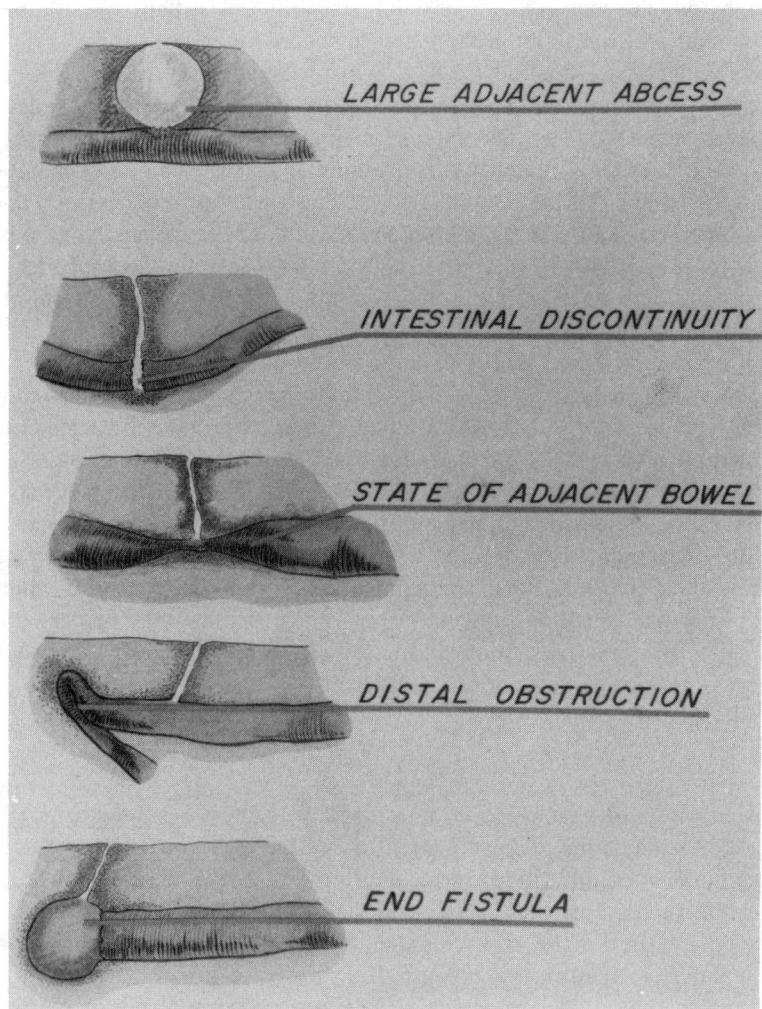

FIG 38–1.
Sinography in patients with fistula. Findings of large adjacent abscesses, intestinal discontinuity, destroyed adjacent bowel, and distal obstruction will almost always mean that operation will be required for closure of the fistula. Even if all of these features are absent, spontaneous closure will occur in some but not necessarily all of the fistulas. (From Fischer JE: *World J Surg* 1983; 7:446–450. Used by permission.)

A few words about antibiotics are appropriate here. Various reviews, including my own (Soeters et al.), have indicated that patients with fistulas often will require eight or nine antibiotics during their course. Consequently, I am willing to accept a low-grade fever of 100° to 101°F provided the patient is not septic, by which I mean decompensated, stressful sepsis. Sepsis is still the most frequent cause of mortality in these patients; consequently, if sepsis is not controlled, early operation is indicated. It is inappropriate to change antibiotics and attempt to control a closed-space abscess with antibiotics; mortality will result.

Given the accurate computed tomography (CT) scanners currently available, it should be possible to identify the locations of abscesses a good percentage of the time. However, if the patient is septic and an intravascular or other source such as pneumonia or urinary tract infection cannot be demonstrated, the patient must be taken urgently to the operating room and the entire abdomen explored. Adhesions should be lysed from the ligament of Treitz to the rectum, and inspection for subphrenic, subhepatic, and lesser sac abscesses carried out. Fistula(s) are resected and end-to-end anastomoses performed. The appropriate drainage and other tubes, such as gastrostomy, needle catheter jejunostomy, or feeding jejunostomy, are placed for adjunctive postoperative management. This operation, popularized by Dr. Claude Welch as a "refunctionalization," was frequently carried out prior to parenteral nutrition in order to create an intact gastrointestinal tract so that patients could be fed. This procedure is rarely necessary at present, but at times it is a useful maneuver in the treatment of severely septic patients. Finally, one should bear in mind that these patients do occasionally get acalculous cholecystitis, a diagnosis that may be very difficult to establish in a scarred abdomen since there is ample reason for abdominal tenderness other than acalculous cholecystitis.

Decision

The decision as to when to operate is usually made when there is no sign of decreased fistula output or closure after four to five weeks of sepsis-free adequate parenteral or enteral nutrition. In patients supported by enteral feedings, fistula output will increase at first, but it will soon be followed by decreased fistula output until closure. The characteristics obtained on sinography are most important in the decision-making process. If distal obstruction, bowel discontinuity, large adjacent abscess, or poor quality of bowel adjacent to the fistula are seen on the sinogram, one should not wait four to five weeks but should proceed with operation as soon as the patient is in the best preoperative shape possible. This is a question of surgical judgment. One can tell when the patient has stopped improving as easily from the end of the bed as one can by measuring a variety of parameters. I believe that a rapid increase in serum short-turnover protein levels is useful as an indication when the liver is recovering from the septic episode and can contribute to the mobilization of protein and energy to heal the wound. Although antibiotics may hold a septic process in check, if the patient is not improving or remains septic, then operation should proceed urgently.

Definitive Therapy

Assuming the patient is not septic and that four to five weeks of adequate nutritional support have elapsed without any significant decrease in fistula output, operation should be undertaken. The abdominal wall should be quiescent so that a good abdominal wall closure may be achieved, a problem in situations in which pelvic irradiation has been complicated by a fistula, either from recurrent malignancy or from radiated bowel.

I prefer to use a different incision, often in a different direction. Thus, if the previous incision has been vertical, I prefer to make a long transverse incision. If there are large defects in the abdominal wall, it is wise to plan with a plastic surgery and reconstructive team the creation of a muscle flap after the abdominal surgeon has finished the initial procedure. This may prolong the procedure by two to three hours, but the most important aspect of the closure is that it be done properly. I take no special pride in ownership of a good closure, especially with a difficult abdominal wall after I have been operating for six to seven hours and am tired.

There is little question that adequate exposure, resection, end-to-end anastomosis, and draining of any abscesses within the abdominal cavity are the sine qua non of success in the treatment of patients with fistula. Other procedures, such as staged procedures or bypass with the bowel in continuity, result in an increased number of complications, with the fistula frequently staying open (Figure 38–2). After an extensive procedure on a patient with fistula, I almost always place a Stamm gastrostomy, not using a Foley (which drains air well, but not liquid) but rather a Robinson catheter placed with two concentric sutures of chromic catgut and attached to the anterior abdominal wall. If the fistula is high, one may want to use a needle catheter jejunostomy for feeding purposes below the anastomosis. I use Penrose drains only in collections of purulent material. In the absence of gross purulence, if one uses drainage at all, closed suction drains are more useful and, at least on a theoretical basis, prevent the "two-way drainage" that could result in abscess.

Healing Phase

Parenteral nutrition is continued in the postoperative period until the patient is taking 1,500 calories by mouth. If there are several suture lines, I will not feed the patient for seven to ten days following the operation until bowel movements are regular and the patient is no longer distended. This is particularly true in patients with inflammatory bowel disease. It may be difficult for patients to eat 1,500 calories in the presence of parenteral nutrition that suppresses appetite. It may finally be necessary to stop parenteral nutrition, keeping the line intact and infusing non-dextrose-containing solutions (such as normal saline) to see if the patient will eat in four to five days. I frequently do not start patients on clear liquids, as is the general practice, but may start them on a soft diet. The patient who has had nothing by mouth for six to eight weeks is unlikely to be attracted, nor their appetites stimulated, by gelatin and the peculiarly vile form of broth that passes for clear liquids in American hospitals. If the patient is elderly and feeding is not enthusiastically resumed, one may want to use the gastrostomy for tube feedings, but one must be careful not to provoke diarrhea, which may disrupt a freshly healed anastomosis.

Antibiotics are continued for five days in the presence of sepsis or septic collections. In the absence of sepsis, the usual prophylaxis following bowel resection is followed, depending on the extent of contamination, and antibiotic therapy may be discontinued after 24 to 72 hours. It is wise to choose perioperative antibiotics based on specific cultures preoperatively; the infectious disease team may be very helpful. Closed suction drainage systems are left in place until the output is less than 25 cc per 24 hours. If grossly purulent material is emanating from the drain, the drain is left in until the tract is securely established (from

OPERATION	TOTAL PATIENTS	FAILURE	COMPLICATIONS
RESECTION 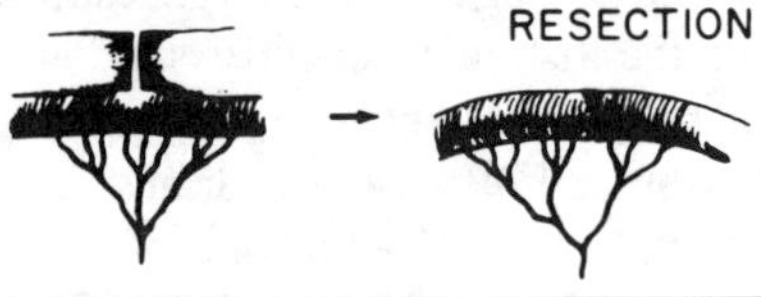	45	2	12
BYPASS 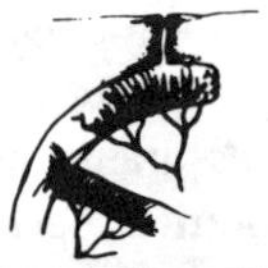	18	5	8
STAGED 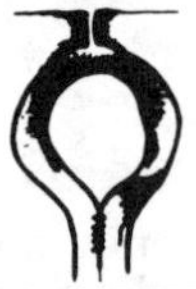	13	6	11

FIG 38–2.
Various operations in the treatment of fistula. Note that resection and end-to-end anastomosis are most likely to result in resolution of the fistula with the fewest complications. Other compromises, including bypass and staged procedures, are less likely to result in a satisfactory resolution of the fistula. (From Freund HR, Bower RH, Fischer JE: The role and effects of parenteral and enteral nutrition in digestive diseases, in Moody FG, Carey LC, Jones RS, et al (eds): *Surgical Treatment of Digestive Disease*, Chicago, Year Book Medical Publishers, 1986, p 57. Used by permission.)

10 to 12 days) and drainage decreases; perhaps it is replaced with a soft Penrose drain.

Other adjuncts that others have described include prolonged nasogastric suction and the passing of a long tube to an area directly above the fistula. In both our own series (Soeters et al.) and that reported by MacFayden and associates, nasogastric suction did not influence final outcome. In addition, we have seen approximately half a dozen patients who have had prolonged nasogastric suction in the presence of a preexistent hiatus hernia and reflux, who sustained significant esophageal strictures and several have required esophageal resection and replacement.

Finally, nutritional support should not be abruptly discontinued, as recently closed fistulas by conservative means may break down with starvation.

SUMMARY

The patient with a gastrointestinal cutaneous fistula represents one of the most severe challenges a practicing surgeon will encounter. Although the situation is complicated, by the system outlined above or by a similar method in which different problems are addressed at different times of the patient's course, it is likely that a successful outcome can be achieved. Care of the patient with a gastrointestinal fistula requires meticulous attention to detail, tenacity of purpose, excellent surgical judgment, and skill in the operating room. These patients are rare challenges, but most will be returned to useful function in society.

BIBLIOGRAPHY

1. Edmunds LH, Williams GM, Welch CE: External fistulas arising from the gastrointestinal tract. *Ann Surg* 1960; 152:445–471.
2. Fischer JE: The pathophysiology of enterocutaneous fistulas. *World J Surg* 1983; 7:446–450.
3. MacFayden VB Jr, Dudrick SJ, Ruberg RL: Management of gastrointestinal fistulas with parenteral hyperalimentation. *Surgery* 1973; 74:100–105.
4. Soeters PB, Ebeid AM, Fischer JE: Review of 404 patients with gastrointestinal fistulas: Impact of parenteral nutrition. *Ann Surg* 1979; 190:189–202.
5. Voitk AJ, Echave V, Brown RA, et al: Elemental diet in the treatment of fistulae of the alimentary tract. *Surg Gynecol Obstet* 1973; 137:68–72.
6. Welch CE: Intestinal fistulas. *Am Surg* 1964; 30:631–634.

39

Acute Ileitis

A 36-year-old woman, who has been previously well, is admitted with right lower quadrant pain, guarding, a fever of 101.5°F and a white blood cell count of 14,000/cu mm. The pain had been gradual in onset and approximately 36 hours in duration. She is nauseated but has not vomited. There is no diarrhea. Exploration of the abdomen reveals a normal appendix, with no Meckel's diverticulum. Approximately 2 in. from the ileocecal valve, a beefy-red, indurated, and edematous terminal ileum is encountered. There is overgrowth of fat over the mesentery that continues for approximately 12 in. proximally, and lymph nodes immediately adjacent to the small bowel are edematous and succulent.

Consultant: Frank E. Gump, M.D.

There are two aspects to be considered in the management of this patient: (1) operative approach, and (2) postoperative course. A number of options are available to the surgeon in the present case. Simply closing the abdomen after establishing the diagnosis and ensuring that there is no perforation of the involved ileum is a reasonable approach and was the standard practice 25 years ago when concern about postoperative complications of all kinds suggested that less was better. A specific concern was the development of postoperative enterocutaneous fistula if the bowel (whether appendix or ileum) was cut. One would expect the least trouble if the wound was simply closed without any further surgical procedures. The disadvantage of this approach related to the chronic nature of Crohn's disease; if another exacerbation came, the fact that the patient was now known to have Crohn's did not eliminate the possibility of appendicitis and the need for reexploration.

This problem constituted a compelling reason to remove the appendix, which would be the second option. Surgeons had originally hesitated to perform an appendectomy in acute ileitis because of concern about postoperative fistulas that appeared in the incision and were thought to come from the appendiceal stump. However, an increasing number of authors reported on the safety of appendectomy in this situation, and the issue appeared to be settled in the mid-1960s after Marx reported that the fistulas came from the diseased ileum and not the appendiceal stump. Our own study confirmed this experience and pointed out that enterocutaneous fistulas in Crohn's disease cannot exit through an intact abdominal wall. We have seen fistulas from the terminal ileum to the buttock, groin, and even the hip joint in patients without abdominal incisions. Once an incision is made, this represents the easiest pathway to the surface. This is relevant to the question of appendectomy, since the surgeon who finds a normal appendix and an involved ileum has already made an abdominal incision. It is this incision and the severity of the disease in the involved ileum that determines whether or not an enterocutaneous fistula will develop. The performance of an appendectomy is irrelevant. Given the clear advantage of managing a Crohn's patient without having to contend with this structure, appendectomy was routinely recommended in acute ileitis by Ferguson in 1970, provided the cecum was not involved.

The third option would be a bowel resection and, practically speaking, this will inevitably require an ileoascending colectomy. While the patient under discussion had 2 in. of normal ileum between her disease and the ileocecal valve, suggesting the possibility of an ileectomy, this is most unusual. Ileitis usually involves the entire terminal ileum, necessitating resection of the cecum. Even if it might be possible in rare instances to do an ileectomy, this procedure has an extremely high recurrence rate, and most authors believe its only role is in the treatment of skip areas.

If we again look back 25 years, ileocolectomy for acute ileitis was unthinkable because it was thought that resection during the acute phase would exacerbate the disease. Furthermore, an anastomosis in the presence of acute disease, to say nothing of an unprepared bowel, was contraindicated for fear of an anastomotic leak. While one could resect and avoid an anastomosis by creating an ileostomy and a mucous fistula, the thought of taking a patient to the operating room with a consent for an appendectomy and having her return to the floor with an ileostomy bag was a major deterrent to this approach.

Thinking about resection started to change because an increasing number of patients with acute ileitis were noted to have one or more perforations. Under these circumstances surgeons were forced to do a resection, and by-and-large an anastomosis followed. It became clear that this approach was not as disastrous as had been expected, and such patients did very well.

The patient under discussion did not have a perforation, and this certainly remains a rare event in acute ileitis. However, there is another indication for resection and, while it is equally rare in acute ileitis, it might apply in the present case. The recommendation to do an appendectomy is always associated with the proviso that the cecum at the base of the appendix be normal. When there is cecal involvement, the surgeon has to choose between option 1 and 3—closing the abdomen without removing the appendix or performing an ileocolectomy. The condition of the cecum was not described; however, since the disease stopped 2 in. from the ileocecal valve, it was probably normal. Therefore, an appendectomy would be done. However, I believe a good case can be made for primary resection if the condition of the cecum rules out an appendectomy. If the local situation and the condition of the patient are favorable, the procedure can be done safely. The only argument against it would be the thought that many patients with acute ileitis will never have further episodes of Crohn's disease; subjecting such patients to an ileocolectomy represents a clear case of overkill. However, as will shortly be discussed, patients that have cecal involvement will inevitably go on to the chronic form of the disease.

To summarize the intraoperative management of the 36-year-old woman presented for discussion, there is general agreement that she should have an appendectomy. Management in case of cecal involvement is more controversial and has to be individualized, but I would favor resection rather than merely closing the abdomen. Since resection implies ileoascending colectomy, the appendix will also be removed.

The words "general agreement" above were carefully chosen since a recent article by Fonkalsrud et al. has questioned the wisdom of incidental appendectomy in acute ileitis. Fonkalsrud and associates do not feel that appendectomy influences the subsequent progression of the disease. Their concern in our patient would be that *if* her disease should progress to involve the cecum, the presence of a wound in the cecum (the appendectomy site) might increase the possibility of a fistula from that area. The authors obviously cannot document this concern, which is based on nine patients, but they do supply suggestive case histories and add to this the fact that acute appendicitis appears to be an uncommon event in patients who were followed up with the diagnosis of Crohn's disease. Their point regarding appendectomy would be: It might hurt and, since the patients will not get appendicitis anyway, the major indication for the procedure is not applicable.

This report may turn back the clock, but at the moment we cannot assume that appendicitis is not possible in Crohn's patients, and the evidence that appendectomy will result in increased fistula formation remains hypothetical at present.

The second issue facing the surgeon in the case presented relates to prognosis. One of the most confusing aspects of acute ileitis is the true incidence of progression to chronic disease. We reviewed the existing reports and our own patients in an effort to explain why some authors found that none of their patients went on to develop Crohn's disease, while in other instances this progression was inevitable. The problem has to do with diagnosis, since pathologic criteria are not available. This reflects the fact that the involved ileum is rarely excised, but even if tissue was available, pathologists have not been able to find any pathognomonic lesions. The foreign body granulomas thought to be characteristic of the disease are found in only about one third of the patients whose Crohn's disease resulted in bowel resection.

The disparity in the incidence of progression to chronic disease noted by different authors reflects the mix of patients entered into each series. On the one hand, there are patients with "real" Crohn's disease that present for the first time because of an acute exacerbation. On the other hand, there are a variety of conditions that result in a red, edematous ileum from whatever cause (food allergy, viral, etc.) having nothing to do with Crohn's disease, and these patients will have no further difficulties once the acute episode has passed. The challenge facing the surgeon in this situation is properly categorizing the patient. Is it Crohn's disease presenting for the first time during an acute episode, or is it some unrelated condition that also results in an abnormal ileum but has nothing to do with Crohn's disease?

At times the history is helpful. Have there been significant intestinal symptoms prior to the acute episode? Has the patient had a perirectal abscess, fissure, or fistula in the past? Such events obviously point to the chronic disease.

Sometimes the operative findings are clear-cut and show chronic changes that could not have developed during the brief symptomatic period that led to exploration for presumed appendicitis. These changes may be in the mesentery, which shows chronic fibrosis and thickening, or in the bowel wall itself. As noted previously, cecal or any large bowel involvement is clear evidence of the chronic disease, and in the present patient the overgrowth of fat could not have taken place in the 36 hours between the onset of symptoms and exploration for presumed appendicitis.

When the operative findings fail to point to a chronic process, it is best to hold off on a final decision regarding the nature of the acute episode until contrast studies can be done in the postoperative period. Some additional questioning about the patient's past history that might have been missed when everyone was thinking appendicitis would also be in order at this time. Contrast studies may show mucosal abnormalities pointing to the chronic disease. A completely normal study would be expected in the other category. Such an approach will identify most patients with the chronic disease, and their prognosis would be no different than any other patient with Crohn's disease. The remaining patients would be expected to do well, since the acute episode that led to exploration is unrelated to Crohn's. While such categorization may not always be clear-cut, it represents a far better way to approach patients regarding their prognosis than simply quoting the published series. These reports are far too variable in the reported incidence of progression to chronic disease to provide any help to an individual patient.

BIBLIOGRAPHY

1. Antonius J, Gump FE, Lattes R, et al: A study of certain features in regional enteritis and their possible prognostic significance. *Gastroenterology* 1960; 38:889–905.

2. Ferguson LK: Surgical viewpoint in regional enteritis. *JAMA* 1957; 165:2048–2052.
3. Fonkalsrud EW, Ament ME, Fleisher D: Management of the appendix in young patients with Crohn's disease. *Arch Surg* 1982; 117:11–14.
4. Gump FE, Lepore M: Prognosis in acute and chronic regional enteritis. *Gastroenterology* 1960; 39:694–701.
5. Gump FE, Lepore M, Barker HG: A revised concept of acute regional enteritis. *Ann Surg* 1967; 166:942–946.
6. Marx FW Jr: Incidental appendectomy with regional enteritis: Advisability. *Arch Surg* 1964; 88:546–551.

Crohn's disease is "incurable". The role of the surgeon is to provide palliation

40

Crohn's Disease

A 23-year-old woman with a six-month history of right lower quadrant abdominal pain and postprandial pain, followed by diarrhea with some mucous, is admitted with a 24-hour history of sudden onset of right lower quadrant pain, fever to 102°F to 103°F, and malaise, anorexia, and occasional vomiting. On physical examination the abdomen is tender, with a mass appreciated in the right lower quadrant of approximately 9 × 5 cm. Bowel sounds are slightly hyperactive. Stool guaiac is negative.

Consultant: George E. Block, M.D.

PRESENTATION

This patient is typical of those suffering from Crohn's disease. There is some confusion as to the nomenclature of this entity, because its original description in 1932 was that of terminal ileal disease. We are now aware that Crohn's disease can be present anywhere in the alimentary canal from mouth to anus. The most common variety of the disease, and certainly the most frequent entity with which surgeons deal, is the ileocolic variety of Crohn's disease. This subset of Crohn's disease primarily affects the distal ileum for varying lengths, and the lesions may extend beyond the ileocecal valve into the right portion of the colon. The ileocolic variety of Crohn's disease has been variously described as terminal or regional enteritis.

The differential diagnosis for lesions of the ileocecal region include colonic cancer in older patients, specific forms of inflammatory bowel disease such as tuberculous enteritis, and such mundane entities as appendiceal abscess.

Although Crohn's disease anywhere in the gastrointestinal tract shares complications in common, the ileocolic variety characteristically comes to the attention of the surgeon because of obstruction or its septic complications—perforation, abscess formation, or fistulas. The role of the surgeon in treating Crohn's disease is that of affording palliation by removing that section of the gut giving rise to the complication. The removal of the involved segment does not imply cure; the disease recurs in the overwhelming majority of patients, although disease-free intervals range from a few months to many years. (*Editor's note:* Some recent studies suggest a slightly more optimistic view, with 25% to 40% of patients free of recurrence at 15 years.)

A form of acute ileitis is occasionally encountered when operating for a suspected appendicitis. In this situation the terminal ileum is inflamed and indurated, and the peritoneal cavity may contain a cloudy exudate. This form of ileitis is not true Crohn's disease and only rarely evolves into the chronic, recurrent enteropathy characteristic of Crohn's. Specific microorganisms have been indicated in its genesis: *Yersinia* or *Campylobacter* may either be cultured or diagnosed by serologic means from the exudate and are treated by specific aminoglycosides.

DIAGNOSTIC PROCEDURES

This patient, while typical for an individual with an acute exacerbation of Crohn's ileocolitis (terminal ileitis), is at risk for harboring an acute perforation or a localized abscess. In order to evaluate the patient's abdominal mass to ascertain if this is a simple flare of the disease or a septic complication of the enterocolitis, I employ a number of diagnostic procedures in addition to careful and serial physical examinations.

A simple flat plate of the abdomen together with upright and lateral decubitus films may often reveal obstruction, the presence of free air indicating a perforation, or gas bubbles that are outside the lumen of the bowel diagnostic of an abscess. Sonography, in my experience, is of limited value in this acute situation because a fluid-filled loop of bowel can usually not be differentiated from an abscess cavity. Computerized axial tomography with contrast media is helpful in identifying abscess cavities or localized perforations. Contrast radiographs, while helpful, may be dangerous in that barium may be released through an occult perforation into an abscess or the peritoneal cavity. If the patient has not been previously diagnosed as suffering from Crohn's disease, a contrast radiograph of the colon and terminal ileum utilizing a water-soluble media may be helpful. (*Editor's note*: The concern about the use of even thin barium in a situation with potential perforation or abscess is well taken. However, it is difficult for even an experienced radiologist to discern mucosal detail with water soluble contrast; thus only gross details will be observed. The vast majority of Crohn's patients referred to me already have the diagnosis established by objective means such as contrast radiographs or endoscopy.)

A sine qua non of accurate diagnosis is the serial examination of the patient that includes a rectal examination. If there is spreading peritonitis, immediate operation is necessary. Mere local inflammation without perforation allows for intensive medical treatment to prepare the patient for operation and the adjuvant support that will enhance the patient's operation and recovery.

PREPARATION FOR OPERATION

My working diagnosis for this patient is that of chronic Crohn's ileocolitis with an acute exacerbation. Of particular concern is whether or not this flare is complicated by a free perforation or abscess formation. Free perforation mandates immediate operation—resection of the perforated segment with exteriorization of the terminal ileum as an ileostomy and the distal colon as a mucous fistula. I may, however, elect to close the distal colonic segment and return it to the peritoneal cavity. This decision will depend upon the amount of contamination present. Another attractive alternative to avoid a second stoma on the abdominal wall is to close the distal bowel, bring it through the anterior rectus fascia through a stab wound, and leave the skin and subcutaneous tissue open. If the closure fails, the luminal contents will discharge through the open superficial wound. If the closure is successful, the open wound will immediately heal over the closed colon.

Occasionally, a small anterior collection of pus is present between the ileum and the anterior abdominal wall, which may be drained prior to addressing the problem of the underlying Crohn's disease. These small, localized collections will not develop into a clinical fistula following drainage and will allow an elective resection of the diseased bowel within a few days. More chronic and larger abscesses require immediate drainage followed by prompt resection of the diseased bowel.

Corticosteroids

Like the majority of her counterparts, this patient will undoubtedly have been treated with corticosteroids. Corticosteroids are not effective against the septic complications of the disease and may well worsen the situation by moderating the patient's inflammatory response and masking clinical progression. Therefore, I do not use corticosteroids in the treatment of an acute flare in these patients. However, if this patient has received large amounts of corticosteroids for a long period of time, she may have an atrophy of her pituitary-adrenal axis and will require exogenous steroids during her acute stress. I utilize physiologic and not pharmacologic amounts of corticosteroids for this purpose. An intravenous preparation of hydrocortisone is my choice, in doses not to exceed 100 mg/day.

Antibiotics

The flare of the patient's disease is essentially a septic complication from a rent in the continuity of the bowel, with fecal contamination of the adjacent bowel and soft tissue. Antibiotics are therefore a logical adjuvant treatment and should be chosen to be effective against the organisms encountered in the gut. Preoperative cultures and sensitivities are usually not available. I assume that the offending organs are enteric, both aerobic and anaerobic, and that a mixed infection exists. Most clinically important anaerobes are susceptible to penicillin, with the exception of the most common organism in the colon, *Bacteroides fragilis*, which is penicillin-resistant. Chloramphenicol, clindamycin, metronidazole, and the newer cephalosporins are effective against *B. fragilis* and most other anaerobic species.

The aminoglycosides are weakly effective against anaerobes, but they represent a wise choice for the aerobic and coliform species suspected to be present. They are effective against most strains of *Escherichia coli, Klebsiella,* enterobacter, and *Proteus*. The use of a penicillin is logical because of its effectiveness against the gram-positive cocci and bacilli commonly found in the gut. Thus, a triple antibiotic program relying on the combination of a penicillin, an aminoglycoside, and an agent effective against anaerobes is my regimen of choice.

Bowel Preparation

I assume that this patient will undergo an intestinal resection in the immediate future and, therefore, strive for some degree of mechanical bowel preparation. Mechanical preparation of the bowel may be difficult. This patient has symptoms of a partial small bowel obstruction characteristic of the fibrosis in the ileum. Large amounts of purgatives are not well tolerated and theoretically may engender perforation. From a practical standpoint these patients have a tender abdomen and a partial small bowel obstruction, so that purgatives and enemas are ill-tolerated and bothersome. Depending upon the severity of symptoms and the timing of operation, preparation may be achieved by placing the bowel at rest with nasogastric suction and allowing nothing by mouth. Alternatively, small amounts of laxatives, usually iso-osmolar electrolyte solution in combination with mannitol, may be given incrementally over a period of several days to obtain an adequate mechanical preparation of the bowel. In patients with an acute flare of Crohn's disease it has been my practice, when anticipating an early operation, to begin small doses of this solution orally and advance to the tolerance of the patient. The majority of patients tolerate this regimen well.

Prior to operation, I proctoscope the patient to ensure that the rectosigmoid is uninvolved with disease and that the far left side of the bowel, at least, will be available for anastomosis.

Parenteral Nutrition

There are no convincing data that total parenteral nutrition (TPN) is specifically therapeutic for Crohn's disease, per se, or its acute complications. (*Editor's note*: I agree that data as to the specific effect of TPN on Crohn's disease are not yet

When planning a surg. incision in a pt c̄ Crohn's be mindful of the possibility of a future stoma.

available. However, TPN associated with other means of treatment may, over a two-week period, sufficiently ameliorate Crohn's disease as to make operation easier and delineation of normal and diseased bowel more apparent.) However, TPN is a convenient tool to utilize in the perioperative period. The patients are often malnourished and may even present with obvious protein depletion. Anabolism, however, will not be achieved by a few days of TPN. It will, however, expand the extracellular fluid and establish relative homeostasis, allowing for a safe anesthesia. The anorexia due to the initial symptoms, the time required for preparation, and the postoperative delay in resumption of feeding cumulatively result in a two-week starvation. Parenteral nutrition, therefore, is a convenient method of support during preoperative preparation and postoperative recovery. I do not utilize enteral feeding for these patients.

TIMING AND PERFORMANCE OF OPERATION

I would proceed to care for this patient based on the working diagnosis of an acute exacerbation of chronic ileocolitic Crohn's disease. If possible, I prefer to operate on patients with a subsiding or resolved acute exacerbation. To this end, I attempt to treat the patient medically in order to decrease the intra-abdominal inflammation. If the patient's symptoms and findings subside with the medical program, I delay operation until maximum resolution is achieved. If there is little or no improvement, or if the process appears to worsen, operation is undertaken immediately. In many cases, five to ten days of medical treatment may be necessary prior to operation to achieve maximum resolution. The medical treatment is taken as preparation to operation so that dissection is easier and, most importantly, the normal bowel adjacent to the inflammatory mass will not be sacrificed unnecessarily because of adhesion to the mass or mistakenly removed because of nonspecific inflammation. Delineation between normal and diseased bowel is made easier by the subsidence of acute inflammation.

OPERATIVE PROCEDURE

I choose my incision with care. One must always bear in mind that all Crohn's disease patients have the potential for a permanent ileostomy. Therefore, the incision must be made so as not to compromise the site of a possible future stoma. I usually employ a transverse infraumbilical incision extending across both rectus muscles. This incision may be lengthened as necessary, gives excellent exposure of the small bowel and colon, is cosmetically acceptable, and is a safe incision through which herniation and evisceration are rare. My alternative to this incision is an infraumbilical midline incision; I never use a paramedium incision.

Prior to commencing my dissection, I explore the bowel to determine the extent of the Crohn's disease. The small bowel is examined from the ligament of Treitz to the diseased bowel. The length of the uninvolved bowel is recorded in the operative note to be available for consideration at the time of the inevitable future recurrence. The extent, if any, of the involvement of the colon is similarly noted, and any adherence or fistulas to the bladder, vagina, or abdominal wall are noted and divided. If there is a purulent process with exudate in the right lower quadrant, such an exploration is delayed until the resection and an abdominal toilet are completed. Large abscesses, if any, are drained extraperitoneally with sump drains through separate stab wounds. I do not use Penrose drains. Smaller abscesses adjacent to the inflammatory process or within the mesentery can usually be removed with the operative specimen.

An initial estimation of the "free margins" are ascertained prior to commencing the dissection. This estimate is made by gross appearance of the bowel and by palpation. The absence of stenosis, creeping mesenteric fat, or a thickening of the bowel are usually accurate determinants between normal and involved bowel. Further evaluation is made following resection. Ideally, I prefer to excise only the bowel involved with the Crohn's lesion, leaving a 2- to 3 in. margin of normal bowel both proximally and distally.

For this patient, with an acute flare of Crohn's disease, I prefer resection to bypass. I rarely, if ever, use bypass procedures at the initial operation for the ileocolic variety of Crohn's disease. Dissection is begun at the root of the mesentery at the posterior aspect of the ileum and carried over the ureter and gonadal vessels and around the cecum. This incision is made within 1 cm of the mesenteric attachment of the bowel. Dissection is carried superiorly up to the right gutter and extended to the hepatic flexure, taking down the duodenal-colic ligament and perhaps an inch or two of the gastrocolic ligament. Following this, the fusion fascia immediately beneath the peritoneum is divided; here several bothersome vessels are encountered and are clipped. Mobilization of the right part of the colon will then demonstrate the ureter and duodenum, which are avoided. After mobilization of the distal small bowel and proximal right part of the colon, the specimen is free to be delivered into the abdominal wound. I then isolate the bowel with packs from the main abdominal cavity.

The dissection of the mesentery is my next step. In the usual Crohn's disease patient the mesentery is thickened, there are numerous hypertrophied lymph nodes in the mesentery, and the uninitiated can have some difficulty in dissecting the mesentery. Because of the thickened mesentery with abundant lymphatic tissue, I routinely incise the peritoneum of the anterior and posterior mesentery and divide the anterior lymphatics between hemostats and ligate these to prevent an oozing of blood and to isolate the ileocolic arcade at the posterior of the mesentery. After these maneuvers, the thickened mesentery is thinned so that the ileocolic arteries and veins are isolated and can be ligated and transected individually. An attempt at mass clamping and dividing of the thickened mesentery will often result in retraction of the vessels with bothersome hematoma formation. There is no advantage to excising all of the obviously inflamed lymph nodes, as this will only result in a high arterial ligation with concomitant sacrifice of normal bowel. All patients with Crohn's disease are at risk for a short gut, so care must be taken to preserve as much normal bowel proximally and distally as possible.

The watchword for the indications and extent of operations for Crohn's disease is *conservatism*. The bowel is transected to be opened in the pathology suite. I personally inspect the specimen prior to making the anastomosis to ensure that both the proximal and distal ends of the bowel are uninvolved by gross lesions of Crohn's disease. Cameron[2] and others[2] have shown that the presence of microscopic disease in either the proximal or distal ends does not influence the frequency or rapidity of recurrence, provided no gross lesions are present. Nonetheless, I prefer to avoid making an anastomosis through gross lesions of Crohn's disease such as linear ulcerations or cobblestone mucosa. I will, however, accept occasional aphthous ulcers, particularly in the proximal segment. This is especially important in patients who are undergoing their second or third operation and are at danger for a short gut. Patients with Crohn's disease will often have aphthous ulcers throughout the distal half of the bowel. Obviously, resection of all of these "abnormal" areas would unnecessarily sacrifice absorptive surface.

I now make the decision whether to do a primary anastomosis or a temporary stoma. I employ an end ileostomy and mucous fistula only in cases of gross contamination of the peritoneal cavity by spreading peritonitis or a giant abscess. In 200 consecutive cases in which contamination was present but not overwhelming in 53% of the patients, my colleagues and I have employed primary anastomosis with almost uniform success. In these patients, postoperative sepsis was manifested in a few patients by wound sepsis (4%), intra-abdominal abscess (3%), and anastomotic leak (2.5%). Either an end-to-end or end-to-side anastomosis is accomplished between the small bowel and colon. I choose the anastomosis based upon the size of the two lumens. If an end-to-side anastomosis is chosen, the blind end of the right part of the colon is closed in layers and the small bowel anastomosed in an end-to-side fashion, leaving a short blind stump of about 2 cm.

Areas of skip disease are treated on their own merit. If the skip disease is immediately adjacent to the main disease and its inclusion in the excision will not result in a short gut, the skip disease is included in the excision. If the skip disease is proximal and is merely stenotic, I employ either a plasty operation as advised by Alexander-Williams and Haynes or I open the bowel through a normal area and dilate the stenosis with dilators. This has been uniformly successful in relieving obstructive symptoms. Areas of skip disease that do not pose problems of obstruction or imminent perforation are left undisturbed.

The mesenteric defect is then closed. The abdomen is copiously irrigated of debris and contamination. I close the abdomen with monofilament stainless steel wire. The skin is then closed primarily; however, if there is gross contamination, the skin and subcutaneous tissue are left open. If a stoma is chosen because of contamination, reanastomosis is accomplished within 90 days.

POSTOPERATIVE CARE

The patient begins to receive a supportive dose of hydrocortisone if steroids were administered prior to operation. This gradually tapered, and the patient is discharged from the hospital taking 35 mg of hydrocortisone/day in divided doses, and is rapidly weaned from this medication. Parenteral alimentation is continued until the patient is consistently eating a normal diet of at least 1,500 calories per day, at which time TPN may be precipitously withdrawn.

Follow-up examination of patients after the usual postoperative visits should include examinations at least twice a year by the surgeon or gastroenterologist to elicit any symptoms of recurrent disease and to examine the perineum for manifestations of perineal Crohn's disease. I monitor the blood cell count and other indices that would reflect either malabsorption or blood loss. If any abnormal values are obtained or if there are significant complaints, appropriate diagnostic measures are then instituted. I would not counsel this female patient to avoid pregnancy after the wound had healed.

BIBLIOGRAPHY

1. Alexander-Williams J, Haynes IG: Conservative operations for Crohn's disease of the small bowel. *World J Surg* 1985; 9:945–951.
2. Pennington L, Hamilton SR, Bayless TM, et al: Surgical management of Crohn's disease: Influence of disease at margin of resection. *Ann Surg* 1980; 192:311–318.
3. Reilly J: Inflammatory bowel disease, in Fischer JE (ed): *Total Parenteral Nutrition*. Boston, Little, Brown & Co, 1976, pp 187–202.
4. Rombeau JL, Barot LR, Williamson CE, et al: Preoperative total parenteral nutrition and surgical outcome in patients with inflammatory bowel disease. *Am J Surg* 1982; 143:139–143.

41

Carcinoid

A 49-year-old man is admitted with chronic recurrent right lower quadrant pain, tenderness over McBurney's point, a white blood cell count of 9,000/cu mm with occasional shifts to the left, and nausea but no vomiting. Stool guaiac is negative. At exploration, the appendix is seen to be mildly infected. However, at the base of the appendix, there is a 1.5-cm rock-hard mass. A lymph node of 1 cm in the mesentery is somewhat firm.

Consultant: Bernard M. Jaffe, M.D.

PRESENTATION AND DIAGNOSIS

This patient presented with classic signs and symptoms of appendicitis. The fact that the leukocyte count was normal should play no meaningful role in discouraging the diagnosis of appendicitis. Normal blood cell counts are frequently (approximately 30% of the time) noted in patients with appendicitis, and falsely elevated white blood cell counts are regularly seen in patients with normal appendices at exploration for presumed appendicitis. The only two ways clinical hematology can be useful are if the leukocyte count is markedly suppressed (below 4,000/cu mm), indicating overwhelming sepsis, and if toxic granulations on polymorphonuclear cells are observed by an experienced hematologist. With right lower quadrant pain and localized tenderness (even in the absence of guarding or rebound tenderness), abdominal exploration using a horizontal or oblique incision is indicated.

OBJECTIVES IN PROPER CARE

Rather than typical appendicitis, this patient had a firm mass at the base of the appendix, with mild inflammation distally. In fact, luminal obstruction of the appendix is important in the pathogenesis of this inflammatory process. While typically a fecalith or lymphatic hypertrophy occludes the lumen, tumors can do so as well. Having recognized a tumor in the base of the appendix, the surgeon must evaluate and execute the objectives of the proper care of the patient. These include: (1) treating the appendicitis per se; (2) establishing the pathologic diagnosis of the tumor; (3) determining the extent of its spread (staging); (4) resection of the tumor with the sites of lymphatic metastases, if appropriate; and (5) developing a plan for subsequent monitoring of tumor progression and treatment of metastatic disease.

Treating the Appendicitis

Removal of the appendix is necessary as one component of the therapy. The mere presence of a tumor should not inherently alter the management of the inflammatory process. As with all cases of appendicitis, the peritoneum should be irrigated and appropriate antibiotics administered. Since there was no appendiceal perforation or purulent collection, drainage would not be necessary.

Establishing the Pathologic Diagnosis

The most common neoplasms of the appendix are carcinoids. While it is common knowledge that these tumors are yellow in color, this characteristic appearance only becomes apparent when they are sectioned. In situ, they appear as noncharacteristic intramural lesions. I will focus most of the subsequent discussion on these tumors.

Adenocarcinomas also occur in the appendix. In general, they are quite virulent lesions that behave exactly like their counterparts in the cecum. While leiomyomas and leiomyosarcomas occur commonly in Meckel's diverticula, they rarely (if ever) start in the appendix. Likewise, the most common tumors at the ileocecal valve—lipomas—are exceedingly rare in the appendix. Thus, assuming the mass is intrinsic to the appendix and not an appendicolith, the differential diagnosis would realistically include carcinoid vs. adenocarcinoma. A biopsy with frozen section examination is necessary in order to make this distinction and firmly establish the diagnosis. If the tumor has grown through to the serosa, a shave biopsy will allow for pathologic diagnosis (Fig 41–1). Assuming it is readily accomplished, appendectomy should be performed and a frozen section of the obstructing lesion obtained. If at all possible, biopsy of the enlarged mesenteric lymph node should be avoided; it may be hyperplastic due to the inflammation and, even if it is involved with metastatic tumor, resection for biopsy would interfere with examination of the final resection specimen. Tissue diagnosis is necessary for the subsequent objectives. For the sake of this discussion, let us assume the diagnosis is carcinoid.

Determining the Extent of Tumor Spread

In planning definitive resection, there are four primary criteria that must be

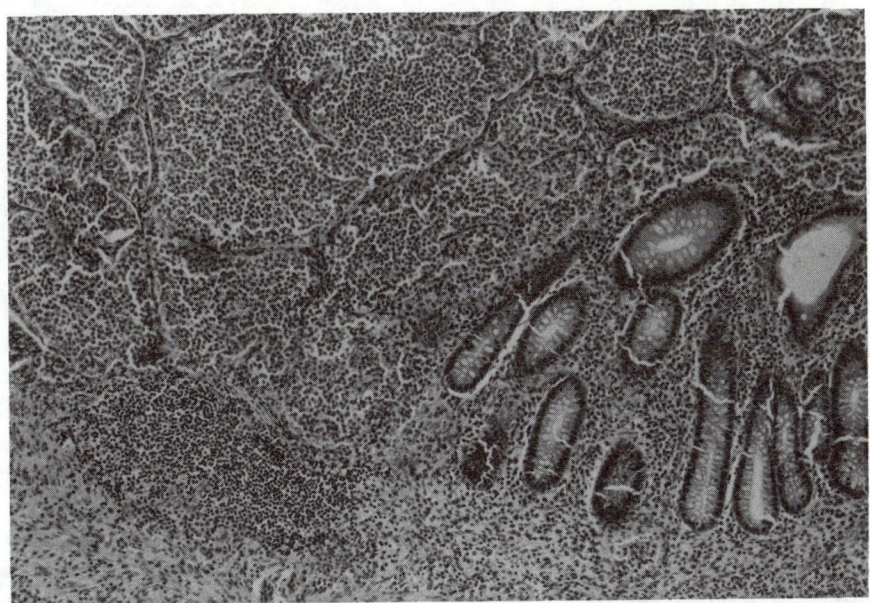

FIG 41–1.
Histology of a carcinoid tumor.

considered: (1) the size of the primary tumor, (2) the depth of its invasion with respect to serosal surface, (3) the presence and distribution of involved lymph nodes, and (4) the presence of peritoneal implants and/or liver metastases. The diameter of the tumor should be accurately measured. It is vital to ascertain if the tumor approaches or broaches the serosal surface of the appendix. Finally, the right part of the colon should be widely mobilized and the mesocolon carefully examined for additional enlarged lymph nodes. Since there is a 35% to 40% rate of multiplicity of carcinoids (two thirds of which are synchronous and one third metachronous), the entire small intestine should be examined for other primary tumors. Since the initial incision was a limited oblique or horizontal one, inspection of the entire peritoneum will be impossible. Nonetheless, it is important that the incision be lengthened to allow the surgeon to palpate the peritoneal surfaces and to examine the surface of the liver. If there is widespread tumor (whether the liver is involved or not), the patient is at increased risk for anesthetic problems. These complications, including unstable blood pressure and pulse, hyperglycemia, and contraction of the extracellular fluid volume, are due to release of a variety of hormones (e.g., serotonin, substance P, enkephalins) from the tumor. In this circumstance, blood glucose levels should be measured at frequent intervals (and abnormal values treated) and hemodynamics carefully tended to. It is important to remember that epinephrine is a potent releaser of *metastatic monitoring: measure levels of blood serotonin & substance P.*

hormones from carcinoids and should not be administered to these patients. If hypotension must be treated pharmacologically, dopamine is quite safe.

Resection of the Tumor

In general, appendectomy alone is adequate therapy if: (1) the serosa is not broached; (2) the tumor is not greater than 1 cm in diameter; (3) there are no suspicious mesenteric lymph nodes; and (4) there is no evidence of widespread disease. If any of these four criteria are not met, more extensive therapy is mandated. There is no question but that the frequency of metastases is directly related to the size of the lesion (but not with the primary site). Statistically, by the time a carcinoid is 1 cm in diameter, there is a 30% to 35% likelihood of metastases; if 2 cm, the likelihood is 98%. Recently there has been a strong tendency to lower the size indication for right hemicolectomy. While traditional teaching has advocated a 2-cm cut-off point, it is now clear that appendiceal carcinoids of 1.5 cm or greater in size should be treated by right hemicolectomy. The difficult range is between 1.0 cm and 1.49 cm, in which the surgeon must make the judgment based on other criteria. With a 1.5-cm lesion and a suspicious mesenteric lymph node, right hemicolectomy (including the mesentery and nodes along the ileocolic vessels) and ileotransverse colostomy are indicated in this patient. While it is very controversial, in my opinion, reanastomosis would not be indicated in the presence of widespread peritoneal contamination with pus or enteric contents (in cases of free appendiceal perforation). If other intestinal carcinoids are identified, they should be resected with their mesenteric node-bearing areas. Sites of metastatic disease should be biopsied, if possible, for histologic confirmation.

Monitoring for Treating Metastases

Assuming there is no clinically apparent metastatic disease and all the gross tumor is resected, a plan must be established to monitor for possible later recurrence. There have been significant new advances in the area. The traditional modality for chemical screening for carcinoid disease has been the measurement of urinary excretion of 5-hydroxyindoleacetic acid (5-HIAA), with the normal value in most laboratories being 12 µg/day. However, this determination is far from ideal. Since there are more than 25 pathways for the degradation of serotonin, only one of which yields 5-HIAA, there is a 30% rate of false negatives. On the other hand, steatorrhea due to any etiology causes elevation in the rate of 5-HIAA excretion. Since loss of terminal ileum and the ileocecal valve predisposes to steatorrhea, there is a strong likelihood of false positivity. Far more specific information can be obtained by direct measurement of circulating levels of serotonin and substance P.

Let me digress briefly to explain the relevance of substance P. Substance P is an 11-amino acid peptide initially discovered by von Euler and Gaddum in the 1930s. Once isolated and chemically characterized in the 1970s, it was rapidly recognized that substance P coexisted with serotonin in enterochromaffin cells. In fact, there is significant suggestion that serotonin and substance P coexist in the same intracellular granules. Because of this relationship, it is not surprising that high concentrations of substance P have been identified in carcinoid tumors and that patients with carcinoid tumors have elevated plasma levels of this peptide. While the physiologic role of substance P is being extensively studied, in carcinoid disease it appears that this peptide is responsible for the hemodynamic abnormalities and flushing.

While measurement by radioimmunoassay of circulatory concentrations of serotonin and substance P is quite specific, there is a potential problem with this modality as well, i.e., the possibility of intermittent hormone secretion and normal basal levels. In view of this, we have characterized two provocative tests, the objectives of which are to stimulate hormone release (measured in plasma) during provocation of symptoms. While calcium (Ca) infusion (4 mEq Ca/kg/hour for three to four hours) works rather consistently, there is significant danger induced by increasing the level of serum calcium to 13 to 14 mg/dl. Hence, we prefer the intravenous injection of pentagastrin (0.5 µg/kg). This technique is quite safe and symptoms are provoked within two to three minutes of injection. The test, with venous blood sampling, is usually completed within ten minutes.

I advocate the use of pentagastrin challenge as the most sensitive and specific method for identifying tumor recurrence. A baseline study should be performed in this patient shortly after his recovery from appendicitis and at six-month intervals thereafter. Conversion from a negative test to a positive one would warrant an extensive search for tumor that may be a metachronous primary or metastasis from the original lesion. If the pentagastrin test became positive, localization studies would include small bowel contrast radiography, ultrasonography, and computed tomography (CT) scanning or magnetic resonance imaging (MRI). Except in the liver, contrast angiography should play no major role in localization. In my experience, peripheral venous sampling with substance P radioimmunoassay (Fig 41–2) has been the most effective technique for identifying intra-abdominal carcinoid disease.

TREATMENT

The fate of patients with carcinoid disease is extraordinarily unpredictable. Some patients develop rapidly progressive disease and succumb quickly, while others seem to live symbiotically with their tumors (even with liver metastases) for many years. This puts the surgeon in a very difficult position. What can one say to a family that adequately describes the uncertainty facing a patient with carcinoid tumor?

Unfortunately, once carcinoid disease becomes metastatic, little if anything can be done to arrest its growth. Standard chemotherapy is of little value. While initial reports of streptozocin use were optimistic, this drug has proved to be rather disappointing. There have been recent reports of the successful use of interferon, but far too few patients have been treated with this drug to allow for a realistic appraisal of its value.

Currently, operative therapy plays a very small role in the management of patients with metastatic carcinoid disease. Only rarely are liver metastases single or confined to one lobe, i.e., accessible to possibly curative surgical resection. There is no role for debulking of carcinoid tumor; it neither reduces symptoms nor prolongs life.

The major aim of the long-term care of carcinoid patients is symptomatic

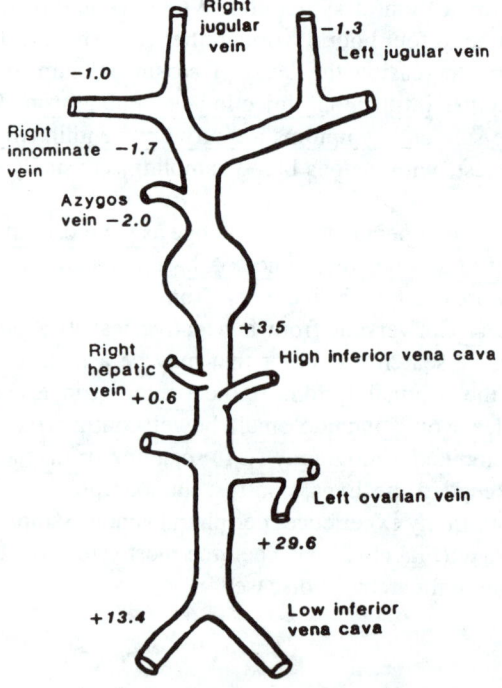

FIG 41–2.
Localization of a carcinoid in the left ovary. The (+) and (−) numbers represent differences in specific venous concentrations of substance P from mean arterial blood levels. Note the step up in the left ovarian vein. (From Strodel WE, et al: *J Surg Oncol* 1984; 27:106. Used by permission.)

control. Regardless of the presence of metastases, there is no indication for therapy other than the disability caused by manifestations of carcinoid syndrome, e.g., flushing, diarrhea, and bronchoconstriction. On the other hand, once a patient becomes symptomatic, reduction of symptoms becomes an important component of care. While hepatic artery ligation previously was commonly utilized in patients with liver metastases, the currently advocated therapy is arterial embolization, which can be repeated successfully several times.

The most exciting recent developments have included the recognition of new agents to control carcinoid symptoms. An analogue of somatostatin (Sandostatin) has been shown to be most effective. It reduces both flushing and diarrhea and, despite its lack of specificity, it has very few side effects. The disadvantage of this agent is that it must be administered subcutaneously. Ketanserin, a new oral 5-HT_2 antagonist, is much more effective in controlling diarrhea than it is flushing. Finally, we have shown that verapamil (the calcium-channel blocker) antagonizes the effects of both serotonin and substance P, and preliminary use of this drug has shown it to be quite effective.

SUMMARY

The management of a patient with carcinoid tumor requires consideration of a great number of issues. By planning and executing a sequentially programmed plan of care such as the one described, the surgeon may provide maximal care for these patients.

There is no role for debulking of carcinoid tumor.

42

Obstruction of Splenic Flexure

A 63-year-old male patient, who was previously well, has noted the gradual onset of obstipation over the past three months. Thirty-six hours prior to admission the patient experienced total constipation without passage of gas or stool, and the abdomen began to be distended. He became nauseated. On physical examination the abdomen was distended, with hyperactive bowel sounds but no tenderness. Stool guaiac is positive. An abdominal x-ray reveals the presence of a column of gas extending to the splenic flexure, where it stops abruptly. An emergency barium enema reveals a constricting lesion at the splenic flexure, without passage of barium.

Consultant: Claude E. Welch, M.D.

What is the proper operation for acute intestinal obstruction due to a cancer of the splenic flexure? Several methods need to be considered. The choice of procedure will vary depending upon several factors of which the most important are the build and fitness of the patient, the skill and familiarity of the surgeon with alternative operations, the anesthetist, and the conditions in which the procedure is carried out.

The primary objective of the operation is to relieve the obstruction. This can be done by a total diversion of feces by colostomy; decompression by cecostomy; or primary resection of the tumor followed either by primary anastomosis or proximal colostomy and distal mucous fistula, with continuity to be restored at a later time.

The second objective is to carry out the most effective procedure to cure the cancer. This will involve a discussion of the amount of colon and surrounding tissues such as the mesentery or adjacent organs that should be removed.

The operation that is chosen should have an acceptable mortality and morbidity rate. Technical features, therefore, are important. Furthermore, other matters being equal, the operation that permits the most rapid return to normal health is desirable. Finally, because colon cancer has a significant incidence both of synchronous and metachronous cancers or polyps that together occur in about

5% of cases, it is desirable to reduce the threat of these lesions at the time of the original operation.

CHOICE OF OPERATION

From a practical point of view, there are several operations used most commonly for acute colonic obstruction due to cancer of the splenic flexure:

1. One-stage subtotal colectomy with primary ileosigmoid anastomosis.
2. Three-stage resection primary transverse colostomy followed by resection of the splenic flexure and anastomosis and, in the third stage, closure of the colostomy.
3. One-stage segmental resection of the splenic flexure with primary colocolic anastomosis. In order to relieve the obstruction and increase safety, the proximal colon must be emptied at the time of operation.
4. Cecostomy followed by segmental resection of the splenic flexure and anastomosis. Since cecostomies usually close spontaneously, this is a two-stage operation.
5. Resection of the splenic flexure with proximal colostomy and distal mucous fistula. Anastomosis is carried out at a second stage.
6. Ileostomy followed by segmental resection and anastomosis of the splenic flexure. This is a three-stage operation.

Every surgeon has his preference for one of these operations. I prefer No. 1, with No. 2 my second choice (Fig 42–1). The advantages and disadvantages of each of the methods must be considered.

Subtotal Colectomy With Ileosigmoid Anastomosis

The advantages of this operation are: (1) both relief of the obstruction and proper operation for the cancer are done at the time of the first operation; (2) unsuspected polyps and cancers of the right and transverse colon are removed simultaneously; (3) if the cecum is enormously distended and about to rupture, that danger is removed; and (4) postoperative development of another cancer in the remaining colorectum or a suture line recurrence can be determined readily by either rigid or flexible sigmoidoscopy.

The disadvantages are : (1) it requires a surgeon familiar with the method; (2) it may not be desirable if the anesthetist or operative conditions are less than optimum; and (3) in old patients most of the sigmoid should be retained to avoid protracted diarrhea.

Every operative procedure designed to give the optimal chance of cure of the cancer must conform with certain standards. Hence, the description that follows is applicable to every resection for obstruction of the splenic flexure.

Deflation of colon may be accomplished by inserting a large chest tube in the distal ileum & passed into the colon.

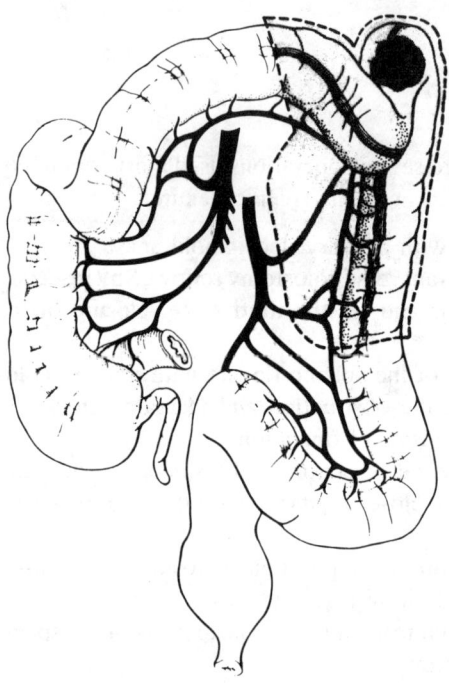

FIG 42–1.
Primary resections and anastomoses for obstructing cancer of the splenic flexure. *Subtotal colectomy.* The resected bowel includes the shaded area, the entire proximal colon and the terminal ileum. Distention of the proximal colon is reduced by means of a 30-cm sump sucker introduced through an incision in the distal ileum. The anastomosis of the ileum to the colon can be 25 cm proximal to the anus in good-risk patients; it should be at the upper level of the sigmoid in old patients to lower the incidence of postoperative diarrhea. *Segmental resection of the splenic flexure.* The extent of the resection is shown by shaded area. This operation is used in poor-risk or very obese patients. The obstruction must have been relieved by previous colostomy or cecostomy, or the proximal colon must be emptied at the time of the resection. After resection, the transverse colon is anastomosed end-to-end with the upper sigmoid. (From Welch CE, et al: *Manual of Lower Gastrointestinal Surgery.* New York, Springer-Verlag, 1980, p 107. Used by permission.)

The amount of colon that is excised should be at least 10 cm both proximal and distal to the tumor. Suture line implantation after resection and anastomosis of the splenic flexure is rare, but chances theoretically are diminished if ties are placed both distally and proximally prior to manipulation; in the presence of marked distention, proximal ligation may not be possible until the colon is deflated.

Deflation is accomplished most readily by means of a special long (30-cm) sump sucker. If the ileocecal valve is incompetent, there will be distention of both the colon and small intestine. The sucker is inserted through the distal ileum and first passed upward, removing the contents of the small intestine; thereafter it is passed through the ileocecal valve. Colonic gas and liquid feces are evacuated so that the diameter of the colon is reduced. The sucker is withdrawn and the opening closed by suture. By this means, excellent exposure of the operative field results.

Ties are placed on the left colic artery and vein midway down the mesentery, and also on the marginal artery proximal and distal to the tumor. The right and transverse colon and then the descending colon are mobilized. The ureter must be protected carefully during the dissection. Finally, the splenic flexure is freed.

As it is usually attached firmly to the lower pole of the spleen, gentle and meticulous dissection is important. It is necessary to emphasize the need to avoid rupture of the bowel or splenic injury during this dissection.

The left colic artery is ligated and divided just distal to the inferior mesenteric artery, and the vein ligated and divided at the same level. The distal ileum is divided between clamps, just proximal to the point in which the sucker had previously been introduced. Distally, the colon is divided between clamps about 25 cm proximal to the anus or at the level of the upper sigmoid in elderly patients.

The anastomosis is the next step. It is not necessary to enter into the arguments of hand-sewn vs. stapler anastomoses in this discussion. Suffice it to say that my personal preference is for a two-layer anastomosis made with interrupted absorbable sutures for the inner layer and nonabsorbable for the outer. Silk or cotton can be used for the outer layer; other nonabsorbable sutures such as Tevdec also are suitable. There is some prejudice against wire because of the dangers involved if any member of the operating team should prick his/her finger.

The final step is closure of the mesenteric defect that has been left following the resection. This is no problem if a subtotal colectomy has been done in which the ileosigmoidostomy lies comfortably inferior to and behind the small bowel, or if a relatively localized segmental resection has been done. It may be impossible if a long segment of the left colon has been removed and an anastomosis is made between the transverse colon and the intraperitoneal rectum; in these cases the large mesenteric trap will have to be left open.

There are several controversial points concerning resection of the splenic flexure for cancer. The first is the extent of the mesenteric dissection and the point of arterial ligation. Some surgeons have argued in favor of ligation of the inferior mesenteric artery at its origin in order to secure a wider resection. However, the inferior mesenteric trunk proximal to the left colic branch is only 2.5 to 3 cm in length in most cases. This additional amount is not of great significance. Furthermore, any enlarged lymph nodes in this area can be excised without disturbing the arterial supply. The problem with removal of the entire left colic artery is that the entire left part of the colon has to be removed and an anastomosis made between the transverse colon and the intraperitoneal rectum. Not only does this add considerably to the difficulty of the operation, but clinical studies have shown no great advantage in removal of the entire inferior mesenteric trunk over the more limited dissection.

The second controversy is concerned with the amount of tissue that should be removed about the splenic flexure. Some surgeons have argued in favor of routine concomitant splenectomy and distal pancreatectomy. It is my impression that if cancer has extended to these viscera, the tumor is incurable. Certainly, removal of the tail of the pancreas involves the possibility of serious postoperative complications. There also is some fragmentary evidence that removal of the spleen with colon resection may add to the number of postoperative complications and mortality. Consequently, the spleen or tail of the pancreas is removed only if there is every reason to believe they are invaded directly by tumor.

The situation is somewhat different if the stomach or small intestine merely appears to be involved by direct extension of the cancer. Here a block dissection of the adherent area along with the splenic flexure is indicated.

Three-Stage Resection

Three-stage resection consists of: (1) transverse colostomy, (2) resection and anastomosis of the splenic flexure, and (3) closure of the colostomy.

The advantages of this procedure are: (1) it allows immediate relief of the life-threatening intestinal obstruction; (2) it is applicable in all situations, but it is particularly desirable if the patient is extremely obese or in poor condition, or if the surgeon is not well-versed in surgery of the colon or operative conditions are poor; and (3) if the patient is in poor condition, better preparation prior to resection is possible.

The disadvantages are: (1) the complications and mortality after this operation in skilled hands are not significantly reduced from those of primary resection and anastomosis; (2) the cancer is left in situ where it theoretically at least can continue to grow or metastasize before the resection is done; (3) because of complications following colostomy, occasionally the cancer never can be removed; (4) the condition of the cecum is difficult to determine unless a long incision is made; (5) the period of disability is much longer than after a one-stage procedure; and (6) the incidence of late ventral hernia at the site of a colostomy closure is common, so that a fourth operation will be necessary in some cases.

The transverse colostomy (Fig 42–2,A) is made well to the right of the midline. The transverse colon is withdrawn and a rod or other device to prevent retraction is passed beneath the bowel. In case of severe colonic distention, the bowel is opened immediately with the scalpel after closure of the incision.

Some technical problems do occur with this operation. Sometimes the mesentery of the transverse colon is so short the colon will not reach the abdominal wall; in this case, colostomy must be abandoned and a cecostomy made. A huge omentum also may require detachment and replacement in the abdominal cavity.

The second stage preferably is carried out 10 to 12 days later. The third stage—closure of the colostomy—is done usually a month after discharge from the hospital after the second stage. A barium enema to be certain the anastomosis is satisfactory is done prior to closure of the colostomy.

One-Stage Segmental Resection and Anastomosis

The main feature of the one-stage segmental resection of the splenic flexure—

aided by intraoperative emptying of the obstructed colon and completed by an anastomosis of the transverse colon to the descending colon—is the removal of gas and solid and liquid feces from the colon so that a primary resection and anastomosis can be performed. Several methods have been devised to empty the colon. A long mobile distended transverse colon may be divided, drawn away from the operative field, and the contents emptied into a bucket beside the operating table. Another way is to tie a large tube into the distended colon and empty it through this conduit. This method has been endorsed most recently by both Dudley and Fielding.

The advantages of this procedure are: (1) the operation is completed in one stage; (2) at the time of the laparotomy, the cecum can be inspected and a wider resection done if there is evidence of vascular damage; and (3) the right portion of the colon is preserved so that postoperative diarrhea is less than after subtotal colectomy (this is important in older patients).

The disadvantages are: (1) the possibility of severe contamination of the abdominal cavity if a clamp should slip or the devices should leak; (2) the right colon may be the site of polyps or another cancer that is not detected; and (3) the anastomosis is made between normal distal colon and proximal colon that may be severely affected by edema or lack of blood supply.

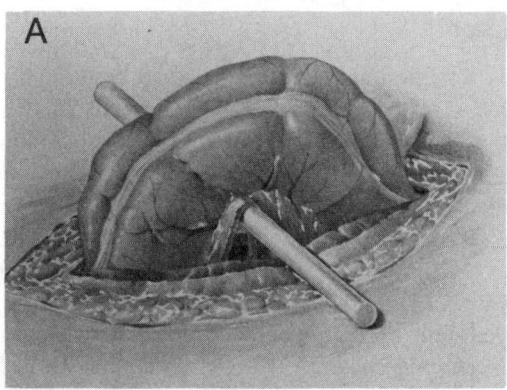
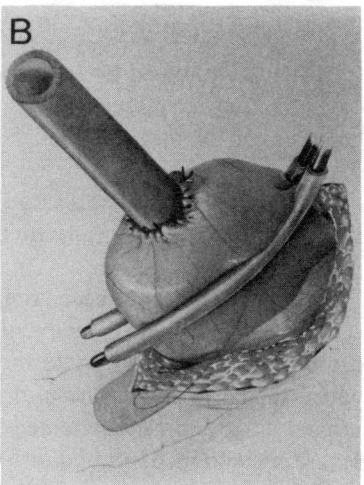

FIG 42–2.
Other methods to relieve acute obstruction. **A,** *transverse colostomy* defunctions the distal colon. **B,** *tube cecostomy* decompresses the distended colon. A soft rubber tube is superior to a Foley or Pezzar catheter. It has numerous holes near the tip. It is inserted into the cecum; the tip lies in the ascending colon. (From Welch CE, et al: *Manual of Lower Gastrointestinal Surgery.* New York, Springer-Verlag, 1980, pp 159 **(A)**, 155 **(B)**. Used by permission.)

Is there objective data?

There is no question that the proponents of this method believe it can be done safely and effectively. However, I have been somewhat dubious about the safety of the procedure if it is done by surgeons who are unfamiliar with the details. The possibilities of fecal contamination are very high, particularly since the most dangerous part of the operation—emptying the distended bowel—is done prior to resection of the tumor, so that contamination could be spread widely during subsequent manipulation.

I also have some theoretical objections to the use of colon for an anastomosis after it has been subject to the damage of edema and possibly vascular compromise from preceding obstruction. It is far safer to use an ileocolic anastomosis. The ileum is easy to use, and it may even be easier to use if it is slightly distended. Blood supply is excellent. The descending colon also has entirely normal blood supply, os that an ileocolic anastomosis has a better chance to heal. Whether or not some experimental proof can be found to substantiate the comparative safety of colocolostomy vs. ileocolostomy in the presence of obstruction, I still would have some qualms considering the fact that most colon resections for cancer are done in older patients, many of whom already have significant vascular problems. In my opinion, this is a method that is not for use by amateurs and even has theoretical disadvantages in the hands of experts.

Cecostomy for Relief of Obstruction

Cecostomy, followed by segmental resection and anastomosis, can be done by either of two techniques. Tube cecostomy (see Fig 42–2,B) succeeds in decompression of the distended colon, and in two thirds of the cases does not require operative closure or repair of a later hernia; this is therefore usually a two-stage operation. The second method of cecostomy, in which the mucosa is sewed to the skin, always requires secondary closure and thus is a three-stage procedure.

The advantages of cecostomy are: (1) it allows immediate inspection of the cecum, so that if there is incipient gangrene or rupture of the muscle the diagnosis can be made and appropriate measures undertaken; (2) it can be done with the patient under local anesthesia if necessary, os that very obese patients or those in poor condition can be treated simply and expeditiously; (3) it will relieve the severe distention of the colon proximal to the tumor; (4) it allows complete mobility of the transverse colon for use in the later resection; and (5) some measure of preparation prior to the subsequent resection can be achieved by antibiotics injected through the cecostomy.

The disadvantages are: (1) the procedure succeeds only in decompression and does not completely defunction the colon, so it is rare for the colon to return to a reasonably normal state prior to resection; (2) the possibility of fecal contamination at the time of resection therefore is greater after cecostomy than after a defunctioning transverse colostomy, since the colon cannot be emptied as effectively; (3) the possibility of intraoperative contamination is greater in the hands of a surgeon not accustomed to the method compared with this possibility with transverse colostomy; and (4) the right and transverse colon remain at risk for other polyps and cancer, either synchronous or metachronous.

Many years ago, there were sharp controversies concerning the value of cecostomy vs. transverse colostomy as the first stage of an operation for obstructing cancer of the left part of the colon. Since then it has become clear that the one-stage resection and anastomosis has become the procedure of choice for all cancers of the right and transverse colon. I believe that with the use of intraoperative decompression, obstructing cancer of the splenic flexure can be treated in the same fashion. For this reason, whether or not colostomy is superior to cecostomy for cancer of the splenic flexure is moot except in a few cases. At present, I prefer transverse colostomy to cecostomy for the above reasons.

Primary Resection

When this operation is done the segment containing the cancer is resected, the proximal end of the retained colon is brought out as a colostomy, and the distal end of the colon is either brought out as a mucous fistula or closed according to the Hartmann procedure.

The advantages of primary resection of the splenic flexure with anastomosis deferred for a second state—are: (1) it allows removal of the cancer at the first stage, increasing the chance for cure from that disease; (2) it may be used in emergency situations, for example, if after resection of the colon the patient's condition suddenly deteriorates; and (3) if perforation of the bowel with peritoneal contamination is found in addition to acute obstruction, this is the procedure of choice.

The disadvantages are: (1) unless some method has been found to evacuate the distended colon, the operation for acute obstruction is likely to lead to numerous technical difficulties such as rupture of the bowel and wide contamination; and (2) the extent of the resection of the cancer is likely to be compromised.

Loop Ileostomy

Loop ileostomy—followed by resection and anastomosis of the splenic flexure, and at a third stage by closure of the ileostomy—is used very rarely and has few advocates. It is useless and dangerous unless the ileocecal valve is incompetent; if the valve is incompetent, it has no advantages over transverse colostomy.

PRINCIPLES OF OPERATION

Certain principles must be followed regardless of the operation that is done for obstructing cancer of the splenic flexure. The obstruction usually is acute and is most common in the aged. Determinations of blood chemistry are important, but they are not likely to be abnormal. Likewise, blood and urine examinations usually are normal. There may be some measure of dehydration, but urine output can be restored readily. A plain abdominal x-ray film is essential and, in most instances, a barium enema should be done to determine the exact site of obstruction. At times, however, the barium enema may not clearly delineate the cancer, but the barium spills over into a greatly dilated transverse colon.

Early operation is essential. Delay may lead to rupture of the cecum, particularly if it is found to be over 13 cm in diameter on the plain film. A nasogastric tube is passed and placed on suction. Preoperative antibiotics such as cephalexin or a combination of clindamycin and gentamicin are given. If the patient's condition is so poor that a general anesthesia cannot be tolerated, either a transverse colostomy or cecostomy can be done with the patient under local anesthesis.

At the time of operation, if the patient is a good risk and operating conditions are satisfactory, a laparotomy is carried out through either a left paramedian or a transverse supraumbilical incision. The great distention of the small bowel and colon should be relieved by use of the long sump sucker. Thereafter the exposure usually is excellent. On the other hand, if the patient is a poor risk, relief of the obstruction continues to be imperative and can be secured either by transverse colostomy or cecostomy.

The choice between a one-stage resection and alternatives often is not easy even for the accomplished surgeon. Surgeons are inclined to overestimate their ability. They must weigh the operating conditions carefully. In case of doubt, the choice should be in favor of a staged operation and the choice made between an initial transverse colostomy and a cecostomy.

Assuming that the operation has been performed in one to three stages and has been successful, the patient should have a total colonoscopy within six months if the right portion of the colon has not been removed. If the operation was resection and ileosigmoidostomy, the anastomosis and remaining colorectum will be accessible to the rigid or flexible sigmoidoscope. Regular follow-ups are scheduled thereafter.

PROGNOSIS

Statistics concerning the morbidity and mortality of competing methods of treatment of this disease vary considerably and can be compared only in very general terms. For example, one-stage resection and anastomoses are lauded by many surgeons who report a mortality of around 15%. The mortality of patients who have three-stage procedures, if deaths after the first stage are included, appear to be higher. Yet it must be recalled that the published articles reflect the most satisfactory results. The figures from large clinics cannot be transposed to community surgeons who must deal with large numbers of severely ill, nontransportable, poor-risk patients.

In general terms, the five-year crude survival rate for cancers of the colon that have been resected for cure is 53% to 60% in large institutions. In most studies the prognosis for patients with obstruction is significantly lower, although a few investigators have found a somewhat better survival rate. If the obstruction is combined with acute perforation, the immediate mortality is very high and five-year survivals extremely rare.

CONCLUSION

The surgeon has to recognize that certain principles must apply in the treatment of obstructing cancer of the splenic flexure, one of the most difficult portions of the colon with which to deal. It is relatively inaccessible and intimately attached to such organs as the fragile spleen. Rough dissection easily can lead to perforation, fecal contamination, and spread of cancer at the time of the original operation.

The surgeon must be prepared to perform any one of several operations. *Expeditious relief of the acute obstruction is the cardinal object.* The second object is to perform an adequate operation for the cancer. With care, in the majority of instances, both can be accomplished in one stage. However, even the most skillful surgeon at times will find it safer to treat the obstruction first and the cancer a few days later.

BIBLIOGRAPHY

1. Corman ML: *Colon and Rectal Surgery*. Philadelphia, JB Lippincott Co, 1984.
2. Fielding LP, Welch JP: Intestinal obstruction, in *Clinical Surgery International Series*. Edinburgh, Churchill-Livingstone Inc, 1987.
3. Goligher JC: *Surgery of the Anus, Rectum and Colon*, ed 4. London, Bailliere Tindall, 1980.
4. Welch CE, Ottinger LW, Welch JP: *Manual of Lower Intestinal Tract Surgery*. New York, Springer-Verlag, 1980.
5. Welch JP, Donaldson GA: Management of a severe obstruction of the large bowel due to malignant disease. *Am J Surg* 1974; 127:492–499.

43

Extensive Villous Adenoma of the Rectum

A 63-year-old woman complains of increased bowel activity and the passage of clear mucus as well as leakage at night. Abdominal examination reveals no abnormality, but rectal examination reveals an easily palpable mass. Sigmoidoscopy reveals what appears to be fronds and a typical villous adenoma lesion that terminates at 5 cm from the anal verge. Multiple biopsies reveal villous adenoma with atypicality. On barium enema the lesion is seen to extend proximally for about 8 cm and is entirely circumferential.

Consultant: Warren E. Enker, M.D.

The case is that of a 63-year-old woman with a villous adenoma of the rectum requiring operative management. Before deciding upon her surgical management, the case should be reviewed and placed into broader clinical context by examining the following factors: (1) location; (2) clinical features of villous adenomas: (3) presence or absence of invasive carcinoma, i.e., the role of biopsy; (4) other colonic neoplasms (benign and malignant); (5) the options of surgical management; and (6) the case in focus.

LOCATION

This villous adenoma is located in the rectum 5 cm from the anal verge. It is annular or circumferential and extends internally up to 13 cm from the anal verge. Location alone raises serious questions regarding management. Whether viewed from the Memorial Hospital approach reported by Quan and Castro (0 to 5 cm) or from the St. Mark's Hospital approach reported by Thompson (0 to 8 cm), the lower end of this tumor is situated within the low rectum.

That a villous adenoma should be located in the rectum is a common finding. Of the 215 cases reported by Quan and Castro, 144 (67%) were located within the rectum, while Christiansen and associates reported that 82% of villous adenomas were located within the rectum. Thompson, in reporting on 121 cases of villous adenoma, divided the rectum into the lower third (0 to 8 cm) and the middle third (8 to 12 cm). At Memorial Hospital the rectum has been defined as the distal large bowel measuring 0 to 11 cm from the anal verge with 0 to 5 cm considered the low rectum and 6 to 11 cm the mid or upper rectum. The portion 12 cm and above is generally considered to be rectosigmoid or some portion of the abdominal colon.

Selection of treatment is heavily influenced by location. Colonic lesions, if small and pedunculated, are usually treated by colonoscopic polypectomy or by resection, depending upon their size and the presence or absence of invasive carcinoma. Rectal lesions represent a more serious problem of management, i.e., sphincter preservation. Location within the rectum, size, annularity, or signs of malignancy may all influence the choice of treatment. If a benign-appearing tumor can be removed transanally or occasionally via a trans-sphincteric approach as a biopsy *in toto*, then this is the first step that is generally applied. In the case of a midrectal mass, especially without signs of cancer, sphincter preservation will be the rule. In a low rectal villous adenoma, especially with clinical signs of cancer, an abdominoperineal resection will be performed, but such procedures are in the minority. Quan and Castro reported that only 34 of 144 cases (24%) of rectal villous adenomas were treated by abdominoperineal resection; 33 of these proved to be cancers. Nivatvongs et al. reported that only one of 11 circumferential villous adenomas of the rectum required abdominoperineal resection, and Thompson was able to perform a sphincter-preserving operation (excision, diathermy, or resection) in 7 out of 8 similar cases. Thus, it would appear that sphincter preservation is the highest priority.

CLINICAL FEATURES OF VILLOUS ADENOMAS

Quan and Castro have indicated that the texture, consistency, or feel of a villous adenoma can indicate malignancy to the experienced examiner. While in the case of "soft" lesions on rectal-digital examination 50% of lesions contained cancer, 17 of 19 intermediate and 9 of 9 firm lesions contained invasive cancer. Nivatvongs and associates are less optimistic about detecting cancer by palpation. While 67% of villous adenomas in their series were located in the rectum, only 17% were even detected by palpation alone due to their characteristically soft, easily missed texture.

Ulceration or induration (in the absence of a previous biopsy) is strongly indicative of invasive cancer. Nivatvongs and associates have demonstrated that when these two features are absent 91% of villous adenomas, regardless of size, are clinically benign, i.e., do not contain invasive carcinoma. All authors agree that invasive carcinoma means invasion through the muscularis mucosa.

Annularity, in contrast to size alone, has greater bearing on malignancy. In

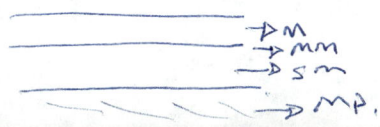

39 instances of annularity, Quan and Castro reported that 30 (77%) contained malignancy as defined above.

PRESENCE OR ABSENCE OF INVASIVE CARCINOMA—THE ROLE OF BIOPSY

The desire for accurate preoperative assessment in villous adenoma frequently leads to the misguided use of biopsy. The preoperative biopsy of a villous adenoma is subject to a high degree of sampling error. Quan and Castro demonstrated that 29 of 52 cases in which the initial or preoperative biopsies were reportedly benign subsequently demonstrated invasive carcinoma after excision or resection, a false-negative biopsy rate of 52%. When an initial biopsy of cancer was obtained, invasive cancer was not present in four cases (11%). Of 35 suspicious cases, 9 (27%) were subsequently proved benign and 24 (73%) malignant. The total rate of accuracy was 36% of all biopsies and, in particular, 52% false negatives. Similar findings were reported by Christiansen et al. Of 76 cases in which biopsy demonstrated a benign villous adenoma, 27 subsequently showed carcinoma invading the muscularis mucosa; a 36% rate of biopsy-related error. More germane is the fact that 92 of 215 cases were clinically managed *without* the use of biopsy; size and location determining treatment. In one respect, biopsy can even interfere with treatment, as when submucosal induration ruins the plane of submucous excision, a technique originated by Sir Alan Parks and one that is now in common use via the transanal approach, as reported by Thompson. The induration that results exclusively from biopsy may confuse or misguide subsequent examiners, resulting in unnecessarily radical treatment.

Where a villous adenoma is suspected on digital examination and sigmoidoscopy, biopsy should be avoided at least until a treatment decision has been made on the basis of size, location, and clinical signs of benign or malignant disease.

OTHER COLONIC NEOPLASMS—BENIGN AND MALIGNANT

Patients with villous adenomas of the rectum or rectosigmoid frequently have benign and malignant disease present elsewhere in the colon; thus, they should be carefully examined. Data are derived predominantly from the precolonoscopy era. However, a general idea of the prevalence of benign diseases or of synchronous benign and malignant neoplasms is available. Quan and Castro reported the following synchronous findings by all means of examination (i.e., sigmoidoscopy, barium enema, etc.) in patients with villous adenomas: 35 invasive carcinomas (16%), 105 adenomas (49%), and 45 cases of hemorrhoids, diverticulosis, etc. Thus 65% of patients had a second neoplasm.

Thompson reported that 30 of 121 patients (25%) with villous adenomas had a synchronous neoplasm. There were 9 cancers and 21 cases of adenomas, 10 of which were single and 11 multiple.

Christiansen et al. reported that 75 of 174 patients (43%) with villous adenomas of the colon and rectum had synchronous tumors; 37 (50%) of these were malignant. Thus, a careful search of the remaining colon is strongly indicated when a patient is found to have a villous adenoma. These figures are in broad general agreement with the axiom that 50% of patients with a rectal adenoma will have a synchronous adenoma in a more proximal colonic location, as reported by Winawer. Total colonoscopy or, at a minimum, flexible sigmoidoscopy and a high-quality double-contrast barium enema are indicated prior to treatment, as the total scope of treatment may include a second neoplasm in a significant number of patients.

OPTIONS OF SURGICAL MANAGEMENT

Villous adenomas are treated according to the same principles as are other lesions of the colon. Benign lesions of the colon, if amenable to colonoscopic polypectomy (i.e., pedunculated), may be excised by snare technique and are submitted for complete pathologic evaluation. If invasive carcinoma is discovered, resection may be necessary depending upon pathologic criteria. Morson et al. would advocate a subsequent resection for pedunculated adenomas with "aggressive histology" (i.e., poorly differentiated disease) or for involved margins of excision. Cooper's data would suggest broader criteria for resection when the adenoma has been based upon a "short stalk" of 1 to 2 mm. In his experience, 20% of such cases with invasive carcinoma have demonstrated lymph node metastases. In the absence of medical contraindications, sessile adenomas with invasive carcinoma are, in our experience, an indication for resection along the usual guidelines of cancer treatment.

Lesions of the rectum may present more of a problem in designing and accomplishing treatment goals. For clinically benign lesions that are not annular, are neither indurated or ulcerated, and are located within reach of the anus, transanal excision of the villous adenoma can usually be accomplished as the first step. Submucous excision as introduced by Parks is the preferred technique. Invasive carcinoma involving the muscularis mucosa can be treated by re-excision of the remaining rectal wall for margins. Invasive carcinoma involving the muscularis propria or deeper will be detected as a positive deep margin, in which case further excision or resection is indicated. Alternatively, a full thickness excision may be accomplished from the outset. Only rarely is abdominoperineal resection appropriate, as previously indicated. While still controversial, large lesions that do not lend themselves to transanal excision may be treated by transsphincteric or transcoccygeal approaches. These approaches should currently be reserved for clinically benign lesions or for patients in whom the morbidity of a major resection would be prohibitive.

Lesions of the mid-rectum, especially if small and clinically benign, may also be treated by cautery snare or by excision until complete pathologic evaluation is available. For larger lesions, for those with clinical signs of malignancy, and especially for annular lesions, resection is indicated on clinical grounds alone, due to the anticipated high rate of invasive malignancy, as well as on technical considerations.

Certain features make it possible to treat villous adenomas of the rectum with sphincter-preserving approaches when abdominoperineal resection would otherwise be considered. Generally, when diagnosed, fewer cancers arising in villous adenomas are extensive, i.e., Dukes B and C stages. Cancer-related five-year and ten-year survival figures of 93% and 70%, respectively, are considerably better than average. Some of these tumors even lend themselves to current treatment by local excision with or without supplemental radiotherapy. When local excision has been performed on clinical grounds, five-year and ten-year survivals of 100% and 94%, respectively, prevail, suggesting that the cancers detected in villous adenomas of the rectum generally represent relatively early disease. In other cases requiring resection in which focal malignancy does not occupy the entire adenoma, closer distal margins may be employed compared to those usually advocated in order to preserve rectal continuity. In this specific instance, biopsy of the distal edge of the adenoma may be helpful in determining a benign border. If a clear margin cannot be obtained after complete mobilization of the rectum (i.e., division of both lateral ligaments, complete dissection of Denonvillier's fascia and of Waldeyer's fascia, thus elevating and straightening the rectum), the mucosa can even be divided via a transanal approach under direct observation. In some cases, portions of the internal sphincter can be preserved. In difficult cases, restoration of continuity has been successfully achieved by modifications of the Soave technique (as reported by Scoma) or by the use of the end-to-end primary coloanal anastomosis (Figs 43–1 and 43–2).

The overall mortality from cancer arising in a villous adenoma is low. Quan and Castro reported 23 deaths due to cancer in 215 patients (11%). In 26 cases (12%), residual villous adenoma required further treatment at various follow-up intervals. In seven cases, locally recurrent cancer developed and claimed six of seven lives. Thompson has reported 26 instances of recurrent benign villous adenoma in 121 cases treated (21%).

THE CASE IN FOCUS

The patient described in this case presentation has an annular lesion with its distal edge located 5 cm from the anal verge. Biopsies, although not entirely representative, show atypia but no invasive carcinoma. Nonetheless, we can expect on clinical grounds alone a 75% incidence of invasive cancer from the data presented, thus indicating the need for resection as opposed to local treatment. In the absence of clinical features of malignancy, sphincter preservation may be achieved by taking a less extensive distal margin and by using the coloanal technique of restoration. If necessary, the distal mucosa may be incised via the transanal approach. A diverting colostomy should accompany this operation.

(Editor's note: This lesion is quite low. Were it higher, any one of a number of techniques might be used. At 5 cm, it is unlikely an anterior resection using a hand-sewn anastomosis from above is possible, even in a thin patient. Thus, one might use either an end-on-end stapler or the coloanal anastomosis described by the author. Whatever the technique of anastomosis, some sphincter dysfunction, which is usually temporary, will result. In my opinion, eversion of the rectum probably injures some of the delicate nerves around the rectum that are involved in continence. Thus, anastomosis should be carried out within the uneverted rectum, an advantage of the coloanal technique. One can retain adequate sphincter function, especially if anastomosis is done at the junction of

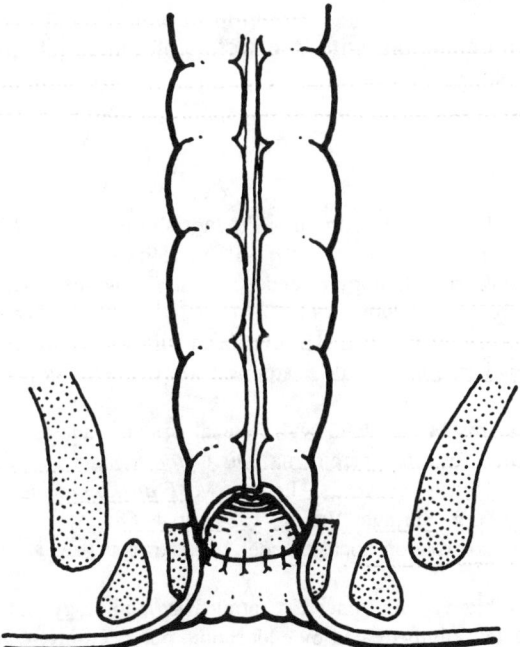

FIG 43–1.
The coloanal reconstruction following low anterior resection provides an end-to-end primary anastomosis, without eversion of the rectum. When operating for cancer, the internal sphincter is divided at the level of the anastomosis, without preservation of a perianastomotic cuff.

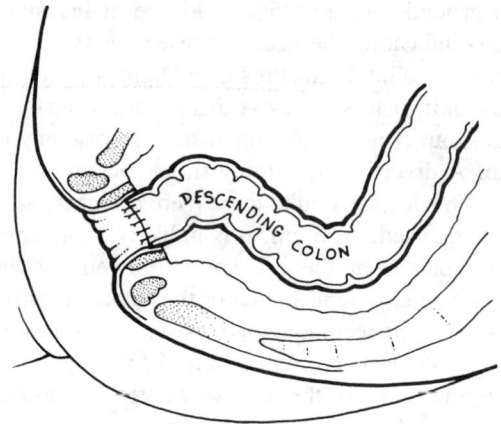

FIG 43–2.
In performing coloanal reconstruction, it is important to preserve the anorectal right angle in order to maintain resting continence. The proximal segment or descending colon must completely fill the sacral hollow in order to ensure faithful reconstruction of the anorectal right angle.

transitional rectal epithelium with true rectal columnar epithelium at the top of the columns of Morgagni.)

BIBLIOGRAPHY

1. Christiansen J, Kirkegaard P, Ibsen J: Prognosis after treatment of villous adenomas of the colon and rectum. *Ann Surg* 1979; 189:404–408.
2. Cooper HS: Surgical pathology of endoscopically removed polyps of the colon and rectum. *Am J Surg Pathol* 1983; 7:613–623.
3. Enker WE, Laffer UTh, Block GE: Enhanced survival of patients with colon and rectal cancer is based upon wide anatomic resection. *Ann Surg* 1979; 190:350–360.
4. Enker WE, Stearns MS Jr, Janov AJ: Peranal coloanal anastomosis following low anterior resection for rectal carcinoma. *Dis Colon Rectum* 1985; 28:576–581.
5. Huber A, von Hochstetter AHC, Allgower M: *Trans-Sphincteric Surgery of the Rectum.* Heidelberg, Springer-Verlag, 1984, pp 1–68.
6. Kraske P: Zur Exstirpation hochsitzender Mastdarmksiebse. *Verh Dtsch Ges Chir* 1985; 14:464–474.
7. Morson BC, Whiteway JE, Jones EA, et al: Histopathology and prognosis of malignant colorectal polyps treated by endoscopic polypectomy. *Gut* 1984; 25:437–444.
8. Nivatvongs S, Nicholson JD, Rothenberger DA, et al: Villous adenomas of the rectum: The clinical accuracy of assessment. *Surgery* 1980; 14:549–551.
9. Oh C, Aufses AH Jr: Local excision of low and mid-rectal villous adenomas (Editorial). *Am J Surg* 1982; 144:291.

10. Quan SHQ, Castro El B: Papillary adenomas (Villous tumors): A review of 215 cases. *Dis Colon Rectum* 1971; 14:267–280.
11. Scoma JA: Management of benign villous adenomas of the entire rectum. *Dis Colon Rectum* 1978; 21:630–632.
12. Thompson JPS: Treatment of sessile villous and tubulovillous adenomas of the rectum. *Dis Colon Rectum* 1977; 20:467–472.
13. Winawer SJ: Colorectal adenomas: Guidelines for detection and follow-up. *Medical Student* 1983; 9:19–20.

44

Sigmoid Vesical Fistula (Diverticulitis)

A 56-year-old man with a previous history of intermittent constipation and diarrhea reports the passage of air upon urination. A spun sediment of urine reveals some vegetable matter. Cystoscopy reveals an area of bullous irritation at the dome of the bladder. Barium enema does not reveal a sigmoid vesical fistula but ample diverticuli.

**Consultants: Richard M. Devine, M.D.,
Robert W. Beart, Jr., M.D.**

When a patient presents with pneumaturia and fecaluria, the physician must assume that the patient has an enterovesical fistula unless proved otherwise. In a patient this age, the most likely cause is a diverticular abscess that has eroded into the bladder. Colon cancer is the second most common cause of enterovesical fistulas in this age group. Crohn's disease is a possible cause, but it usually occurs in a younger patient (20 to 30 years old) and there is usually a history of Crohn's disease prior to a fistula developing. Crohn's disease is the most common cause of fistulas from the small intestine to the bladder, and 1% to 5% of patients with Crohn's disease will develop an enterovesical fistula. Other, less common causes include appendiceal abscess, trauma, surgical injuries, ingested foreign bodies that have perforated the bowel, the perforated Meckel's diverticulum. In more recent reports, fistulas secondary to radiation therapy, often in women with gynecologic malignancies, are a small but difficult group.

Enterovesical fistulas are more common in men by a 2:1 or 3:1 margin. The exceptions to this are fistulas secondary to radiation therapy. The interposition of the vagina and uterus between the colon and bladder lowers the incidence in women.

DIAGNOSIS

Unexplained, recurrent urinary tract infection failing to clear with appropriate antibiotic therapy is the most common way patients with enterovesical fistulas present. The common symptoms are those associated with bladder infection, i.e., suprapubic pain, dysuria, frequency, and urgency. Pneumaturia is present in approximately 60% of patients and fecaluria in less than half. Pneumaturia is considered pathognomonic for an enterovesical fistula, but it may rarely be due to bladder infection with gas-producing organisms, recent bladder catheterization, or other manipulation. The pneumaturia is described as a hiss and occurs at the end of voiding, simply because the air rises to the dome of the bladder and is expelled as the bladder empties.

Patients may have the fistula for months before the diagnosis is confirmed. If a patient presents with pneumaturia and fecaluria, the physician is obviously alerted to the possibility of a vesicoenteric fistula. If these symptoms are absent, however, the diagnosis can be difficult and in some cases is not made until surgery. If a patient presents with recurrent urinary tract infections that are not cleared by antibiotic therapy, an enterovesical fistula should be in the differential diagnosis, and appropriate tests should be done to document the fistula. In less than 20% of patients, there is no history of the original illness causing the fistula; when there is, it tends to be minor and does not require hospitalization. Minor abdominal pain and alteration in bowel habits are the most common intestinal symptoms. Urine usually does not leak from the bladder to the bowel, so it is uncommon to have patients passing urine from the rectum, although it does occur. Sometimes a patient will present with gram-negative sepsis and shock, either from an intra-abdominal infection or an ascending urinary tract infection.

Patients whose fistulas are secondary to Crohn's disease do not have more bowel symptoms than Crohn's patients without fistulas. They are, however, more likely to have a palpable mass on physical examination.

Routine urinalysis is abnormal in most cases and usually shows pyuria and bacteruria as well as hematuria. Results of urine cultures will be positive in the majority of patients, but they may be negative at times, especially if the patient had a recent course of antibiotics. *Escherichia coli* is the predominant organism, with other gram-negative enteric organisms cultured less frequently. Dietary fiber seen in a urine specimen is diagnostic for the fistula.

Proctoscopy has the lowest yield in demonstrating the presence of a colovesical fistula. In a patient with diverticulitis the sigmoid is often fixed and angulated, and it is unusual to be able to pass a rigid proctoscope to the area where the fistula originates. Most patients whose cases were reported in the literature were evaluated prior to the widespread use of flexible sigmoidoscopes. Even though a flexible colonoscope may be passed more readily into the sigmoid, it is doubtful that the fistula could actually be visualized in many cases. This does not detract from its use, as it is important in diagnosing colon cancers and assessing the rectum and sigmoid prior to surgery. There has been one report of doing flexible sigmoidoscopy and cystoscopy concurrently, injecting dye through the sigmoidoscope near the suspected site of the fistula and watching

Get IVP in pt c̄ cancer, Crohn's & previous radiation therapy.

for its appearance in the bladder. The authors of that report did not indicate how many patients had been evaluated with this technique.

Barium enema will demonstrate some abnormality (usually diverticulitis) in almost all patients, but it will demonstrate the fistula in only 20% to 50% of patients. In some cases the barium enema will show extravasation but no definite connection to the bladder. If a patient is suspected of having an enterovesical fistula and the barium enema is normal, Crohn's disease should be considered and confirmed with a small bowel series.

Cystoscopy should be done to evaluate the bladder for cancer. The cystoscopist will actually see the fistula in less than 50% of cases but will often see a focal area of granulation tissue and edema that suggests a fistula is present in 80% of patients. Cystoscopy will also rule out bladder calculus, which occurs in up to 10% of patients due to their chronic urinary infection and the presence of fecal material in the bladder. A completely normal cystoscopy occurs in 20% of patients, but it does not rule out the diagnosis.

Intravenous pyelography is important in evaluating the urinary tract. It is particularly important in patients with primary or recurrent cancer, patients with previous radiation therapy, and patients with Crohn's disease because these patients are more likely to have associated urinary tract pathology, such as hydronephrosis, that may affect surgical management. Cystographs rarely show a deformity in the bladder wall, either an extrinsic mass or triangular elevated portion of bladder wall corresponding to the point of attachment of the fistula.

Computerized tomography (CT) is currently being used to evaluate these patients. If the diagnosis is established by other tests, CT scan is probably unnecessary. Findings on CT scans include the detection of small amounts of intravesical air, the detection of orally or rectally administered contrast in the bladder or bladder wall, adjacent bowel wall thickening near the site of the fistula, and an extraluminal mass that may contain air.

If a fistula cannot be demonstrated by x-ray films or endoscopy, other less direct methods may be used to prove a fistula is indeed present. There have been two reports (Amendola et al. and Krco et al.) of examining the patient's urine after barium enema that have shown a 95% sensitivity for proving a fistula is present. After a barium enema, the patient's urine is carefully collected and centrifuged. An x-ray film is then taken of the test tube, and amounts of barium as small as 0.001 ml can be detected. Urine samples should be collected up to 24 hours if the first sample does not demonstrate any barium. Charcoal has also been used in much the same manner as barium.

Methylene blue has been used by injecting it into the rectum and then checking for the blue dye in the urine. After seeing several patients who had a positive test but no fistula, Deshmukh demonstrated that the dye is absorbed by the colonic mucosa in normal subjects and then excreted into the urine. Its use in this manner should be discontinued. (*Editor's note*: A very sensitive diagnostic test involves the use of ^{14}C polyethylene glycol (PEG), orally or as a retention enema, and subsequent counting of the radiation in the urine by liquid scintillation spectrometry. Use of ^{14}C-PEG, which is not absorbed, may be difficult in view of the current paranoia with respect to even beta radiation.)

TREATMENT

The treatment of an enterovesical fistula can range from medical management alone to surgical treatment with either a single or multistage procedure. In the past, surgical treatment usually consisted of three stages: (1) a diverting colostomy, (2) resection of the diseased bowel with anastomosis, and (3) colostomy closure. Currently, a single-stage approach is more common in appropriate patients. Appropriate patients would be those in whom a bowel prep has been completed and there is an absence of generalized intra-abdominal infection, with normal bowel at the site of the anastomosis. If an anastomosis cannot be done safely, a two-stage procedure is preferred in which the septic focus is removed at the first stage with an end colostomy followed at a later date by colostomy closure. Colostomy alone may be appropriate as a palliative procedure in patients with recurrent pelvic malignancies.

These fistulas rarely close spontaneously, and those with the greatest chance of closing by themselves are secondary either to trauma or surgical misadventure. Colostomy alone will not cause these fistulas to heal, nor will it prevent recurrent urinary infections.

At surgery, a lower midline incision is made, and any small bowel that is stuck in the pelvis is mobilized and retracted. The best way to approach the fistula is to mobilize the colon proximal and distal to the fistula. Usually the area between the rectum and the base of the bladder will be relatively free of adhesions, with the sigmoid stuck to the dome of the bladder. In the patient with a fistula caused by diverticulitis, the colon can be "pinched" off the bladder, dividing the fistula at the same time. This blunt dissection is safer and usually less bloody than sharp dissection. The actual tract cannot always be found at the time of surgery. The area of the fistula on the bladder is closed with two layers of interrupted absorbable sutures. The diseased bowel is resected and either a colostomy or anastomosis created. If there is suitable omentum, it is placed between the bladder and the bowel wall and tacked in place. A catheter is left in the bladder for 10 to 14 days.

Patients who have a fistula secondary to cancer are more difficult to treat. These patients can be divided into two groups, those who have fistulas at the time the cancer is diagnosed and those who have fistulas that develop with either a recurrence or as a result of treatment of the cancer. The first group is easier to manage than the second; the fistula tract and a portion of the bladder wall must be resected. A large portion of the posterior bladder wall and dome of the bladder can be resected and primarily closed, with the remaining bladder eventually expanding to give an adequate capacity. The bladder is repaired in two layers with absorbable sutures. Permanent sutures and staples should probably not be used in the bladder, as they can act as a nidus for the formation of subsequent bladder stones. If the cancer involves the trigone, a total cystectomy should be done. In more than half of these patients, the operation is considered palliative because of invasion into surrounding structures or distant metastasis. Those who are resected for cure have an acceptable five-year survival rate of 56% (as reported by Aldrete and ReMine).

Patients whose fistula is the result of recurrent cancer or treatment of the primary cancer (i.e., radiation therapy) can be very difficult to treat, and the results are poor. Looser et al. described 30 patients with colourinary tract fistulas secondary to cervical cancer, with an overall survival rate of only 16%. In deciding how to manage these patients, it is important to determine whether recurrent disease is present and, if present, how extensive it is. Those patients without recurrent disease who have a reasonable life expectancy should be approached aggressively. In those patients with a poor life expectancy, any procedure that can alleviate their suffering should be done, such as a colostomy with or without urinary diversion.

PROGNOSIS

Because enterovesical fistulas result in recurrent bladder infections, it is feared that pyelonephritis, renal failure, and systemic infection will occur. In practice, these complications are rare. There are a few patients in several recent reports who have been followed for many years with medical therapy and have had no serious complications. Most patients with fistulas can have surgical correction with minimal morbidity and mortality. There is no question that surgery is the treatment of choice to correct colovesical fistulas. It is not an absolute indication for surgery, however. In the debilitated, high-risk patient with minimal symptoms or complications from the fistula, medical management may be a reasonable alternative to surgery. Patients who have urinary obstruction may be more susceptible to develop ascending renal tract infection and may require either relief of the obstruction or repair of the fistula.

SUMMARY

The most common causes of enterovesical fistulas are diverticulitis, cancer, and Crohn's disease. The patients present with recurrent urinary infection. Evaluation should include endoscopy of the colon and bladder, and x-ray films of the colon and urinary tract. Surgery can usually be done electively, and a one-stage resection with primary anastomosis of the bowel is the preferred treatment, but it should be done only in appropriate patients. Medical management is acceptable in patients who are poor surgical candidates.

BIBLIOGRAPHY

1. Aldrete JS, ReMine WH: Vesicocolic fistula: A complication of colonic cancer. *Arch Surg* 1967; 94:627–637.
2. Amendola MA, Ayha FP, Dent TL, et al: Detection of occult colovesical fistula by the Bourne test. *AJR* 1984; 142:715–717.
3. Deshmukh AS, Bansal NK, Kropp KA: Use of methylene blue in suspected colovesical fistula. *J Urol* 1977; 118:819–820.
4. Krco MJ, Jacobs SC, Malangoni MA, et al: Colovesical fistulas. *Urology* 1984; 23:340–342.
5. Looser KG, Quan SHQ, Clark DGC: Colourinary tract fistula in the cancer patient. *Dis Colon Rectum* 1979; 22:143–148.

In debilitated pts that are high-risks c̄ ↓ symptoms, medical management is a reasonable alternative.

45

Ulcerative Colitis

A 27-year-old woman with known ulcerative colitis undergoes routine colonoscopy. Multiple areas of dysplasia are seen. No frank malignant degeneration is seen. Activity has been intermittent over the past ten years, with satisfactory control with varying doses of steroids and sulfasalazine (Azulfidine).

Consultant: Lester W. Martin, M.D.

Dysplasia refers to microscopic changes observed on the biopsy specimen from a patient with ulcerative colitis and is regarded as a premalignant condition and, consequently, an indication for urgent operation. Colonoscopy has proved to be the preferred method of following patients with ulcerative colitis. It is believed that colonoscopy with multiple biopsies gives a more precise indication of premalignant potential than does simple radiographic examination with barium enema. With the patient's history of ulcerative colitis for ten years, it is a well-known fact that her chances of developing malignancy within the next ten years are approximately 30%.

The operation that we do at the present time consists of a total colectomy, a mucosal proctectomy, construction of a neorectal reservoir from terminal ileum, and anastomosis of this reservoir to the anorectal canal (Fig 45-1). The objective is to eradicate the disease and yet preserve anorectal continence. Because of the multiple suture lines within the pelvis, there is an increased risk of leak that would result in pelvic sepsis. To prevent this catastrophic complication, we protect the anastomosis with a proximal diverting ileostomy, completely dividing the bowel, closing over the distal end. We attach the closed distal end to the underneath surface of the peritoneum adjacent to the ileostomy. The ileum, proximal to the ileostomy, is sutured to the anterior abdominal wall. The ileostomy stoma is matured with a Brooks turnback technique.

Prior to operation it is important to exclude Crohn's colitis as a diagnosis. If performed for Crohn's colitis, we believe the operation is doomed to failure because of the fact that Crohn's is a full-thickness disease and will continue as an inflammatory process within the wall of the bowel, leading to fistula formation

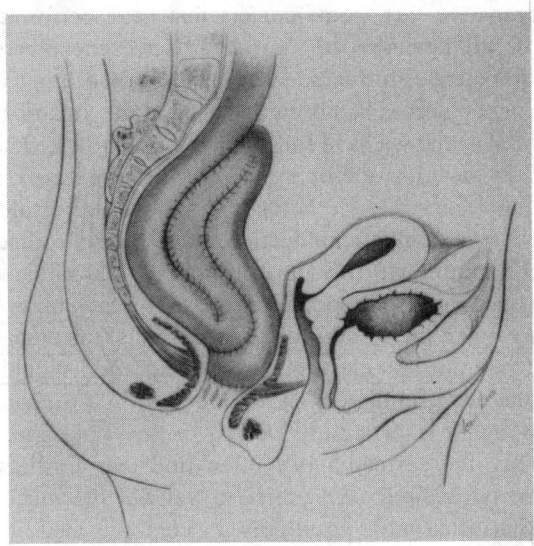

FIG 45–1.
Diagram of neorectal reservoir positioned entirely within pelvis with anastomotic line at top of anorectal columns.

in surrounding structures. We cannot exclude this diagnosis in 100% of the cases. We rely rather heavily on the multiple colonic biopsies that have been obtained by forceps at the time of colonoscopy. We also obtain the small bowel contrast radiographic examination to exclude skip areas involving the small intestine that would be indicative of Crohn's. If the upper gastrointestinal (GI) radiographic (with small bowel) study is normal and the colon biopsies are consistent with the diagnosis of ulcerative colitis, we are willing to accept the patient for operation for the sphincter-preserving type of procedure.

In order to strip the mucosa from the muscular wall of the rectum, it is necessary that the mucosa be intact, in other words, not ulcerated. If the mucosa is inflamed, bleeding will be more active. Therefore, it is desirable to have the mucosa of the rectal area as free of active disease as possible at the time of operation. We accomplish this by means of an intense preoperative regimen, employing steroid enemas and/or steroid suppositories, along with systemic measures directed at the control of the general disease process of ulcerative colitis.

Since ulcerative colitis is primarily a mucosal disease, it is possible to eradicate the disease completely by removing the mucosa only. We generally begin the mucosal dissection just below the peritoneal floor. If one removes the entire thickness of the rectum down to the level of the anorectal junction, there is concern that damage would result to the nerves going to the bladder and the reproductive organs. In fact, some centers that have performed the operation with removal of full thickness of the rectum have encountered an incidence (albeit low) of impotence, retrograded ejaculation, and urinary retention, suggesting that the pelvic nerves had been damaged at the time of operation. In our experience, the males that we have followed up have indicated no problems with sexual function. In fact, just the opposite, they have reported improved sexual function following recovery from the debilitating disease of ulcerative colitis.

At the time of operation, after induction of anesthesia, we spend considerable time irrigating the rectum with 1% kanamycin in normal saline via a large rectal tube. Following opening of the abdomen, we place a heavy tie around the sigmoid colon and again irrigate the rectum, through the rectal tube that had been left in place, in order to minimize soilage in case a perforation should be made in the mucosa during the mucosal dissection. We prefer to do the mucosal dissection from above, although it is difficult to identify the level of dissection. When half the team moves to the perineum, we often find that considerable additional mucosal excision is required. We prefer to transect the mucosa from below, since it can be transected more accurately. Accuracy is also improved with the aid of large retracting sutures that can be placed through the anal verge and sutured laterally and anteriorly. The incision is made at the top of the anorectal columns around the entire circumference, and the mucosa is elevated until the line of dissection meets that from above and the mucosal sleeve can be completely removed.

Various types of reservoirs have been designed. We prefer the S-shaped reservoir constructed from 12 in. of terminal ileum so that the entire reservoir is 4 in. in length, with one limb being antiperistaltic and two limbs being isoperistaltic. The reservoir will hold approximately 200 cc. It is anastomosed directly to the anorectal canal and must lie completely within the pelvis so that it can be evacuated voluntarily by the patient. We have used the J-shaped reservoir for six patients when the anatomical arrangement of the blood supply to the terminal ileum was such that we were not able to create the S-shaped reservoir. These patients have had a distinctly greater stool frequency than with the S-shaped reservoir, but otherwise the J-shaped pouch functions well and is satisfactory. We have performed the isoperistaltic lateral reservoir on only one occasion. Actually, it was a revision that had been performed elsewhere and the patient was referred to us because of complications. We revised the reservoir and left it as an isoperistaltic lateral reservoir. Again, the stool frequency was greater than with the S-shaped reservoir. We are convinced that positioning of the reservoir is of greater importance than its configuration. The reservoir should be attached to the top of the anorectal columns and should lie below the peritoneal floor. We believe it is important to preserve the transitional epithelium that covers the anorectal columns, since this provides the sensory limb of the involuntary reflex arc that keeps the patient from having soilage at nighttime, when asleep, or when attention is diverted otherwise.

Of our 135 patients operated upon over a 20-year period, there have been no deaths, while four have permanent ileostomies because of complications that occurred during the early stages when we were developing the details of the operative procedure. In the last 75 patients, we have encountered minimal complications and very few postoperative problems. Four patients out of the entire series have developed stenosis at the anorectal suture line and have required resection and reanastomosis. This incidently can be accomplished by the transanal route. We use a meticulous mechanical bowel-preparation preoperatively in addition to systemic antibiotics and have the patients receive total parenteral nutrition for one week following the operation when it has been required to allow the rectum to become quiescent.

For the patient with toxic megacolon, hemorrhage, perforation, or fulminant disease, we recommend that a subtotal colectomy be performed, with the rectum closed as a Hartmann pouch and the reservoir created at a later date when the patient is in better physical condition.

Patients with ulcerative colitis are generally highly intelligent, hard-working, over-achieving individuals. Many patients with ulcerative colitis are professionals. They are most appreciative and it is a gratifying segment of society with which to work. The results have been excellent, with restoration of the patient to a status of complete continence and a reasonable bowel function.

The most distressing and most frequent complication that other surgeons are encountering elsewhere is nighttime soilage. This occurs when the surgeon fails to preserve the transitional epithelium above the dentate line.

BIBLIOGRAPHY

1. Martin LW, LeCoultre C, Schubert WK: Total colectomy with mucosal procterectomy and preservation of continence in ulcerative colitis. *Ann Surg* 1977; 186:477–480.
2. Martin LW, Fischer JE: Preservation of anorectal continence following total colectomy for chronic ulcerative colitis. *Ann Surg* 1982; 196:700–704.
3. Martin LW, Fischer JE, Sayers HJ, et al: Anal continence following Soave procedure: Analysis of results in 100 patients. *Ann Surg* 1986; 203:525–530.

46

Familial Polyposis Coli

A 29-year-old patient with a family history of familial polyposis is sigmoidoscoped. Between 50 and 100 polyps, varying between 0.5 and 1 cm in diameter, are seen. No evidence of malignancy is encountered. Barium enema reveals moderate polyposis throughout the colon as well.

Consultant: Keith A. Kelly, M.D.

DIAGNOSIS

The history suggests that this patient has familial polyposis coli, an autosomal-dominant, inheritable condition in which adenomatous polyps appear throughout the large intestine. With this in mind, careful physical examination should be accomplished, looking especially for epidermoid cysts, fibromas, or lipomas of the skin; osteomas (especially around the jaw or in the skull); and desmoid tumors. The eye should be examined for the deposition of black pigment in the retina.

Before proceeding with treatment, the diagnosis should be confirmed by biopsy of several of the polyps via the proctoscope. The polyps in familial polyposis are adenomatous polyps and not hyperplastic polyps, inflammatory polyps, or pseudopolyps. Nonadenomatous polyps indicate the presence of another disease that may or may not require operation. Upper gastrointestinal endoscopy should also be done to look for gastric or duodenal polyps. Gastric polyps are found in 50% to 70% of patients with familial polyposis coli, and duodenal polyps are found in a similar percentage of patients. The gastric polyps and the duodenal polyps should both be biopsied to ascertain whether or not these polyps are hyperplastic or adenomatous. The gastric polyps are more likely to be hyperplastic polyps than are the duodenal polyps, which are most commonly adenomatous. Even so, gastric adenocarcinomas have been associated with the hyperplastic gastric polyps. An increased likelihood of duodenal carcinoma is present in patients with duodenal polyps. Should the gastric or duodenal polyps be localized and few in number, they should be removed endoscopically. A carpeting of polyps in the stomach or duodenum does not allow this possibility.

*The ano-rectal area should be carefully assessed for sphincteric function. When questionable obtain manometric studies.

The management of diffuse polyposis of the stomach or duodenum is not clear at this time. Most surgeons await definite evidence of malignancy before advising operative excision.

The anorectal area should also be carefully examined to assess the anal sphincter and to ascertain the degree of anorectal continence for stool. Anal sphincteric damage from past anal disease or previous anorectal operations, such as hemorrhoidectomy, anal fissurectomy, or anal fistulotomy, should be investigated with anorectal manometry. An incompetent anal sphincter precludes an ileo-anal operation. A history of fecal incontinence should be assessed by infusing 154 mM of sodium chloride NaCl at 50 ml/minute into the rectum until 1,000 ml has been inserted. If the patient can tolerate this rectal infusion without transanal leakage, he/she likely has a satisfactory mechanism of anal continence.

NEED FOR OPERATION

The next question is whether this patient should be advised to have operation. The answer is yes. Nearly all patients with familial polyposis will develop a large bowel malignancy if followed long enough. The polyps usually first appear in the teenage years. The longer the patients have the polyps, the more likely they are to develop malignancy, so that by late adulthood nearly all patients will have developed an adenocarcinoma.

CHOICE OF OPERATION

The two operations commonly considered today for familial polyposis coli are ileal pouch/anal anastomosis or colectomy and ileorectostomy. I favor the ileal pouch/anal anastomosis. The operation completely excises the cecum, the colon, and the proximal rectum, and it removes all diseased mucosa from the distal rectum. A rectal reservoir or pouch is constructed from the terminal ileum, and transanal fecal flow is restored by anastomosing the pouch to the dentate line endorectally. The restoration of intestinal continuity obviates the need for a permanent ileostomy. Because the rectal dissection is done mainly from within the lumen of the rectum via the perineal approach, the chance of damage to the innervation of the urinary bladder and sexual organs is minimized. Thus, postoperative dysfunction of these organs is unlikely. Another advantage of the technique is that no perineal wound results from the procedure, a wound sometimes difficult to heal.

Colectomy and ileorectostomy is a less attractive operation because it leaves in place the rectal mucosa that can subsequently develop rectal adenocarcinoma in the years after the operation. In our own series of ileorectostomies done at Mayo, about 40% of the patients developed a carcinoma in the rectum after a

20-year interval. The incidence of carcinoma, therefore, is sufficiently high to warrant resection of the rectal mucosa at the initial procedure.

Some authorities have recommended resecting the rectal mucosa only if there are more than 10 to 20 polyps in the rectum. Usually the rectal mucosa is covered with myriads of polyps, as was true in the case presented here, so that retaining the rectum is not an option. Even in patients in whom polyps may not be visible macroscopically, however, microadenomatosis of the rectal mucosa may be found when rectal biopsies are taken. Thus, a premalignant epithelium is present and should be resected.

Patients who have already developed a carcinoma at the time of operation can still be considered for the ileal pouch/anal anastomosis, providing the carcinoma does not involve the mid or distal rectum and providing the lesion can be completely excised grossly at the time of operation. The standard cancer-curative operation can be done for proximal rectal carcinomas or carcinomas involving the colon and cecum. The mesentery and lymph drainage should be taken widely and en bloc with the resection of the bowel, and the ileoanal anastomosis done. In those individuals who have mid or distal rectal carcinomas, a proctocolectomy should be accomplished with either a Brooke ileostomy or a Kock pouch. When a colonic or proximal rectal tumor has already metastasized to the liver or elsewhere in the peritoneal cavity so that the entire tumor cannot be encompassed by the resection, the primary tumor should be resected and an ileocolonic or ileorectal anastomosis performed.

ILEOANAL OPERATIVE TECHNIQUE

In the ileoanal operative technique, the patient is placed in the modified lithotomy position, and a vertical midline abdominal incision is made. (*Editor's note:* Some surgeons use Lloyd-Davies stirrups in which the thighs are lower, thus giving more unobstructed access to the abdomen.) The presence of familial polyposis coli is confirmed and the existence of other diseases or abnormalities in the abdomen carefully ascertained by inspection and palpation. The presence or absence of desmoid tumors in the small intestine mesentery or mesenteric fibromatosis should be carefully noted. Some surgeons believe that these conditions mitigate against the ileoanal anastomosis, but I believe that the decision depends on the severity of the condition. Providing the ileum can be brought down satisfactorily to the dentate line for the ileal pouch/anal anastomosis, the presence of mesenteric fibromatosis does not always contraindicate the operation.

Once the diagnosis is confirmed, the cecum, the entire colon, and the proximal rectum are resected and the distal rectum stapled shut. A J-shaped pouch is then made from the terminal 30 cm of ileum (Fig 46–1). The anterior and posterior walls of the pouch are closed in two layers using 2-0 chromic catgut. The ileal mesentery is freed from the retroperitoneum all the way to the

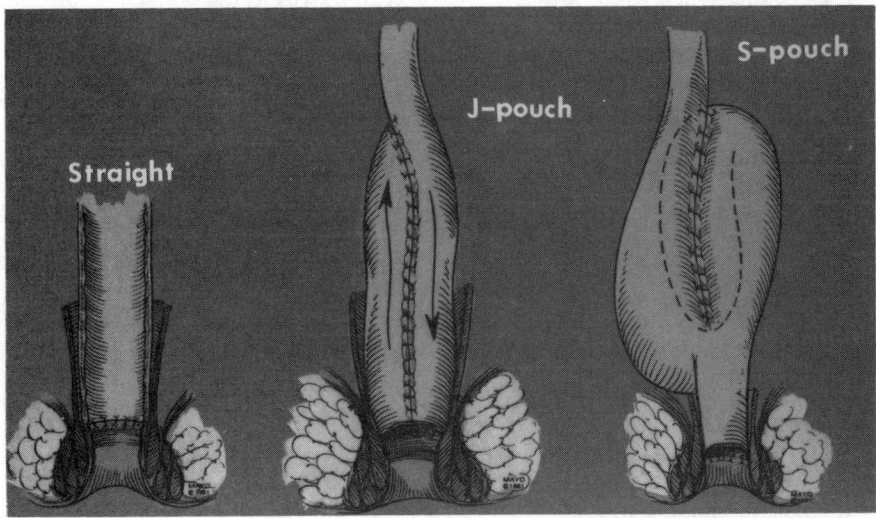

FIG 46–1.
Diagram of straight ileal-anal anastomosis *(left)*, ileal J-shaped pouch/anal anastomosis *(center)*, and ileal S-shaped pouch/anal anastomosis *(right)*.

pancreas, and the superior mesenteric vessels are "skeletonized." The ileocolic artery and vein are divided to allow increased mobility and laxity of the ileal mesentery. This allows the ileum to stretch down to the dentate line. The bottom of the J-pouch should project approximately 2-3 cm beyond the pubic tubercles to allow it to reach to the dentate line. (*Editor's note*: In addition to skeletonizing the superior mesenteric vessels, particularly as they cross the third portion of the duodenum, mobilizing the ligament of Treitz is very helpful in giving additional length, enabling the ileum to reach.)

Should it appear that the ileal mesentery is so short that a J-pouch would not reach the dentate line, the surgeon should consider using an S-shaped pouch. The S-shaped pouch has an efferent limb approximately 2 to 3 cm in length, an additional length that is sometimes just sufficient to allow the pouch to reach the dentate line. (*Editor's note*: Dr. Lester Martin and I prefer the S-pouch, believing that fewer stools result as compared with a J-pouch. However, in our hands the efferent limb is very short, only 1 cm. Experienced surgeons may differ, each believing in the correctness of his/her approach.) The third alternative would be to use the straight ileum for the anastomosis. The ileum itself gives the most mobility and allows for the most distant reach. However, construction of the anastomosis with a straight segment of ileum means that in the early months and years after operation, the patient will have more diarrhea than with a pouch.

Once the pouch is constructed, the surgeon moves to the perineal approach and, using an endorectal dissection, removes the distal rectal mucosa. The excision begins at the dentate line and proceeds in a proximal direction for approximately 5 cm. A dilute solution of epinephrine injected beneath the rectal mucosa elevates it from the underlying rectal tunica muscularis and facilitates the dissection. The proximal rectum can also be everted through the anal canal to facilitate the removal. Once the rectal mucosa has been freed from the dentate line to a point 5 cm proximal to the dentate line, the mid-rectum can be transected at this point and more orad portions of rectum removed.

The previously constructed ileal pouch is then brought down endorectally for the anastomosis. A small incision is made in the apex of the pouch and the anastomosis made, sewing the open end of the pouch to the dentate line and the underlying anal sphincter with interrupted and continuous 3-0 chromic catgut. The surgeon then returns to the abdomen and anchors the ileal mesentery to the retroperitoneum, beginning at the pouch and proceeding to the pancreas. The closure of this space prevents herniation of small intestine behind the mesentery in the postoperative period.

In most patients a loop ileostomy is then created in the right lower quadrant. The loop ileostomy allows the anastomosis to heal prior to the passage of fecal content through it, thus decreasing the possibility of a leak or a perianastomotic infection. However, in some individuals, especially in those with no concurrent disease, in whom the dissection goes smoothly and the anastomosis is made without tension and with good blood supply, the operation can be done as a single-stage procedure without the ileostomy. If the ileostomy is used, it is closed at a second operation approximately two months after the initial procedure. Just before the ileostomy is closed, the ileal pouch and ileoanal anastomosis are examined radiographically using barium sulfate to ascertain that healing is complete.

EARLY POSTOPERATIVE COURSE

Once intestinal continuity is restored, the patient is kept on a fiber-free diet for approximately six weeks. This allows the gastrointestinal tract to accommodate to its new arrangement and to dilate prior to the introduction of bulky foods. Psyllium husk (Metamucil) and loperamide HCl (Imodium) are useful in thickening the bowel content, slowing transit, and improving absorption.

The main postoperative complications of the operation are intestinal obstruction and infection. Pelvic and wound infections decrease with the experience of the surgeon. A surgeon familiar with the procedure should have an incidence of sepsis below 5%. Intestinal obstruction appears in about 10% of patients and may be somewhat more likely in patients operated upon for familial polyposis coli than for ulcerative colitis. The presence of mesenteric fibromatosis with polyposis enhances the likelihood of intestinal obstruction. (*Editor's note*: The frequency of intestinal obstruction in my own personal series has been markedly decreased by my suturing the diverted (Brooke ileostomy) ileum, above and below the ileostomy to the anterior abdominal wall, thus effectively dividing the abdomen into right and left compartments.)

RESULTS OF OPERATION

By six months after operation, patients can expect approximately five bowel movements during the day and one bowel movement at night. This pattern stays constant at least over a period of five years, the length of Mayo's current follow-up. Continence is usually excellent, especially during the day. About 25% to 30% of the patients will have slight fecal spotting at night. By spotting is meant a spot of fecal staining on a perineal pad occurring once or twice a week during sleep. Fecal spotting does decrease as the interval from operation lengthens. At five years after operation in our series, it had virtually stopped. At any rate, fecal spotting has not been disabling.

Sexual and urinary function are well maintained. Protection of the sympathetic nerves as they course over the sacral promontory during the mobilization of the rectum will preserve sexual function. The endorectal approach for the removal of the distal rectal mucosa also protects urinary and sexual innervation. Female patients can anticipate normal sexual responses, normal fertility, and the delivery of an infant through the usual vaginal route. The quality of life of individuals after recovery from the operation differs little from that of healthy subjects.

LONG-TERM FOLLOW-UP

Long-term follow-up includes the use of upper gastrointestinal endoscopy at intervals of two to three years to ascertain the nondevelopment of polyps in the stomach or duodenum. As mentioned above, these individuals are at risk for the development of adenocarcinomas, especially of the duodenum. To date, megaloblastic anemia from the inability to absorb vitamin B_{12} has not appeared in our patients at Mayo; thus, routine injections of cyanocobalamin are not currently recommended. The ileal pouch and distal ileum should be endoscoped at three-year intervals to check for the development of ileal polyps.

BIBLIOGRAPHY

1. Bess MA, Adson MA, Elveback LR, et al: Rectal cancer following colectomy for polyposis. *Arch Surg* 1980; 115:460–467.

2. Heimann TM, Bolnick K, Aufses AH: The results of surgical treatment for familial polyposis coli. *Am J Surg* 1986; 152:276–278.
3. Metcalf AM, Dozois RR, Kelly KA, et al: Ileal J pouch-anal anastomosis. *Ann Surg* 1985; 202:735–739.
4. Stevenson JK, Reid BS: Unfamiliar aspects of familial polyposis coli. *Am J Surg* 1986; 152:81–84.

47

Acute Diverticulitis With Intramesenteric (Pericolic) Perforation

A 63-year-old man was admitted to the hospital with a history of several months' duration of alternating diarrhea and constipation, culminating with the onset of gradually increasing left lower quadrant pain of 24 hours' duration. The patient complained of nausea but had not vomited. Physical findings included a pulse rate of 110 beats per minute, rectal temperature of 101.4°F, and pallor, accompanied by slight diaphoresis. There was voluntary abdominal wall guarding, with rebound tenderness in the left lower quadrant but no significant tenderness in other areas of the abdomen. Peristaltic sounds were noted to be somewhat hyperactive, and rectal examination, including a stool guaiac, was negative. The white blood cell count was 14,000/cu mm, with 78% polymorphonuclear leukocytes and 3% bands.

Consultant: Robert J. Baker, M.D.

DISCUSSION

Left lower quadrant pain in a male patient at this age and with the suggestive history of alternating diarrhea and constipation most often represents one of the several complications with which acute sigmoid diverticulitis can present. Diverticulitis is a relatively modern disease, and although earlier anatomical descriptions of colonic diverticulitis were published in the mid- and late 19th century, this disease has become a common cause of acute symptoms in the 20th century. The high prevalence of the disease in industrialized Western nations and the rarity with which it is encountered in underdeveloped nations are noteworthy. The role of diet in the genesis of colonic diverticula has been subject to interesting and extensive debate, but little significant data exist on which to base definite conclusions.

As with other inflammatory gastrointestinal disease, the basic treatment of uncomplicated sigmoid diverticulitis is nonsurgical; the use of bed rest, intravenous fluids, gastric suction, and judicious (or selective) antibiotic therapy has been the standard mode of treatment of patients with acute diverticulitis for several decades. Over one third of patients will recur, however, and 90% of those will be within five years of the original attack. On the other hand, the complications of perforation, hemorrhage, obstruction, fistula formation, or recurrent attacks (intractability) comprise the major reasons for surgeons to be asked to render care to patients with acute diverticulitis, and the surgical management of each of these complications has been under considerable scrutiny and evolution in the past two decades.

DIFFERENTIAL DIAGNOSIS

Differential diagnosis of left lower quadrant pain is not as difficult as that of pain located in the right lower quadrant. Patients with acute diverticulitis present with severe lower abdominal pain, primarily in the left lower quadrant, but often extending to the midline and occasionally even located primarily on the right side of the abdomen. There is usually acute tenderness in the area of the pain, and voluntary or involuntary guarding is frequently encountered. Approximately 75% of patients will present with a mass; this will often be a well-defined mass, especially if a large pericolic abscess is present, but in the majority of patients the mass is ill-defined, and there is a "fullness" or a suggestion of a mass. Rigidity or voluntary guarding may mask the presence of the inflammatory mass, and peristaltic sounds vary from absent to somewhat hyperactive, depending on the degree of reaction or obstruction caused by the inflammatory process.

With acute diverticulitis and localized perforation, there will be fever, tachycardia, and often nausea, with or without vomiting. Occasionally diarrhea will accompany the acute process, and there may be a minimal amount of blood or mucus in the bowel movement. Patients may feel more comfortable with the hip joint flexed and may even be found to lie on the right side with both hips flexed; this is a manifestation of the larger pericolic phlegmon or abscess that causes secondary inflammation of the left psoas muscle, producing a psoas sign analogous to that found on the right side with retroperitoneal appendicitis.

The most common diagnostic errors are made when this lesion is confused with left-sided inflammatory and neoplastic lesions of the tube and/or ovary; also confusing are Meckel's diverticulitis, acute appendicitis, Crohn's disease, and mesenteric vascular occlusion. It is of interest that most series that address the question indicate that 10% to 20% of patients who are operated upon and prove to have diverticulitis are initially explored by the gynecologic service, with the diagnosis of ovarian or tubo-ovarian disease suggested by the mass, fever, and tachycardia. Approximately 40% of women with acute sigmoid diverticulitis has been misdiagnosed in their hospital course as having a palpable gynecologic lesion; the failure to investigate the colon in patients with what is presumed to be overt disease of the tube and ovary leads to the frequent errors discovered at laparotomy.

Approximately one third of patients with acute sigmoid diverticulitis will have microscopic hematuria, a manifestation of inflammatory involvement of the adjacent ureter and bladder. Urinary frequency and dysuria are encountered in 20% of patients with acute diverticulitis; these occur primarily in male patients in whom the inflamed sigmoid lies on the dome or left side of the bladder. For 50% of patients with acute diverticulitis, the attack requiring hospitalization is the initial manifestation of the disease process. Rarely, Crohn's colitis may coexist with diverticular disease and, in fact, Crohn's disease may precipitate acute diverticulitis when diverticula are present in the same area.

DIAGNOSTIC STUDIES

Radiography

Radiologic evaluation of the patient with acute left lower quadrant pain due to localized perforation of sigmoid diverticular disease ordinarily commences with routine supine and upright films of the abdomen. These films rarely offer specific diagnostic information unless the diverticulitis has caused colonic obstruction or the pericolic collection of purulent material has been accompanied by a significant amount of air from the lumen, in which case tiny bubbles of air or even an air-fluid level may be visible on the upright and supine films. (*Editor's note*: Occasionally one may follow the air column from the left column toward the sigmoid and see narrowing as the mass is approached.)

Real-Time Sonography

Numerous findings suggestive of sigmoid diverticulitis have been reported using real-time sonography. Most commonly, these findings are thickening of the wall of the inflamed segment of colon, specifically seen on oblique scanning. Perimural and adjacent abscesses have also been detected, but the specificity of this examination is open to question. Obviously, if sonography is to be done, it should be performed prior to contrast studies of the colon in order to prevent confusion in interpretation.

Contrast Studies

Several radiographic studies have been reported advocating the instillation of water-soluble dye into the colon in the presence of acute sigmoid diverticulitis. A recent study by Wexner and Dailey of 71 patients admitted with left lower quadrant peritonitis, fever, and leukocytosis purported to demonstrate that barium enema or water-soluble contrast enema was specific, and that the water-soluble study was the most accurate and most cost-effective modality available. On the other hand, a study by Parks et al. some years ago emphasized that radiologists reviewing colon films experienced 38% disagreement in diagnosis of diverticulitis vs. diagnosis of diverticulosis on barium enema study. Because of this, and since only one of seven patients with pericolic or intramesenteric perforation of the sigmoid colon will demonstrate extramural dye on barium enema, it seems impractical to rely on contrast studies in the acute state to delineate the nature of the disease process. Most surgeons view barium enema in the face of acute inflammatory complications of colonic disease with something less than enthusiasm since it is possible, and perhaps likely, that the instillation of contrast may precipitate a perforation of the inflammatory lesion or, more commonly, cause a localized intramural perforation to break down and develop into spreading peritonitis. The general dictum that patients with significant acute abdominal pain should not be subjected to intraluminal contrast studies of the lower gastrointestinal tract is valid and one that is not likely to be abandoned because it is possible "to get away with it" most of the time.

Computerized Tomographic Scanning

Computerized tomographic (CT) scans have proved to be extremely useful in acute sigmoid diverticulitis as well as other acute abdominal conditions. A recent report by Morris et al. of 20 patients with acute diverticulitis who had barium enemas resulted in 60% positive findings; 24 patients had CT scans in a parallel group, 63% of whom had positive findings of thickening of the colonic wall, increased density of pericolic fat, and diverticular or peridiverticular abscess. Although the cost is considerably higher with CT scanning, it is important to emphasize that there is no risk to the patient of worsening the process by CT scanning in contrast to the small but finite percentage of patients who will be poorly served by some form of contrast. Several recent experiences on our surgical service indicate the considerable value of CT scans in delineating the disease process as well as in demonstrating the presence of a lesion that occasionally can be effectively treated by percutaneous catheter insertion with CT control (Figs 47-1 to 47-3). Furthermore, monitoring the progress or regression of the lesion with repeat scanning is often very helpful.

Another application of the CT scan is in percutaneous drainage of abscesses that are localized in the pelvis or in the pericolic tissues, thereby allowing the acute process to subside. If nonoperative management succeeds, the patient may be operated upon in six to eight weeks and is dealt with as any elective sigmoid resection, whereas an emergency operation to drain the pus would, in the current surgical climate, cause the surgeon to embark on the resection of unprepared colon, with the necessity for a staged procedure.

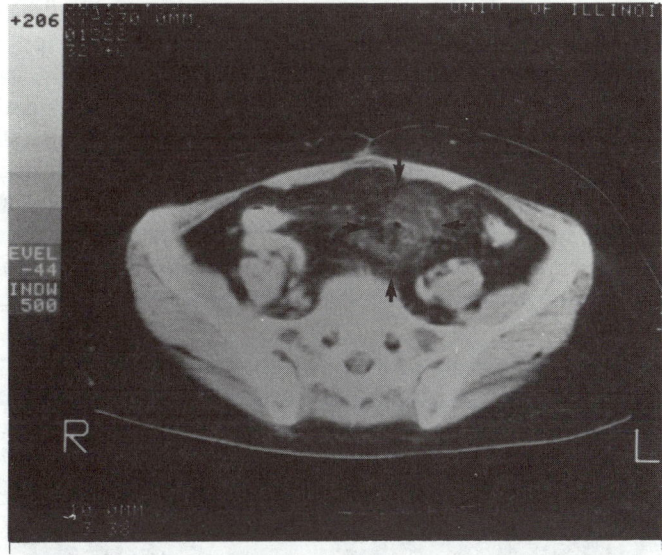

FIG 47–1.
A 64-year-old man presented with pain in the left lower quadrant and suprapubic area, tenderness, and low-grade fever. After 24 hours in the hospital, his pain was unimproved, his temperature rose to 102°F, and his white blood cell count increased. The CT scan demonstrated the narrowing of the sigmoid colon, edema of the wall of the sigmoid, and considerable mesenteric edema, characteristic of acute sigmoid diverticulitis without perforation. Further observation of the patient and continued intravenous antibiotic therapy resulted in resolution of the acute process.

Endoscopy

Endoscopy with fiberoptic instruments generally yields little or no useful information, except to assist in ruling out perforated carcinoma or other mucosal lesions of the colon. With perforated diverticulitis, mucosal edema, luminal narrowing, and mucus or blood may be seen, but the intramural and perimural location of the inflammatory process precludes any specific diagnostic conclusions from signoidoscopy in the vast majority of instances.

OPERATIVE TREATMENT

Basic treatment of localized perforation of sigmoid diverticulitis is expectant, with close monitoring of temperature, pulse rate, abdominal tenderness, size of mass, and loss of peristaltic sounds. With deterioration or failure of response in 24 to 48 hours, operation should be undertaken. Management of perforative sigmoid diverticulitis has evolved over the past 30 years from the performance of a colostomy as the first stage of a lengthy three-stage procedure to one of three currently favored operations that require resection of the diseased colon (Fig 47-4). The mortality from the three-stage operation—consisting of diverting colostomy and drainage, elective sigmoid resection in eight weeks, and closure at some later date—has ranged from 10% to 25% in years past. Furthermore, approximately one third of patients subjected to colostomy for diverticulitis never have the colostomy closed, either because the patients are too infirm after their episode of perforated diverticulitis to undergo definitive resection, or because definitive resection is performed but, for a number of reasons, the patient is not a candidate for closure of the colostomy. The only reasonable indication for this operation currently is in elderly or debilitated patients with intestinal obstruction due to diverticulitis.

In the past 15 years the frequency with which colostomy and drainage of a local peridiverticular abscess has failed to cause prompt resolution of the inflammatory process has engendered a more aggressive approach to acutely perforated sigmoid diverticulitis, even when there is a significant collection of pus

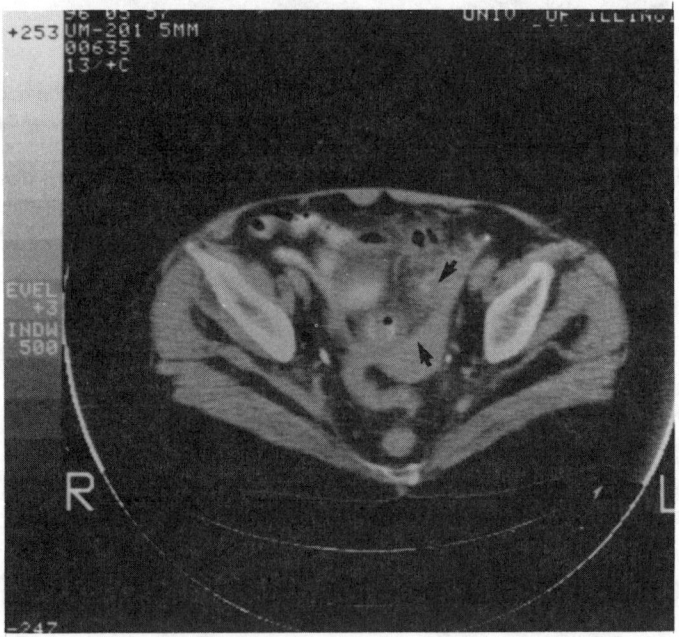

FIG 47-2.
A 59-year-old woman was admitted to the surgical service with pain in the suprapubic area, extending somewhat to the left of midline. Her temperature was 99.8°F and white blood cell count was 11.6/cu mm, with 74% polymorphonuclear leukocytes. No mass was detectable. The CT scan showed extensive perisigmoidal edema and adjacent fluid-filled loops of bowel. A pericolic phlegmon was diagnosed.

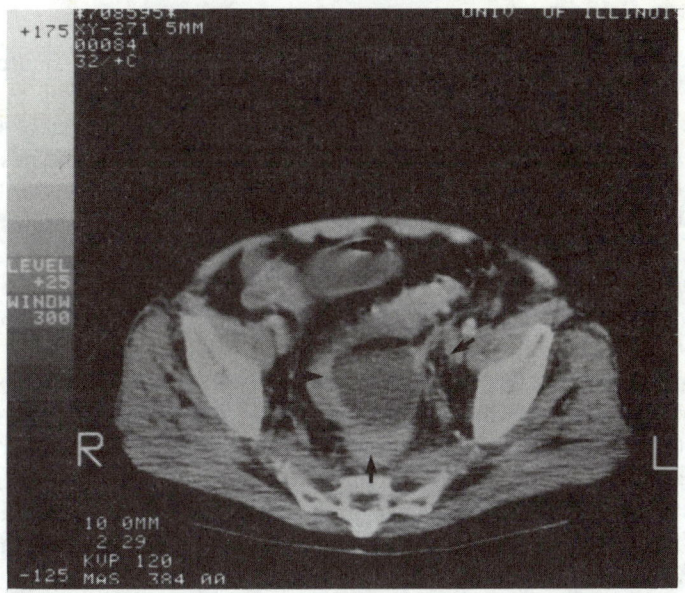

FIG 47–3.
This 72-year-old patient was admitted to the surgical service with a five-day history of nausea, vomiting, abdominal distention, and suprapubic pain radiating to the left lower quadrant. No mass was palpable, but CT scan showed a well-developed pericolic abscess, with marked thickening of adjacent intestine and walling off of the process. Immediately superior to the abscess several out-pouchings in that loop of sigmoid colon can be seen, representing diverticula.

and colon content. Three procedures are currently advocated for this type of acute diverticular disease, including resection of the diseased colon in all three instances (see Fig 47–4).

Exteriorization of Proximal and Distal Limbs

The simplest procedure available is to resect the diseased colon to noninflamed margins, exteriorize the proximal limb, and mobilize the distal limb to the point where it is possible to bring it to the skin. This procedure is useful primarily in thin patients and results in a significant segment of distal sigmoid colon (above the rectum) remaining in situ. If the distal colon is not involved with the inflammatory process, it should still be resected at the time of reestablishment of colonic continuity, since 7% to 10% of patients have recurrences following the incomplete excision of distal sigmoid.

Hartmann Procedure

This procedure—exteriorization of proximal descending colon, suture or staple closure of distal rectosigmoid—has proved to be the most useful operation in the face of acute localized sigmoidal perforation. There is invariably substantial edema and difficulty in mobilizing the distal limb, precluding the possibility of exteriorization of the distal limb, and closure of the distal limb can be readily accomplished with a stapler or a single row of full-thickness sutures. The advantage of the Hartmann procedure in avoiding an anastomosis is clear, but subsequent reestablishment of intestinal continuity may prove to be a more extensive procedure than the surgeon who performs the operation occasionally anticipates. The distal limb can be adequately localized for the surgeon by the insertion of a large-caliber rectal tube into the distal segment prior to undertaking the operation, after the induction of anesthesia. An alternative that also works well is to have a cooperative assistant insert a colonoscope after the abdomen is opened and adhesions are lysed, allowing identification of the distal limb in a dramatic way as the colonoscopic light shines through the rectosigmoid wall at the site of closure. In the event that an appreciable length of sigmoid colon remains, it should be removed at the second operation.

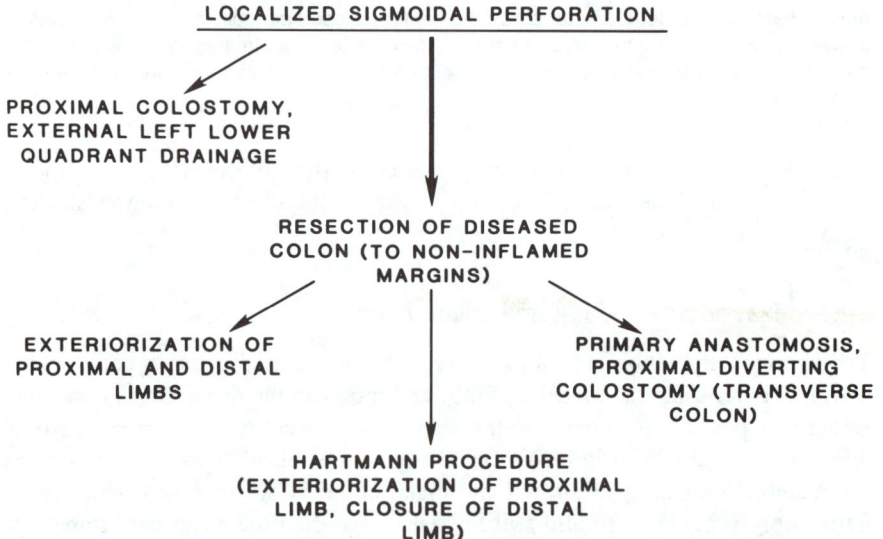

FIG 47–4.
Surgical treatment of intramesenteric or pericolic perforation of sigmoid diverticulitis.

Primary Anastomosis With Proximal Diverting Colostomy in Transverse Colon

There has been recent enthusiasm for performing a more definitive procedure at the time of operation. Some surgeons essay the courage to reanastomose the intestine without protecting the suture line, while most who perform primary anastomosis want a proximal diverting colostomy in the circumstances of operating upon an acute localized perforation. (*Editor's note:* Even more so because anastomosis is being carried out in unprepared bowel.) In general, this procedure is more difficult than the Hartmann since the intestinal wall is frequently very edematous and the sutures placed may tear through the intestinal wall. The same criticism holds for staple closure of the anastomosis performed with an end-to-end anastomotic stapler (such as EEA instrument). Nevertheless, if the perforation is small or the purulent material is intramural or in a very localized area, it may be possible to perform this procedure, which does not require the second extensive laparotomy that closing a Hartmann colostomy does. Obviously, even the marginal-risk patient will usually tolerate the closure of a loop or double-barreled colostomy that, properly performed, will provide excellent diversion. Loop colostomies must be opened widely on the operating table to provide the required diversion, and it is current practice to mature the colostomy at the time it is formed so that both lumina are separated and easily seen.

The question of drainage of the area from which the colon has been resected with any one of the three resective procedures is generally resolved by the truism that "it is not possible to drain the peritoneal cavity." On the other hand, some surgeons like to provide short-term drainage of the area of an abscess; therefore, if a significant collection of pus has been encountered, a sump drain may be useful for 72 to 96 hours. In the event that a primary anastomosis is performed, it is generally wise not to place drains close to the suture line.

SUMMARY

The diagnosis of intramesenteric or pericolic perforation of acute sigmoid diverticulitis in patients over 40 years of age is not difficult, especially with CT scanning and/or oblique ultrasound studies. If symptoms subside or improve promptly in 24 to 48 hours, operation is undertaken electively at eight to ten weeks. When no improvement or even deterioration occurs, urgent operation most often entails resection with Hartmann closure of the distal limb, while exteriorization of both limbs or primary resection with proximal colostomy are occasionally appropriate. With current perioperative supportive measures, operative mortality should not exceed 4%.

BIBLIOGRAPHY

1. Himal HS, Ashby DB, Duigan JP, et al: Management of perforating diverticulitis of the colon. *Surg Gynecol Obstet* 1977; 144:225–226.
2. Meyers MA, Alonso DR, Morson BC, et al: Pathogenesis of diverticulitis complicating granulomatous colitis. *Gastroenterology* 1978; 74:24–31.
3. Morris J, Stellato TA, Haaga JR, et al: Utility of CT in colonic diverticulitis. *Ann Surg* 1986; 204:128–132.
4. Parks TG, Connell AM, Gough AD, et al: Limitations of radiology in the differentiation of diverticulitis and diverticulosis of colon. *Br J Surg* 1970; 2:136–138.
5. Rodkey GV, Welch CE: Changing patterns in the surgical treatment of diverticular disease. *Ann Surg* 1984; 200:466–478.
6. Sweatman CA Jr, Aldrete JS: Surgical management of diverticular disease of colon complicated by perforation. *Surg Gynecol Obstet* 1977; 144:47–50.
7. Wexner SD, Dailey TH: Initial management of left lower quadrant peritonitis. *Dis Colon Rectum* 1986; 29:635–638.

48

Diverticular Bleeding

A 65-year-old man is admitted with the sudden onset of hematochezia, postural hypotension, and syncope. Previous history is unremarkable. On physical examination, bowel sounds are slightly increased; there is no tenderness or masses, and the abdomen is not distended. There is bright-red blood on the finger. Over the next three hours, 2 units of blood are required to maintain positive vital signs, and angiography is undertaken that reveals a bleeding point in the hepatic flexure.

Consultant: David L. Nahrwold, M.D.

DISCUSSION

We are presented with a case that requires application of the principles necessary to properly manage gastrointestinal hemorrhage and that exposes the controversial areas surrounding this subject. The patient has gastrointestinal bleeding to the extent that cardiovascular collapse has occurred; he is in danger of dying if the hemorrhage persists. Emergency surgical intervention may be necessary to stop the bleeding, and in order to carry out the correct procedure, its cause and location must be determined as quickly as possible. Paradoxically, an emergency procedure meant to be lifesaving is fraught with high mortality and morbidity in an elderly man, but the risk can be reduced by careful, rapid preoperative preparation. A plan also needs to be set forth if the bleeding stops. Decisions must be made as to whether elective surgery is indicated and, if not, what medical therapy will be instituted and how the patient will be monitored.

Thus, acute massive gastrointestinal hemorrhage is a complex problem. As with any complicated situation, management is best determined by breaking the problem down into progressively more simple components. In the case of gastrointestinal bleeding, the primary components are resuscitation and assessment, diagnosis, and therapy.

RESUSCITATION AND ASSESSMENT

In the emergency department, the surgeon must prepare to resuscitate the patient even as a history is being taken and certain elements of the physical examination are being performed. The skin, which usually manifests the first signs of blood loss, should be examined for pallor, coolness, sweating, and slow capillary filling. Blood pressure and pulse rate should be taken with the patient in the supine position and, only if they are normal, in the sitting position. A fall in pressure of more than 10 mm Hg and/or an increase in pulse rate of more than 10 beats per minute are indicative of a loss of at least 1,000 ml of blood. Our patient would be expected to have had a loss of at least 1,500 ml based on his history of syncope, but older individuals do not always manifest an increased pulse rate during shock. Older patients, who often know their usual blood pressure, should be asked about a history of hypertension, because a "normal" blood pressure in an elderly person may actually be hypotension. After the baseline vital signs have been measured, they should be taken and recorded every five minutes.

The next step is to obtain intravenous access with a large-bore line; initially, we use an antecubital vein and place a subclavian line later, if necessary. Blood should be obtained for typing and crossmatching blood, complete blood cell count, and determination of serum electrolytes, blood glucose, blood urea nitrogen, and creatinine. Thereafter, rapid infusion of Ringer's lactate solution should be initiated. The rate of infusion can be decreased when vital signs become normal or, if they are normal, when urine output is adequate. A Foley catheter and a nasogastric tube should be placed, the latter to ascertain that bleeding is not from the upper gastrointestinal tract; thus, it should be left in place.

The history should be taken as resuscitation proceeds. Some measure of the acuity of bleeding can be made by asking when the syncopal episode took place, whether or not the patient has been weak or has had episodes of dizziness in recent days, and whether or not melena preceded the present hematochezia. Specific characteristics of the syncopal episode should be elicited to establish that it was not a transient ischemic attack, although this is unlikely. The history should also focus on the cause of the hemorrhage. Details of any present or past abdominal pain, previous bleeding episodes or melena, change in bowel habits, or any symptoms of obstruction should be sought. Especially important is any history of duodenal or gastric ulcer disease, esophageal hiatus hernia and/or reflux, cirrhosis, diverticulitis, Crohn's disease, ulcerative colitis, polyps, or a coagulopathy. Present and past medications must be noted, with special emphasis on anticoagulants, aspirin, and over-the-counter drugs that contain aspirin, nonsteroidal anti-inflammatory drugs, and acetaminophen.

Physical examination can be done as the history is being taken. The lips and buccal mucosa should be checked for the pigmented lesions associated with Peutz-Jeghers syndrome. The hands should be examined for palmar erythema and/or Dupuytren's contracture. The heart and lung examinations are important to check for congestive heart failure and arrhythmias, for which immediate therapy may be necessary. The trunk should be inspected for spider angiomata or telangiectasia. Details of the abdominal examination must include inspection for distention by bowel or ascites, determination of the size of the liver and spleen, and palpation for masses or tenderness. The bowel sounds will be hyperactive due to the cathartic effect of blood in the gastrointestinal tract. In this patient, rectal examination revealed gross blood on the examining finger. Careful palpation for masses should be done, but the examiner must keep in mind that a bleeding villous adenoma may not be felt because of its softness and velvety surface, and that a bleeding pedunculated polyp slips away from the examining finger.

At this juncture an assessment of whether the patient is bleeding from the upper or lower gastrointestinal tract must be made, and a differential diagnosis formulated. This will result in selection of the most appropriate diagnostic tests and avoid waste of time and needless expense. The nasogastric tube should be irrigated with normal saline to see if gross or occult blood is present. When the stomach contains gross blood, immediate esophagogastroduodenoscopy is indicated. Hematochezia may occur in massive upper gastrointestinal bleeding, but during active bleeding the absence of blood in the stomach virtually rules out a lesion in the esophagus, stomach, or proximal duodenum. We shall assume that our patient had no blood in the stomach.

DIAGNOSIS

A differential diagnosis can be formulated at this point. In the absence of blood in the stomach, we can assume that the site of bleeding is in the small intestine or colon. Although they are rare, about one third of all benign small bowel tumors and one fourth of malignant small bowel tumors present with bleeding. Those especially prone to bleeding are leiomyomas, hemangiomas, adenocarcinomas, and lymphosarcomas. Other small bowel lesions that may cause bleeding in older patients are Crohn's disease, the hamartomatous polyps associated with the Peutz-Jeghers syndrome, and vascular ectasia (angiodysplasia). Benign and malignant small bowel tumors and Crohn's disease frequently cause cramping abdominal pain after meals because of their tendency to obstruct. The absence of previous abdominal symptoms and of the perioral pigmented lesions associated with the Peutz-Jeghers syndrome mitigates against these diseases in our patient, but does not rule them out. Vascular ectasia of the small bowel, which presents with bleeding but produces no other symptoms, is a definite diagnostic possibility.

Colonic lesions that may bleed massively include vascular ectasia (angiodysplasia), diverticula, polyps, carcinoma, ulcerative colitis, Crohn's disease, ischemic colitis, and other less common conditions (Table 48–1). Massive hemorrhage from Crohn's disease of the colon with no prior history is extremely rare. Although ulcerative colitis can present with massive hemorrhage even in

TABLE 48–1.

<u>Causes of Colonic Bleeding</u>

Diverticular disease
Vascular ectasia (angiodysplasia)
Adenomatous polyp
Villous adenoma
Carcinoma
Crohn's disease
Ulcerative colitis
Ischemic colitis
Radiation enteritis
Antibiotic-associated colitis
Bacterial colitis
Coagulation disorders
Solitary ulcer

---

older individuals, this too is exceedingly rare in the face of a history completely negative for diarrhea and other abdominal complaints, as well as a normal physical examination. Ischemic colitis, which does occur in our patient's age group, usually is accompanied by diarrhea, abdominal pain, and tenderness, none of which he displayed. Bleeding from villous adenomas, pedunculated polyps, and carcinomas is common, but it usually is chronic and slow, unlike the rapid bleeding seen in our patient. Nevertheless, these lesions may cause massive hemorrhage. Both colonic diverticula and vascular ectasia are notorious for causing massive lower gastrointestinal hemorrhage without antecedent or concomitant symptoms. Therefore, our differential diagnosis must include bleeding from a diverticulum, vascular ectasia, polyp, or carcinoma, with diverticulum and vascular ectasia the most likely. In fact, these two conditions cause most episodes of lower gastrointestinal bleeding in elderly persons.

Having established a differential diagnosis, we now should choose the most efficacious diagnostic tests. The diagnostic procedures will entail transport of the patient to another area, and we must maintain the ability to continue resuscitation there. Adequate personnel, equipment, and supplies must be available. At this point, cross-matched blood is probably available and its rapid infusion should be initiated. Blood passed per rectum should be measured.

We prefer to do routine sigmoidoscopy on all patients bleeding from the lower gastrointestinal tract. The rectum and rectosigmoid colon are relatively inaccessible to inspection and palpation at operation, but lesions are easily identified and sometimes easily treated via the rigid sigmoidoscope. The mucosal changes of ulcerative colitis as well as lesions such as villous adenomas, pedunculated polyps, rectal cancers, and granulomatous ulcers can be diagnosed. The importance of identification of a bleeding lesion within the reach of the standard rigid sigmoidoscope is that the need for a transanal surgical approach can be identified, and laparotomy can be avoided.

Assuming a normal sigmoidoscopy with the rigid scope, opinions differ as to the wisdom of colonoscopy. We believe that colonoscopy should be done unless the hemorrhage is so severe as to preclude adequate visualization. A precise diagnosis can be made in about half of patients who have colonoscopy.[3] In our patient, who has required 2 units of blood to maintain normal vital signs, we may assume that the amount of blood he is passing per rectum precludes colonoscopy. However, if the bleeding ceased at this point, colonoscopy would definitely be indicated. Barium enema should not be done unless colonoscopy is negative and the patient is no longer bleeding, because the presence of barium precludes angiography and scintigraphy.

Some recommend scintigraphy as the next step after a normal sigmoidoscopy or colonoscopy. When the patient is bleeding actively, ^{99m}Tc sulfur colloid should be used. Red blood cells labeled with ^{99m}Tc have a much longer half-life in blood and are best used for intermittent bleeding, since repeated scintigraphy can be done over a 24-hour period. The sensitivity of ^{99m}Tc sulfur colloid scintigraphy is very high; rates of bleeding as slow as 0.1 ml/minute can be detected. However, the transposition of a suspected bleeding site on the scintigram to a specific anatomical site within the gastrointestinal tract is fraught with error; therefore, the practical value of scintigraphy is questionable.

The definitive diagnostic procedure in our patient is angiography, which detects bleeding at a rate of 0.5 ml/minute or more, and which successfully identifies the site of lower gastrointestinal bleeding in about two thirds of patients. The superior mesenteric artery should be catheterized and injected first, followed by the inferior mesenteric. The pathognomonic sign for diverticular bleeding is pooling of the contrast in the diverticulum; this is found in approximately 75% of patients[4] (Fig 48–1). The principal findings in vascular ectasia are a dilated, tortuous intramural vein that empties slowly, a vascular tuft, and an early-filling vein; these three signs may occur singly or in combination (Fig 48–2).

In our patient, pooling of contrast was seen in the hepatic flexure. Almost all vascular ectasias occur in the right part of the colon; however, we shall assume that none of the radiologic signs of ectasia were present. Although most diverticula are located in the left portion of the colon, those that bleed are most frequently found in the right side. (*Editor's note*: Agreed. The reason for the propensity of a diverticulum in the hepatic flexure is unknown, but it is a feature of almost all cases. It argues for subtotal colectomy in treatment of bleeding diverticular disease, if operation is required.) Thus, the most likely diagnosis in our patient is hemorrhage from a diverticulum in the hepatic flexure of the colon; however, vascular ectasia, carcinoma, polyp, and some of the rare lesions previously listed (see Table 48–1) cannot be ruled out with certainty.

THERAPY

By history and physical examination, our patient has lost at least 1,500 ml of blood and needs at least this amount for resuscitation. We also know that the 2 units of blood he has received have been essential to maintain his vital signs. What then are the indications for operation in lower gastrointestinal bleeding? Although opinions differ, we believe operative intervention is necessary when: (1) 1,500 ml of blood are necessary for resuscitation and bleeding is continuing; (2) 2,000 ml of blood are necessary to maintain vital signs during a 24-hour period; (3) bleeding continues for 72 hours, irrespective of the amount; and (4) rebleeding occurs within a week of cessation of a significant hemorrhage. The elderly tolerate blood loss less well than young individuals; therefore, early surgical intervention is mandatory in older patients. Considering the age of our patient and the severity of hemorrhage, we would operate as soon as possible.

If this patient's bleeding had abruptly stopped on admission, colonoscopy should have been carried out and, if nondiagnostic, should have been followed by a barium enema. Obviously, a polyp should be removed at colonoscopy, if possible. Early experience with argon laserization of vascular ectasias is encouraging. A carcinoma requires mechanical and antibiotic bowel preparation, followed by elective colon resection. If a vascular ectasia is identified, elective resection of the colon is indicated after bowel preparation because of the high incidence of rebleeding from this lesion. Once bleeding from a diverticulum has ceased, colonoscopy and barium enema usually reveal nothing other than the presence of diverticula. We do not advocate elective partial or total colon re-

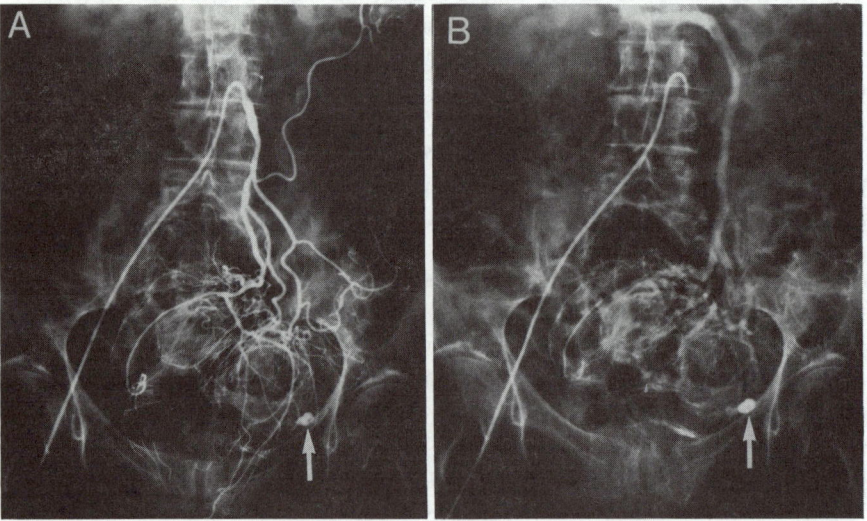

FIG 48–1.
Arterial **(A)** and venous **(B)** phases of an inferior mesenteric angiogram showing pooling in a bleeding diverticulum in the sigmoid colon *(arrows)*.

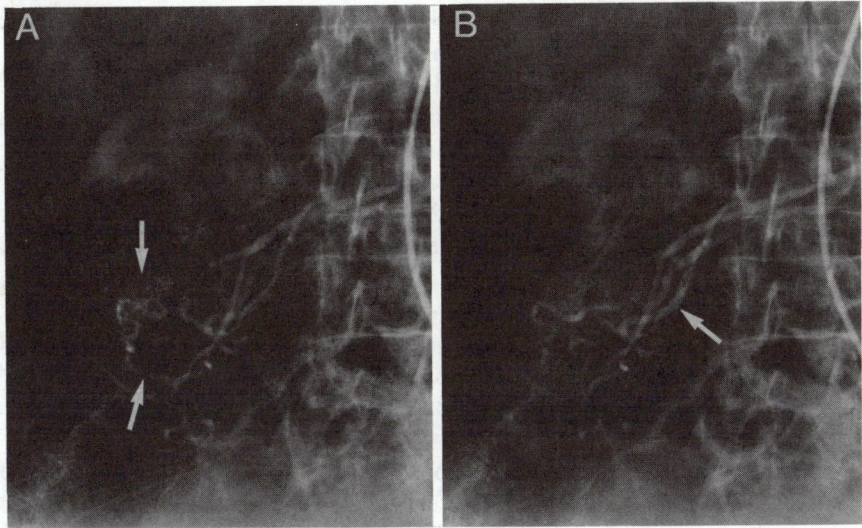

FIG 48–2.
Two phases of a superior mesenteric angiogram that demonstrates a vascular ectasia in the cecum. On **A,** note the vascular tuft *(arrow pointing downward)* and the tortuous intramural vein *(arrow pointing upward).* On **B,** note early filling vein *(arrow).*

section in this situation. (*Editor's note*: Not all authorities agree. Some would advocate elective subtotal colectomy for a single significant bleed in a patient with bleeding diverticulosis, even if that patient stops bleeding spontaneously.)

The use of selective arterial catherterization and of infusion of vasopressin in diverticular bleeding has been studied extensively by Baum and his associates.[1] Using a specific regimen for infusion, they found that immediate control of bleeding could be obtained in a high percentage of patients, but the incidence of rebleeding was significant. This technique is useful in high-risk patients if facilities and expertise are at hand, but it may delay and increase the risk of operation when immediate control is not possible or when early rebleeding occurs. We do not routinely use selective arterial infusion of vasopressin in patients with hemorrhage from a diverticulum or vascular ectasia.

In the bleeding patient, preparation for an operation should proceed even though a final decision to operate has not been made. Results of blood coagulation studies, including bleeding time, platelet count, prothrombin time, and partial thromboplastin time, should be monitored and corrected with appropriate therapy. The volume of blood transfused should exceed the minimum necessary to maintain normal vital signs. When the decision to operate is made, a Swan-Ganz catheter should be placed in elderly individuals such as our patient, in young patients with cardiac or pulmonary disease, and in patients who are unstable despite seemingly adequate volume replacement. Finally, intravenous antibiotic prophylaxis should be administered immediately before the operation.

Our patient should have abdominal exploration through a midline incision. In addition to the usual abdominal exploration, the entire gastrointestinal tract from the upper stomach to the rectum should be carefully inspected and palpated. Sometimes the mesenteric tissue surrounding a bleeding diverticulum is slightly inflamed, giving the sensation of a small mass on palpation, but usually the surgeon cannot identify the site of a bleeding diverticulum or vascular ectasia.

When the site of bleeding has been localized, preoperatively or at surgery, a segmental resection should be done—in our patient, a right hemicolectomy. Primary anastomosis can be carried out safely because the cathartic action of the blood prepares the colon adequately. Although we prefer a two-layer sutured anastomosis, a functional side-to-side anastomosis using stapling devices is an acceptable alternative.

A more vexing problem is when none of the diagnostic studies localizes the bleeding, and the severity of hemorrhage mandates operation. Careful inspection and palpation of the colon should be done, and a colotomy should be made in the area of any suspected lesion to confirm it as the source of hemorrhage. Therapy appropriate for the lesion should then be carried out, usually a segmental resection. Isolation of segments of the colon with noncrushing clamps is occasionally helpful, and others have used intraoperative colonoscopy to transilluminate the colon. More often than not, these maneuvers are not helpful. Total abdominal colectomy with ileoproctostomy should be done when the site of bleeding cannot be identified.[2] This is effective in most patients, but it is necessary less frequently than in the past.

The importance of preoperative sigmoidoscopy is apparent when total abdominal colectomy is necessary, in that the surgeon can be confident that the site of the hemorrhage is not distal to the anastomosis.

REFERENCES

1. Baum S, Athanasoulis CA, Waltman AC: Angiographic diagnosis and control of large-bowel bleeding. *Dis Colon Rectum* 1974; 17:447–455
2. Drapanas T, Pennington DG, Kappelman M, et al: Emergency subtotal colectomy: Preferred approach to management of massively bleeding diverticular disease. *Ann Surg* 1973; 177:519–526
3. Forde KA: Colonoscopy in acute rectal bleeding. *Gastrointest Endosc* 1981; 27:219–220
4. Welch CE, Athanasoulis CA, Galdabini JJ: Hemorrhage from the large bowel with special reference to angiodysplasia and diverticular disease. *World J Surg* 1978; 2:73–83

49

Rectal Prolapse

A 71-year-old woman with chronic constipation is evaluated because of protrusion of tissue from her anus. The perineal musculature is relatively intact. There is, however, a 3-cm protrusion of apparently normal rectal mucosa. The patient is continent of solid stool but does note leakage of mucus. Stool guaiac is negative.

Consultants: Ann Lowry, M.D.
Stanley M. Goldberg, M.D.

OVERVIEW

Long-recognized by the medical profession, rectal prolapse remains a fascinating but poorly understood condition. Since its first description in 1500 B.C. in the Ebers Papyrus, many etiologic theories and corrective procedures have been proposed and discarded. Still today, little agreement exists about the etiology and optimal therapy.

The usual complaints of a patient with procidentia were well described by a patient in 1825 (as cited by Frederick Salmon):

> In September of 1825, I was much annoyed by frequent call to the water closet. Upon inspection of what passed from me, I discovered it was principally composed of slime and blood . . . the constant desire to go to stool still remained and it frequently happened that I could not reach the night stool before the evacuations would pass . . . I observed, likewise, that whenever I went to stool the gut used to come down and I was frequently obliged to put it back with my finger.

This description remains a typical history of a patient suffering with prolapse.

Prolapse occurs most commonly in young children and the elderly. It is more frequent in women in a ratio varying from 3:1 to 10:1. The presenting symptom is usually the protrusion of tissue from the rectum. Early, it may occur only with defecation and spontaneously reduce. With time, it may be noted with lifting, coughing, or assuming an upright position. The sensation of incomplete evacuation or tenesmus are frequently present. Pain, mucus discharge, and bleeding may accompany persistent prolapse. Other patients may seek help for incontinence, unaware of underlying procidentia. Many patients report a long history of constipation and straining. Chronic straining may be a result of slow-transit constipation, inappropriate puborectalis syndrome, or diet-related constipation and other presently unidentified causes.

The current theory of the pathogenesis of rectal prolapse is that intussusception of the midrectum occurs with straining in certain predisposed patients, eventually resulting in complete prolapse. Broden and Snellman, using cinedefecography, documented a circumferential intussusception originating 6 to 8 cm inside the rectum; other investigators have confirmed this. Whether predisposing anatomical features need be present for prolapse to occur is not clear. There are certain anatomical features commonly seen: an abnormally deep cul de sac, lax musculature of the pelvic floor, absence of normal rectal-sacral fixation, and redundant rectosigmoid. However, it is uncertain if they precede or follow the onset of procidentia.

Symptoms of incontinence commonly accompany rectal prolapse, with an incidence varying from 26% to 80% of patients. The symptoms range from leakage of mucus and gas to incontinence of solid stool. Manometric studies frequently reveal low resting tone, perhaps representing internal sphincter dysfunction secondary to constant rectal distention by the intussuscepted bowel. In patients with major incontinence, both resting and squeeze pressures are low. Electromyography (EMG) and histologic studies have revealed evidence of denervation of the puborectalis and external sphincter muscle. Parks believed that over time the chronic straining and prolapse led to a stretch injury of the pudendal nerves, with this neuropathy resulting in incontinence. Loss of the anal rectal angle probably also contributes to the development of incontinence.

Some investigators believe that an initially hidden intussusception progresses to complete procidentia. The constant rectal distention leads to a decreased resting tone, clinically manifested by minor incontinence of gas and mucus. With persistence of the prolapse, stretch injury to the pudendal nerves occurs, resulting in more significant incontinence. Other authors believe that procidentia with incontinence has a different etiology than prolapse occurring without incontinence. For instance, some suggest that straining with childbirth may cause pelvic floor neuropathy leading to both prolapse and incontinence. On the other hand, slow-transit-time constipation may result in prolapse without incontinence. Further investigation, including longitudinal studies, will be necessary to resolve this issue.

EXAMINATION

When examining a patient with a history of protrusion of tissue, it is important to demonstrate the prolapse. Often it can be elicited easily, but it may be necessary to examine the patient immediately after he/she has strained on a commode; the prone jackknife position is the least satisfactory. Complete prolapse must be differentiated from mucosal prolapse, as therapy is very different. In procidentia, concentric furrows will be seen in the prolapsed tissue that may protrude as far as 20 cm. Palpation reveals the thickness of two rectal walls and may reveal the presence of an enterocele anteriorly. The anus if often patulous, but it is in the normal position. In mucosal prolapse, the anus will be everted. Radial grooves are present on the protrusion that is rarely longer than 5 cm.

All patients with procidentia should undergo a digital rectal examination and sigmoidoscopy. Proctosigmoidoscopy will frequently reveal inflammation or ulceration of the anterior rectal wall 6 to 8 cm from the anal verge. Further evaluation of the colon by barium enema or colonoscopy should also be performed. Although prolapse is rarely a presenting symptom for carcinoma or a polyp, those possibilities must be excluded.

Patients with a lengthy history of severe constipation should undergo a transit-time study to exclude slow-transit constipation. We routinely evaluate patients with anal manometry, particularly those with incontinence. We believe the studies are useful as a baseline reference and as an investigational tool. Hopes that preoperative anal manometry could predict the response to rectopexy have not yet materialized. Cinedefecography has been utilized to visualize a difficult-to-demonstrate prolapse and to delineate associated problems such as enterocele.

SURGICAL PROCEDURES

Over 100 procedures have been described for the treatment of rectal prolapse. All of these procedures can be divided into two categories by their approach—abdominal or perineal. Overall, the abdominal procedures have been more successful in correcting the procidentia and in restoring continence. However, the requirement of general anesthesia and the magnitude of the procedure represent more risk to the patient. The perineal procedures are well-tolerated by elderly and high-risk patients. However, in most series the recurrence rate is higher and the improvement in continence is less.

To determine which procedure is appropriate for this patient, we would assess her medical risk factors. Her age alone would favor a perineal approach, but all medical factors must be considered. In addition, the degree of incontinence, clinically and through objective testing, as well as the extent to which the incontinence troubles the patient, must be assessed. A poor-risk, 71-year-old patient who regards incontinence as a minor nuisance would be offered a perineal approach. An otherwise healthy 71-year-old woman who finds incontinence very limiting and is willing to accept the risk of an abdominal procedure would be advised to undergo an abdominal repair. Obviously, many cases will be less clear-cut. Careful discussion with the patient about her symptoms and the risk of the procedure is necessary.

Of the myriad of abdominal procedures described, we advocate abdominal proctopexy with sigmoid resection. We avoid the use of synthetic mesh to reduce the incidence of infections and obstructive complications. Sigmoid resection eliminates the redundant colon and may decrease the incidence of recurrence. Additional benefits are improved bowel management in patients with chronic constipation or diverticular disease. It also eliminates the possibility of sigmoid volvulus after rectopexy. Low anterior resection is avoided because of the increased risk of complication. If preoperative transit-time studies reveal slow-transit constipation, we recommend subtotal colectomy with rectopexy if anal sphincter function is normal.

Prior to the procedure, the patient undergoes a full mechanical bowel preparation and receives both oral and intravenous antibiotics. After induction of general anesthesia, a Foley catheter is inserted. The patient is placed in modified lithotomy position; this position permits a second assistant to stand between the patient's legs and allows perineal access to the rectum for use of an intraluminal stapler if desired. Through an infraumbilical transverse incision, the abdomen is explored. A Balfour retractor with a bladder blade is inserted. The left portion of the colon from the level of the mid-descending colon to sacral promontory is mobilized. The presacral space is entered in the avascular plane, avoiding the presacral plexus. This dissection is continued to the levator ani muscles. The anterior peritoneum is incised, and the rectum is dissected free from the structures anterior to it. The lateral stalks are preserved. After the rectum has been mobilized, the rectopexy sutures of 2-0 silk or Prolene are placed. The sutures are placed through the lateral stalks near the bowel wall, then through the presacral fascia and returned through the lateral stalks. Care should be taken to avoid the midline of the sacral promontory where the middle sacral artery lies. Two sutures are usually placed on each side at approximately S1 and S3. When all the sutures have been placed, they are serially tied. The result should be that the rectum is taut and firmly fixed in the sacral concavity. In addition to fixation of the rectum, the rectopexy helps restore the anal rectal angle. If a constricting band is noted after tying the sutures, the offending sutures must be removed. A standard resection of the redundant rectosigmoid is then performed, followed by a single-layer hand-sewn anastomosis. Alternatively, the intraluminal stapler can be used, but the anastomosis should be completed prior to tying the rectopexy sutures. If not done in this sequence, placement of the staples through the fixed rectum may be impossible or may disrupt the rectopexy sutures. Usually, no attempt is made to close the diastasis in the levator ani muscle nor to obliterate the deep cul de sac (Fig 49–1).

We recently reported on 102 patients who underwent abdominal rectopexy and sigmoid resection. After a mean four-year follow-up, the recurrence rate

For high risk pts a perineal recto-sigmoidectomy.

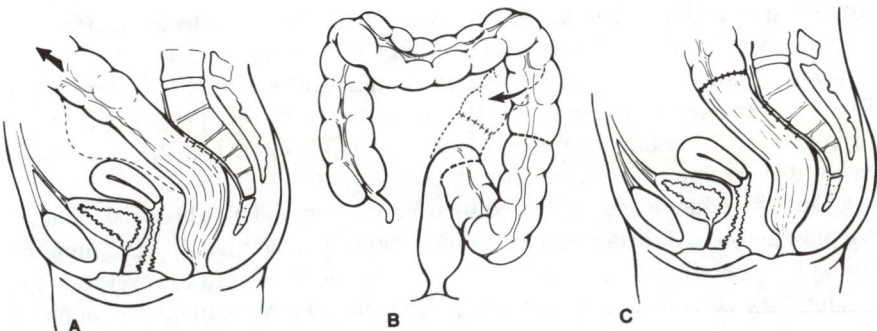

FIG 49–1.
Presacral rectopexy and sigmoid resection. After mobilization of rectum, it is fixed to the sacrum (**A**). Standard resection of redundant sigmoid colon is then performed (**B**). In authors' opinion, the combination is the optimal procedure (**C**). (From Wassef R, Rothenberger DA, Goldberg SM: *Curr Probl Surg* 1986; 23(6):402. Used by permission.)

was 1.9%. There were no deaths and only 4% morbidity. Preoperatively, 63% of patients complained of constipation. Of these, 56% reported improvement in their symptoms postoperatively.

Nine patients underwent subtotal colectomy and abdominal proctopexy. Seven patients believed their results were good to excellent, with significant improvement in their bowel management problems. The two patients with poor results had significant incontinence. Presently, we recommend subtotal colectomy only for patients with no clinical or manometric evidence of sphincter dysfunction and evidence of an atonic colon (abnormal transit-time).

For elderly and high-risk patients, we recommend a perineal rectosigmoidectomy. After full mechanical and antibiotic bowel preparation and preoperative antibiotics, the patient is brought to the operating room. The procedure may be easily performed with the patient under caudal, spinal, or local anesthesia with sedation, as well as general anesthesia. The patient is placed in a modified lithotomy position or prone jackknife position, depending upon the preference of the surgeon and anesthesiologist. With gentle traction applied to the prolapsed rectal wall, an epinephrine solution is injected in the area of the proposed incision. A circumferential incision is then made through the outer tube of rectal wall, exposing the inner tube and its mesorectum. There is some debate as to whether leaving a cuff of 2 to 4 cm of anorectal mucosa improves postoperative rectal sensation and continence. The mesorectum of the redundant bowel is serially divided and ligated. Once the mesorectum has been safely divided, a section of the bowel (usually 15 to 25 cm in length) is removed. Primary anastomosis with either sutures or staples is performed between the sigmoid colon and anal mucosa. Altemeier, whose name is associated with this procedure, described obliterating the peritoneal cul de sac, which he believed represented a sliding hernia sac. We have not obliterated the cul de sac, since prolapse is an intussusception and not primarily a sliding hernia. Altemeier and associates also recommended approximation of the levator ani and puborectalis muscles. Again, because we believe its value is debatable, we have not routinely approximated those muscles. There is some recent evidence by Prasad et al., however, that there is more improvement in continence if the levators are approximated. If that is substantiated, that portion of the procedure should be routine (Fig 49–2).

This procedure is well tolerated by even the very elderly, high-risk patient. We have performed this procedure on 66 patients with no mortality and minimal morbidity with no recurrences. The follow-up period is short, however, and the true incidence is unknown. Others have also reported zero mortality and minimal

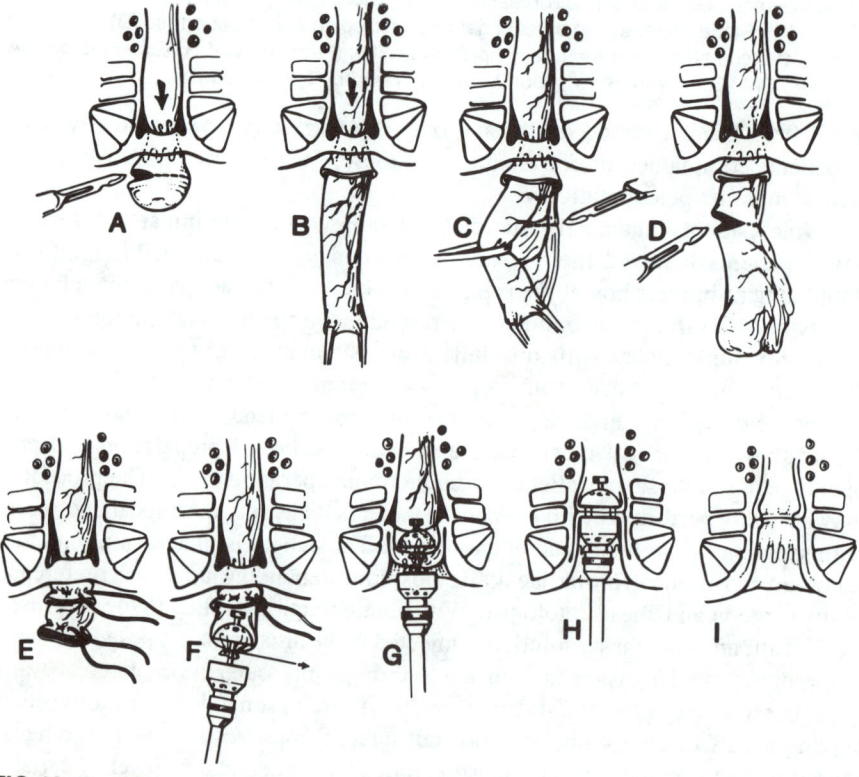

FIG 49–2.
Perineal rectosigmoidectomy. With the rectum prolapsed, the outer tube is incised circularly (**A**) and divided (**B**). The mesorectum is serially ligated and divided (**C**). When all redundancy has been removed, the inner tube is divided, completing the resection (**D**). The anastomosis may be performed with the intraluminal stapling device (E–I) or may be hand sewn. (From Wassef R, Rothenberger DA, Goldberg SM: *Curr Probl Surg* 1986; 23(6):402. Used by permission.)

morbidity. What does vary widely is the reported recurrence rates, ranging from 0% to 60%. There is no obvious explanation for this wide variance.

Occasionally a patient will present with an irreducible rectal prolapse. If there are no signs of systemic illness and the bowel appears viable, sugar may be applied to the prolapsed tissue to reduce the edema. Often it is then possible to reduce the prolapse and later perform an appropriate elective procedure. However, if the bowel appears gangrenous, an emergency perineal rectosigmoidectomy should be performed.

POSTOPERATIVE COURSE

It is clear that correction of procidentia can be performed safely with an acceptably low recurrence rate. The still discouraging aspect of treating rectal prolapse is the frequent persistence of bowel dysfunction. Both constipation and incontinence often persist as major problems postoperatively. While abdominal procedures have been more successful than perineal procedures, the incidence of postoperative incontinence still varies from 20% to 60%. The incidence of postoperative constipation has not been documented.

Improvement in incontinence may require 6 to 12 months to occur; thus, patients should be encouraged to wait for at least one year before any intervention. Regulation of bowel habits with dietary manipulations and bulk agents may help. Mucosal prolapse, which occurs in approximately 10% of patients postoperatively, may contribute to minor incontinence. This can usually be managed by rubber-band ligation, but rarely it may require excisional proctoplasty.

If all of the above measures fail, improvement has been reported after the Parks' postanal repair. This technique involves plication of the levators, puborectalis, and external sphincter muscles through a postanal intersphincteric approach. The object is to recreate an acute anal rectal angle and lengthen the anal canal. Keighley and associates reported an 80% success rate in restoring continence for patients with persistent incontinence after abdominal rectopexy. We have not had as much success with this procedure, but no better alternative has been described.

The relatively minor incontinence experienced by this patient would, hopefully, be significantly improved with correction of her prolapse. At her age, our emphasis would be on dietary management and bulk agents rather than on surgical intervention if her incontinence persists.

BIBLIOGRAPHY

1. Altemeier WA, Culbertson WR, Schowengerdt C, et al: Nineteen years' experience with the one-stage perineal repair of rectal prolapse. *Ann Surg* 1971; 173:993–1006.

2. Broden B, Snellman B: Procidentia of the rectum studied with cineradiography: A contribution to the discussion of causative mechanism. *Dis Colon Rectum* 1968; 11:330–347.
3. Keighley MRB, Matheson DM: Results of treatment for rectal prolapse and fecal incontinence. *Dis Colon Rectum* 1981; 24:449–453.
4. Keighley MRB, Shouler PJ: Abnormalities of colonic function in patients with rectal prolapse and faecal incontinence. *Br J Surg* 1984; 71:892–895.
5. Neill ME, Parks AG, Swash M: Physiological studies of the anal sphincter musculature in faecal incontinence and rectal prolapse. *Br J Surg* 1981; 68:531–536.
6. Prasad ML, Pearl RK, Abcarian H, et al: Perineal proctectomy, posterior rectopexy and postanal levator repair for the treatment of rectal prolapse. *Dis Colon Rectum* 1986; 29:547–552.
7. Salmon F: Practical observations on prolapses of the rectum. *Dis Colon Rectum* 1984; 27:138–145.
8. Wassef R, Rothenberger DA, Goldberg SM: Rectal prolapse. *Curr Probl Surg* 1986; 23(6):402–451.
9. Watts JD, Rothenberger DA, Buls JG, et al: The management of procidentia: 30 years' experience. *Dis Colon Rectum* 1985; 28:96–102.

50

High Fistula-in-ano

A 57-year-old man, in previous good health and with no history of diarrhea, presents with a perirectal abscess that is drained. Over the next three months, conservative therapy reveals persistent drainage and a fistula-in-ano. Sigmoidoscopy and physical examination revealed the site of entrance to be above the internal sphincter, approximately 5 cm from the anal verge. Palpation of the area reveals induration high along the rectal wall.

Consultant: Philip H. Gordon, M.D.

It is understandable, and perhaps beneficial to the patient, that a surgeon presented with a fistula-in-ano characterized by a high internal opening would be intimidated by the problem. Although nonoperative methods of treatment have been attempted through the ages, it is generally accepted that the only form of treatment that affords any reliable prospect of cure is an operation. Recognizing that the reputations of some surgeons have been jeopardized because of the outcome of operations for fistula-in-ano, it becomes incumbent upon the surgeon to make every effort to assess the relationship of the fistulous tracks to the sphincter mechanism. The concern, of course, is the potential double jeopardy of the sequelae of subsequent recurrence and/or impairment of anal continence. Although most fistulas are simple to treat, complicated fistulas challenge the ingenuity, knowledge, and technical skill of the surgeon.

Prior to embarking upon an operation for a fistula-in-ano, it is essential that the surgeon develop an understanding of the anatomy of the pelvic floor as well as the pathogenesis of the fistula-in-ano in order to appreciate the origin and ramifications of fistulas. Current evidence suggests that infection of the anal glands is probably the most common cause of a fistulous abscess. Obstruction of these ducts, whether secondary to fecal material, foreign bodies, or trauma, will result in stasis and secondary infection. Once established, the most common course for a fistula to pursue is from the mid anal canal downward in the intersphincteric plane to the anal verge. Infection may overcome the barrier of the external sphincter muscles, thereby penetrating the ischiorectal fossa, or it

R/o IBD { Sigmoidoscopy, BE, SBFT } only if necessary

may extend upward in the intersphincteric plane. In addition to upward and downward, tracking of pus may pass circumferentially in one of three tissue planes, the most common being the ischiorectal fossa. Horseshoeing may also occur in the intersphincteric plane or in the supralevator plane.

PREOPERATIVE EVALUATION

Given the history of this patient, an extensive evaluation is not necessary. The patient clearly has a persistent fistula-in-ano. A history should be taken to rule out symptoms of inflammatory bowel disease, and sigmoidoscopy should be performed to rule out the presence of inflammatory bowel disease as well as identifying other internal openings. Should any suspicious symptoms be present, a barium enema or even an upper gastrointestinal (GI) and small-bowel follow-through may be indicated. For the most part, fistulography is not necessary, although in a patient with recurrent disease, or if the history is suspicious of an intra-abdominal or pelvic source of sepsis, a fistulogram may prove of value.

PATIENT PREPARATION

In preparation for the operation, a simple cleansing enema is all that is necessary. No shave preparation is required. It is probably wise to explain to the patient the nature of the problem, since muscle will require division with the ever-present potential for alteration in continence.

APPROACHES TO OPERATIVE MANAGEMENT

In approaching a patient with a fistula-in-ano, several guidelines should be kept in mind. According to Goodsall's rule, if there is an opening posterior to the coronal plane, the fistula probably originates from the dorsal midline; however, if anterior, the fistula probably runs directly to the nearest crypt. Openings seen on both sides of the anal canal are likely to arise from the midline posterior crypt with a horseshoe-type fistula. An external opening adjacent to the anal margin may suggest an intersphincteric track, while a more laterally located opening would suggest a transsphincteric, suprasphincteric, or even extrasphincteric fistula. The further the distance of the external opening from the anal margin, the greater is the probability of a complicated upward extension. When the track is fairly low in the sphincter mechanism, palpation of the skin between the secondary opening and the anal canal will reveal a cord structure. Within the anal canal, one might be able to palpate a pit indicative of an internal opening. If traction is placed on the external opening, the crypt of origin may retract into a funnel, thus identifying its location. Following introduction of a probe into the track, the angle the probe makes with the anal canal is helpful in determining the type of fistula. A low fistula will pass toward the anus at an angle of approximately 30 degrees to the skin. Passage of a probe at an 80-degree angle to the skin or almost parallel to the anal canal reveals the presence of a high extension.

The objective of fistula surgery is simple: cure the fistula with the lowest possible recurrence rate, with a minimum of any alteration in continence, and do so in the shortest period of time. To approximate this ideal, a number of principles should be observed: (1) the primary opening of the track must be identified; (2) the relationship of the track to the puborectalis must be established; and (3) division of the least amount of muscle in keeping with cure of the fistula should be practiced.

Over the years, many classifications of fistulas in and about the anorectal region have been described. The aim of any such classification should be to help the surgeon in the operative cure of the disease. In this regard, the classification described by Parks and associates, although very detailed, gives an accurate description of the anatomical course of the fistulous tracks. This knowledge acts as a guide to the operative treatment and has proved of value to me.

With the foregoing background, the patient presented suggests four scenarios that may be found at the time of operation. These have been illustrated diagrammatically in Figures 50–1 and 50–2. Each scenario will be described individually and the appropriate therapy outlined.

Intersphincteric Fistula

During examination of a patient with a fistula-in-ano, a high internal opening may be noted. By high is meant an opening that is above the level of the puborectalis. When faced with such a patient, the surgeon may initially be concerned that this fistula represents a very complex problem; however, examination with the patient under anesthesia may better define the course of the fistulous track and, in fact, this may only represent an intersphincteric fistula that has burst back into the rectal ampulla (see Fig 50–1,A).

Under these circumstances treatment is made up of division of the overlying tissue, which consists of the anoderm, mucosa, and internal sphincter, from the high internal opening to the lower end of the internal sphincter. Search should be made for side branches. The surgeon may initially believe that the track courses outside all of the muscles of continence, but this is not true in the case of intersphincteric fistulas.

After unroofing, the track is curretted of its granulation tissue. Hemostasis is obtained using cautery, and I have marsupialized the track with a continuous 3-0 chromic suture.

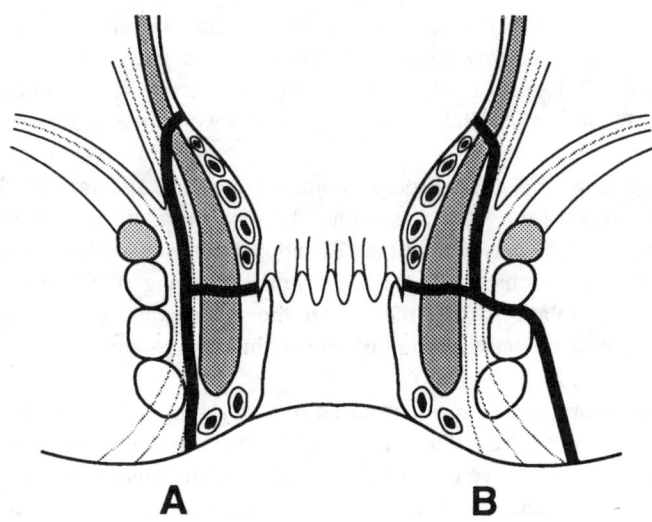

FIG 50–1.
A, relationship of fistula track to sphincter mechanism in intersphincteric fistula. The track is entirely in the intersphincteric plane. **B,** relationship of fistula track to sphincter mechanism in transsphincteric fistula with a high intersphincteric component. The track crosses the external sphincter and descends to the perineum as well as a track ascending in the intersphincteric plane breaking back into the rectum.

Transsphincteric Fistula With a High Intersphincteric Component

In the scenario of the transsphincteric fistula with a high intersphincteric component (see Fig 50–1,B), the level at which the track crosses the external sphincter determines the ease or difficulty encountered in treatment. Most cross at a low level, so that laying open the fistula would result in division of only the lower portion of the internal sphincter and the lower half of the external sphincter. The upward extension in the intersphincteric plane is then laid open and the tracks are managed as described above.

In order to preserve function, fistulas with tracks crossing at higher levels may be treated by division of the lower half of the internal sphincter, creating adequate drainage of the fistulous track, dividing only a portion of the external sphincter, and inserting a seton. This effectively stages the repair, but it is believed that sequential division of the muscle diminishes the chance of incontinence. After insertion of a seton, it is anticipated that division of the sphincter will be followed by scar formation proximal to the ligature, thus holding the muscle fibers together. A nonabsorbable suture such as silk can be passed through the fistulous track and tied loosely. The patient may be instructed to manipulate the seton and, indeed, this may cut through the muscle spontaneously. If not, the seton-contained muscle can be divided at a second stage six to eight weeks later. If the wound does heal well, the seton can be removed without division of the contained muscle, but this policy may result in a higher incidence of recurrence although it will almost certainly result in a lower incidence of alterations in continence.

For patients whose fistula crosses the sphincter muscle at a high level (e.g., transsphincteric and suprasphincteric), there is always the concern that division of the muscle below the track will result in significant alterations in continence. In these circumstances the renewed interest in the advancement rectal flap technique, as reported by Aguilar et al., is appealing. The principles of repair include: (1) excision of the internal opening in the anal canal, (2) excision or currettage of the main track, (3) advancement of a flap of mucosa and submucosa of rectum beyond the original internal opening, and (4) suture of the flap to the anal canal distal to the original opening. Several authors have reported encouraging results using this technique.

Extrasphincteric Fistula Secondary to Transsphincteric Fistula

The extremely rare situation of a high rectal opening associated with an extrasphincteric fistula presents a most challenging task (see Fig 50-2,A). It may arise in a patient with a transsphincteric fistula with a high extension that may burst spontaneously into the rectum, although this is very rare.

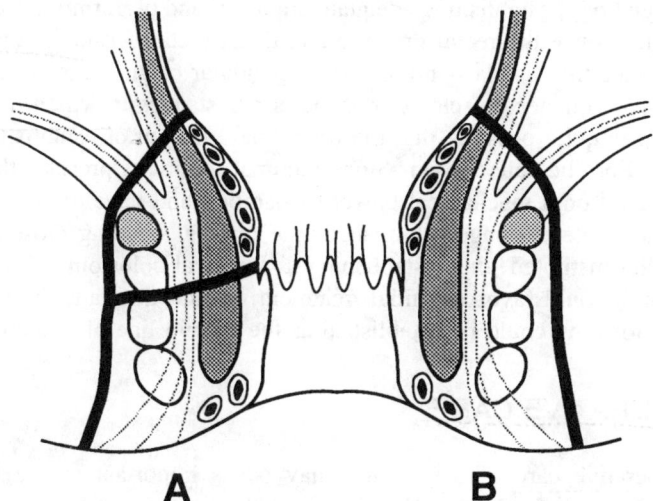

FIG 50-2.
A, relationship of fistula track to sphincter mechanism in extrasphincteric fistula secondary to transsphincteric fistula. The track originates at the dentate line, crosses the external sphincter, and passes through levator muscle and rectal wall as well as descending to the perineum. **B,** relationship of fistula track to sphincter mechanism in extrasphincteric fistula secondary to trauma. The track passes above all the muscles of continence.

In this circumstance two factors perpetuate the existence of the fistula: (1) the infected anal gland in the intersphincteric plane, and (2) the intraluminal pressure that forces mucus and debris through the fistulous track. Both factors must be taken into consideration during the treatment. The infected anal gland in the intersphincteric plane is treated by division of the lower half of the internal sphincter. The secondary fistulous track is curretted and adequate drainage provided, while the internal opening in the rectum is closed with nonabsorbable suture. The patient should be treated with an elemental diet, as reported by Gordon, in order to give the internal opening a chance to heal. Should healing not occur, consideration should be given to the establishment of a temporary diverting colostomy.

Extrasphincteric Fistula Secondary to Trauma

A traumatic extrasphincteric fistula may be caused in two ways (see Fig 50–2,B). A foreign body may penetrate the perineum and enter the rectum, but no such history was given in the patient described. Alternatively, a swallowed foreign body (e.g., fish or chicken bone) may reach the rectum, straddle the sphincters, and be forced through the rectal wall, levator muscles, and ischiorectal fossa, and reach the perineum. Under these circumstances the principles of trauma must be invoked and such fistulas are treated with adequate debridement, removal of the foreign body, establishing adequate drainage, and performing a temporary colostomy to reduce the rectal pressure and distal rectal washout. It should be noted that since this fistula is not of cryptoglandular origin, it is not necessary to divide any sphincter muscle. Under the circumstances in which this patient presented, it is quite possible that the traditional wisdom of establishing a colostomy need not be called upon. Since minimal trauma is present, the patient could be placed on a mechanical bowel preparation and have the foreign body removed, adequate drainage established, the internal opening closed, and an elemental diet instituted, thus establishing a "medical colostomy." This is the method that I would favor as initial treatment; should this fail, the temporary diverting colostomy could be established as the second line of treatment.

POSTOPERATIVE CARE

The postoperative care of the wound may be as important as the operative procedure. The prime goals are healing from the depths of the wound as well as prevention of contact and premature healing of opposed skin edges. Patients are placed on a regular diet (with the exception of those with extrasphincteric fistula) and analgesics are administered as needed. Warm baths are taken two to three times a day for cleansing and comfort purposes. A bulk-forming agent is recommended until wound healing has been completed.

CONCLUSION

Based on the belief that the pathogenesis of 90% of fistula-in-ano is infection of the anal glands, the key to successful treatment consists of eradication of these infected anal glands. Despite the fact that it was noted in the case history that an internal opening was present above the anorectal ring, it must be recognized that in most circumstances this is a secondary opening and that search must be made for the primary opening at the level of the dentate line. Failure to do so is the most common cause of recurrence.

The dilemma facing the surgeon is how to obtain adequate treatment of the fistula without causing a disturbance of sphincter function. Too much division may cause incontinence. Where there is doubt regarding the competence of the sphincter, it is wise to divide it in stages at successive operations, with careful assessment being made of its state in the conscious patient between each stage. (*Editor's note*: Conventional wisdom has it that low rates of incontinence (less than 5%) can be expected if the sphincter is divided in one area. If reoperation is necessary, extreme care in dividing only one half of the internal sphincter—as stressed by the author—and in the scarred area, if possible, is mandatory.) It must be accepted, however, that to obtain cure in many complex fistulas some loss of function is inevitable; the aim is to minimize it.

BIBLIOGRAPHY

1. Aguilar PS, Plaisencia G, Hardy TG, et al: Mucosal advancement in the treatment of anal fistula. *Dis Colon Rectum* 1985; 28:496–501.
2. Fazio V: Complex anal fistulae. *Gastroenterol Clin North Am* 1987; 16:93–114.
3. Goldberg SM, Gordon PH, Nivatvongs S: Anorectal abscess and fistula-in-ano, in Goldberg SM, Gordon PH, Nivatvongs S (eds): *Essentials of Anorectal Surgery*. Philadelphia, JB Lippincott Co, 1980, pp 100–127.
4. Parks AG, Gordon PH, Hardcastle JG: A classification of fistula-in-ano. *Br J Surg* 1976; 63:1–12.

51

Acute Perforated Diverticulitis

A 69-year-old woman is admitted with a sudden onset of left lower quadrant pain, fever, and prostration. She was previously reported to have alternating diarrhea and constipation and has taken psyllium for several years. Physical examination reveals an elderly woman in acute distress complaining of severe abdominal pain from a distended abdomen. There is guarding and rigidity in all four quadrants, maximal in the left lower quadrant, and bowel sounds are diminished. Rebound tenderness is present.

Consultant: Victor W. Fazio, M.D.

OVERVIEW

The patient presented here is suffering from peritonitis. The differential diagnosis therefore includes quite a number of conditions, the most likely being that of perforation of the left side of the colon due to diverticulitis coli, although carcinoma cannot be ruled out even in the absence of a history of rectal bleeding. A flat film of the chest and abdomen that shows a pneumoperitoneum confirms the presence of a ruptured viscus, and laparotomy will be performed unless the patient is moribund. The decision to operate will then focus the clinician on resuscitation and preparation of the patient for surgery. This includes restoration of hydration and treatment of shock to the extent possible. A central venous line is placed and maintained. (*Editor's note*: Some may wish to pass a Swan-Ganz catheter for perioperative monitoring. Information gained from left atrial pressure measurements and cardiac outputs are very useful in the treatment of sepsis.) A nasogastric tube is passed, and urine output is assessed with an indwelling bladder catheter. A blood culture is taken and intravenous antibiotics given; preparations effective against gram-negative aerobes and anaerobes are appropriate, such as gentamicin and metronidazole. If not already done, a flat film of the abdomen is taken as well as a chest x-ray film, and cardiogram; determination of complete blood cell count, SMA analysis, and prothrombin, and partial thromboplastin time is accomplished. Blood is typed and crossmatched, and transfusion is begun if the patient is anemic. Any electrolyte or coagulation abnormality is treated as well as any underlying medical condition such as diabetes mellitus, arrhythmia, and chronic, obstructive pulmonary disease. The principle addressed here is that those metabolic or systemic abnormalities or conditions that can be improved or corrected in the *short term* (within one to two hours) are treated. The surgeon recognizes that fecal peritonitis is a highly lethal condition and that urgent correction of the cause is the most efficacious way of correcting the patient's overall condition.

PREOPERATIVE APPROACH

Radiographic Studies

Chest x-ray film will probably show gas under the diaphragm and confirm the presence of a pneumoperitoneum. A subtle form of this may be evident on the plain abdominal film—a small air leak manifesting itself as a strip of gas on the under-border of the transverse colon. This occurs when the sigmoid perforation is small and partly sealed by omentum. Air fluid levels in the small bowel may also be present.

Barium enema is contraindicated. This may well show the site of the perforation, but barium that has leaked into the abdominal cavity and has mixed with colonic content is a particularly lethal combination. Even an enema with diatrizoate meglumine (Gastrografin) is contraindicated; it is time-consuming and will add little to the information obtainable at laparotomy. (*Editor's note:* Little mucosal detail is usually appreciated from water-soluble dye enemas. In addition, it is dangerous, as the dye is very hypertonic and irritating.)

Computerized tomography (CT) has been used in selected cases of perforative diverticulitis. The term "perforative" requires definition. In a sense, all cases of diverticulitis are perforative, that is, a small, usually localized inflammation around a diverticulum resulting from a sealed perforation. Intramesenteric abscess and paracolic or pelvic abscess secondary to contained or sealed perforation of sigmoid diverticulitis are the next stages of perforation, in order of severity. Here, the signs are those of localized tenderness or peritonitis, as opposed to the present case with generalized peritonitis. With these localized abscesses, in patients *without* generalized peritonitis, CT scanning may be helpful in localizing an abscess. If the location (e.g., extraperitoneal) lends itself to CT-guided needle catheter drainage, this may well allow for detoxification of the patient so that, with antibiotics and a waiting period of one to two weeks, a one-stage resection and anastomosis can be done. In the case under discussion, with generalized peritonitis, there is no role for CT scanning.

Colonic Endoscopy

My practice is to perform proctosigmoidoscopy in the operating room just prior to laparotomy. This will exclude a distally placed, unsuspected cancer and inflammatory bowel disease involving the rectum.

Bowel Preparation

Apart from intravenous antibiotics, no bowel preparation is used.

Stoma Marking

Stoma marking is desirable, but it is frequently overlooked in the heat of the moment. One must consider that a number of elderly patients who survive surgery for perforated diverticulitis will *never* have their colostomy closed. Accordingly, it behooves the surgeon to take the minute or so required to mark out the alternative sites for an end-descending colostomy—away from scars, creases, and body prominences, and within the surface marking of the rectus abdominus muscle.

Position of the Patient

My preference is the lithotomy/Trendelenburg position using Lloyd-Davies stirrups.

Incision

A midline incision is used and can be extended as needed. Upon entering the abdomen, swabs are taken for Gram staining and culture. Attention is directed to identify the perforation; this is then "controlled" by tying linen tapes around the bowel, proximal and distal to the perforation. The peritoneal cavity is then cleansed; this involves removal of all macroscopic debris and irrigation/aspiration of the cavity, including the subphrenic spaces, until a clean return of the warm saline irrigant is obtained.

CHOICE OF OPERATION

Historical Note

It is somewhat surprising that no randomized prospective trials of surgical treatment for diverticulitis have been published in the literature. This stems from the relatively small numbers of cases that an individual surgeon or institution accumulates (regarding perforative diverticulitis) in the short term. Also, the exact definition of perforation, the varying degrees of soiling of the peritoneal cavity, and the numerous methods of management make the conducting of a trial a formidable task. Still, there have been many publications on the subject (nonrandomized studies), and certain trends and concepts are emerging.

In 1942, Smithwick popularized the operation of loop transverse colostomy and drainage of the perforated site. This was done initially for paracolic abscess but was also applied to free perforation with generalized peritonitis. Clearly, different results can be obtained in terms of mortality and morbidity if this operation is applied to a series composed mainly of localized, sealed perforations vs. a series made up predominantly of patients with free perforation. In this latter case, continued fecal contamination of the peritoneum occurs as the stool in the left part of the colon, distal to the transverse colostomy, continues to empty through the perforation. Smithwick had reported mortality rates of 17.1% following resection and 9.8% following colostomy. Thus, he advocated a staged procedure involving a preliminary colostomy followed by resection of the diseased segment with anastomosis. Colostomy closure was the third-stage operation. At least six other studies have reported less favorable results with the three-stage procedure, varying from 22% to 47% mortality. Greif and colleagues reviewed a combined literature experience of 363 patients. In patients with localized peritonitis, mortality was 2% with resection, compared to 12% with colostomy. Mortality rates in patients with generalized peritonitis were 12% and 29%, respectively. (*Editor's note:* The author has made a very good case against transverse colostomy, with which I agree. In my opinion, there is still occasionally a place for transverse colostomy, especially using local anesthesia, in an elderly patient in whom, despite adequate antibiotic and other therapy, the diverticulitis without abscess on CT scan refuses to subside.)

Laparotomy and drainage alone should never be used in patients with generalized peritonitis secondary to colonic perforation. Even in patients with localized peritonitis due to contained perforation, drainage alone is associated with a subsequent colocutaneous fistula rate of 22%.

Exteriorization of the perforation enjoyed a certain popularity. However, the disadvantages were soon realized and the procedure became more or less obsolete. These disadvantages included the fact that the perforated segment was often difficult to manage or exteriorize, and the stoma thus made was quite large and difficult to pouch.

In 1957, Belding advocated sigmoid resection without anastomosis for patients with free perforation. No patients in his series died. At least seven other series have reported very favorable results with this procedure, in which the source of inflammation is removed and there is no risk of anastomotic leak or continued contamination of the peritoneal cavity. Only two stages are involved in the definitive management and intestinal tract reconstruction. When done with reasonable planning, retroperitoneal sepsis is not a significant problem. Details of this procedure will be discussed in the following section.

Resection and primary anastomosis for perforative diverticulitis has been advocated by a number of authors in recent years. Madden, one of the leading spokesmen for the procedure, claims that the operation can be done with a mortality rate similar to that of resection without colostomy. The rationale of the procedure (with anastomosis) is that once the inflamed segment is out, the anastomosis is easier to make, rather than at a later period when adhesions are considerable and the rectal stump is difficult to find. However, the procedure is time-consuming, and patients in this group are usually quite ill and poorly tolerate any prolongation of anesthesia. A wider resection has to be done (than for the Hartmann operation), as definitive operation calls for removal of the perforated inflamed segment, resection of any proximal colon with muscle hypertrophy, and resection of *all* sigmoid with colorectal anastomosis. This could mean a need for splenic flexure mobilization with opening up of tissue planes for retroperitoneal contamination. The bowel is edematous, obstructed, and frequently loaded with stool. On-table lavage of the colon (as for obstructed left-colon cancer resection) is time-consuming and messy. Fecal fistula occurred in 29% of Killingback's series and in 22% of Madden's series. Eng and colleagues reviewed the literature and found a 10% mortality with one-stage resection and anastomosis, compared to 9.1% if no anastomosis was used. However, almost all cases represented perforation *without* general peritonitis or fecal peritonitis.

In summary, there may be an occasional place for one-stage resection in specific cases of perforative diverticulitis *without* general peritonitis. If the patient is otherwise fit and tolerating surgery well, then the operation, possibly combined with a temporary colostomy, is appropriate. Subsequent closure of the temporary colostomy is an easier undertaking than bowel restoration after a Hartmann operation.

We have reviewed our experience with diverticulitis for the period 1970 to 1984. Free perforation with generalized peritonitis occurred in 29 patients of 590 undergoing surgery. Of these 29, 23 patients underwent a two-stage procedure; there was one anastomotic leak and four deaths. Of five patients undergoing a three-stage procedure, there were three leaks and no deaths. The only patient with a one-stage resection and anastomosis did well, without a leak. Overall mortality was 13%, with a leak rate of 13%. A further 241 patients of the 590 had perforation with localized abscess; mortality was 2.9% in this group.

CONDUCT OF THE OPERATION

From the foregoing, it is apparent that I favor resective surgery without anastomosis for patients with generalized peritonitis secondary to perforated diverticular disease. Statistically, the factors that favor high mortality are (1) surgery being done in the elderly and (2) conditions that demand urgent surgery.

Given the urgent nature of the case under discussion, there are certain rules or guidelines that a surgeon should follow:

1. *Remove/resect the perforated segment.*
2. *Do not do more than you have to do.* Definitive resection for diverticulitis involves resection of a 30- to 35-cm segment to get above muscle hypertrophy and distally get down to the rectosigmoid junction at the promontory of the sacrum. Remember why you are there! There will (hopefully) be another opportunity to do definitive surgery. Therefore, a short resection of 10 to 15 cm may be ample.
3. *Do not open up further avenues of sepsis by extensive peritoneal dissection.* As it happens, most perforations occur in the midsigmoid. That being the case, resection of the segment without high ligation of the vessel is appropriate; it is unnecessary and indeed inadvisable if the distal sigmoid colon remains. Initially, the perforation may seem to be low in the pelvis, but gentle digital dissection will allow retraction of the midsigmoid (and the perforation site) back into the abdomen.

It is inadvisable and rarely, if ever, necessary to dissect in the presacral space. Similarly, the splenic flexure is best left alone and not mobilized. What about perforation of the proximal sigmoid in an obese patient? Following resection, it can be impossible to get the descending colon out as a colostomy. This can be solved by the unusual approach of double-stapling the proximal colonic end that would normally be the site chosen for colostomy. A distal loop transverse colostomy is then performed; the rectosigmoid segment is stapled across and brought to the anterior abdominal wall.

What about distal sigmoid perforation? Here, the only way the rectal segment can be exteriorized is by presacral dissection. Since this practice breaches retroperitoneal planes, it is better to staple the rectal stump at the promontory of the sacrum; I usually add a further suture layer beyond the TA-55 autosuture closure. The stump is then anchored to the promontory with a Stout No. 1 Prolene suture.

4. *Don't make a mucous fistula.* In most cases, the distal sigmoid can be stapled across and delivered to the lower end of the abdominal wound. The loose edge of the anterior peritoneum can be tacked to the colonic serosa and mesentery, just below the staple line. This in effect places the stump in an extraperitoneal plane so that, in the rare event that the stump leaks, a small mucous fistula will develop. The fascial sutures in the lower end of the wound are placed with a generous 1-in. gap opposite the stapled stump; the stump is easy to find at secondary surgery. If a mucous fistula is deliberately made, dressings must be used constantly and, in certain cases of profuse mucous output, a second pouch has to be applied.

5. *Examine the opened specimen before closure of the abdomen.* Rarely, one may find that the perforation has been caused by cancer. In that event, the

surgeon will confer with the anesthetist and make a judgment on the wisdom of further surgery at this time. In most cases, this can be done. The wider resection of the mesentery with high ligation of the inferior mesenteric vessels may still be done without necessarily breaching the presacral space or splenic flexure. The left ureter must be identified.

OTHER CONSIDERATIONS

Peritoneal Toilet

Earlier mention was made of this. Copious warm saline irrigation is employed (10 to 20 L) to dilute the inoculum. Moist sponges or forceps are used to painstakingly remove any fecal or vegetable matter. Opinion is divided concerning the role of antibiotic irrigation and continued postoperative irrigation of the abdominal cavity. I do not use this routinely in my practice. (*Editor's note*: Several studies are currently in progress concerning the randomized prospective use of antibiotic irrigation vs. warm saline alone.)

Drains

There may or may not be a residual phlegmonous "nest," either extraperitoneal or attached to the parietes of the left lower quadrant or pelvis. Delayed suppuration of this kind of tissue may occur. If this is present, a Latex rubber drain or Penrose drains are sutured to the surface of the "nest" and brought out through a lateral drainage incision, well away from the colostomy site. The drain site needs to be an aperture the size of two to three fingers; concern about a later incisional hernia is misplaced. If drains are to be used, then *adequate* drainage must be provided.

If no phlegmonous tissue remains, I will place two large Jackson-Pratt-type closed-suction drains into the pelvis. A certain amount of irrigation fluid and blood and exudate will gravitate to the pelvis. These drains may minimize the development of a late pelvic abscess.

Abdominal and Wound Closure

In most cases, figure-of-eight sutures of a short nonabsorbable suture (e.g., No. 1 Prolene) are satisfactory. Rarely are retention sutures required. The skin is closed for a distance of 2 in. opposite the end colostomy to allow for easy pouching of the stoma. The incision above and below are left open. Delayed closure may be effected in seven days. (*Editor's note*: Delayed primary closure certainly gives the lowest incidence of infection. Wound infection rates almost as low may be achieved by closing the wound primarily over subcutaneous drains (in the presence of antibiotics). Drains are left in eight to ten days, since that is when suppuration occurs.)

Late Surgery

Delayed intra-abdominal abscesses may occur and are treated by appropriate drainage, frequently using CT guidance.

For later anastomosis, one must recall that definitive surgery for diverticulitis has *not* been done. It will be necessary to excise all residual sigmoid at the second-stage procedure, as well as any hypertrophied colonic muscle proximal to the colostomy. A stapled or hand-sewn anastomosis can be done. A left ureteric stent is helpful in identifying the left ureter.

When the rectal stump is oversewn and left *in situ*, a number of techniques have been described to facilitate reconstruction. My preference is to have the patient in the Lloyd-Davies stirrups and to identify the rectum by passage of a rubber dilator per anum. Once identified, the rectum can be dilated up to accommodate a Size 29 or 31 stapler, and a circular stapled anastomosis is performed.

BIBLIOGRAPHY

1. Belding HH: Acute perforated diverticulitis of the sigmoid colon with generalized peritonitis. *Arch Surg* 1957; 74:511–515.
2. Eng K, Ranson JHC, Localio SA: Resection of the perforated segment: A significant advance in treatment of diverticulitis with free perforation or abscess. *Am J Surg* 1977; 133:67–72.
3. Greif JN, Fried G, McSherry CK: Surgical treatment of perforated diverticulitis of the sigmoid colon. *Dis Colon Rectum* 1980; 23:483–487.
4. Smithwick RH: Experiences with the surgical management of diverticulitis of the sigmoid. *Ann Surg* 1942; 115:969–985.

52

Regional Enteritis With Stricture

A 35-year-old woman was referred with a history of ill-defined abdominal symptoms since adolescence. She had an appendectomy for a "grumbling appendix" at the age of 17. A university graduate at 23, she had conceived two children by the age of 30. She has had occasional bleeding from "piles" for five years and for three years has had attacks of colicky abdominal pain becoming more severe and with shorter remissions. Salads, vegetables, and fruit "upset" her, and she is more comfortable if she remains on a liquid or blended diet. Her bowels are open four to six times per week. Her abdomen is distended and noisy, but she has lost weight. No abnormalities or diagnostic clues are to be found on direct inquiries into the menstrual, urogenital, familial, or social history. On examination she is seen to be well nourished. The abdominal distention and borborygmi are confirmed, and there is a vague impression of a mildly tender fullness in the right lower quadrant. Anal inspection shows skin tags and a mildly tender induration of the anal canal; rectoscopy shows a normal mucosal appearance. The only abnormalities detected on standard hematologic and clinical chemical screening are a hemoglobin of 11.0 gm/L, a serum albumin of 29 gm/L, and a sedimentation rate of 20 mm in the first hour. Contrast radiography shows a normal upper gastrointestinal (GI) tract, but the terminal ileum shows at least one terminal ileal stricture with several filling defects in the lumen that could be pseudopolyps (Fig 52–1). An air double-contrast barium is normal, apart from some swelling of the ileocecal junction and little reflux into the ileum.

Consultant: John Alexander-Williams, M.D.

Question: How would you manage her?
Answer: Surgically, and what kept you so long?

COMMENTS

First, let me comment on the diagnosis, which was standing out a mile (1.6 km). The woman has almost certainly had Crohn's disease for at least 20 years, which shows what a benign disease it usually is. It is interesting to note that the diagnosis was not appreciated when her appendix was removed 18 years ago; however, as it was done through a "key-hole" incision, that is not surprising.

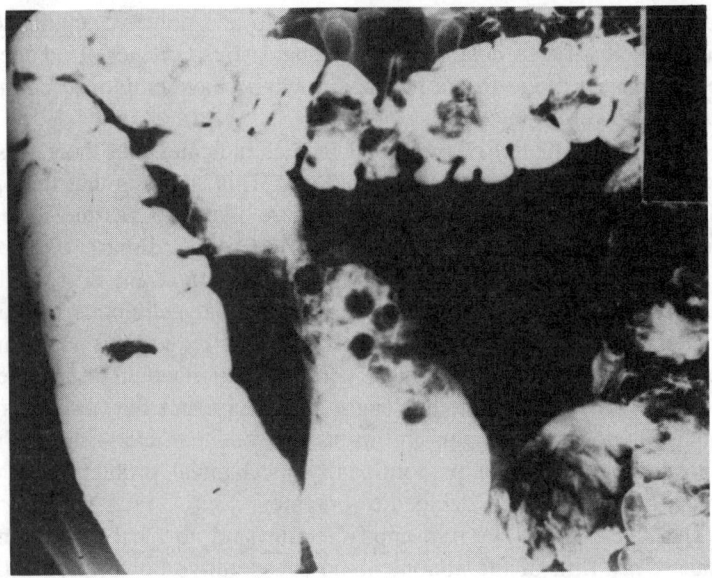

FIG 52–1.
Barium follow-through examination of the terminal ileum showing strictures and filling defects.

Perhaps, in retrospect, it is as well that it was not diagnosed earlier, for this might have provoked inappropriate medical and surgical therapy, turning a gentle natural history into an iatrogenic jungle. At least she has avoided immunosuppressive and steroid therapy and has managed two successful pregnancies without complication or exacerbation.

Her anal lesions, incorrectly labeled as "piles" as they are so often, should have alerted her doctors to the right diagnosis. A biopsy of the skin tag or of the rectal mucosa would probably have led to histologic confirmation of the diagnosis. This might have led to her being spared expensive and uncomfortable overinvestigation. If we have the diagnosis confirmed histologically, why document its geographical location unless this information will alter management policies, which it will not.

The indications for operation are clear from the history. The slow progression of the chronic disease now interferes with the quality of life, that is, she cannot enjoy normal food. The per-oral contrast study suggested multiple ileal lesions, but their localization was too imprecise to guide the surgeon, who will find more precise information at laparotomy. The "pseudo-polyps" are probably not polyps but undigested particles of food. These are often recognizable at operation as having been ingested days or even weeks before. Occasionally there are enteroliths found between the strictures.

I believe that the barium enema examination was unnecessary, particularly in the absence of diarrhea; it was so unlikely to add policy-changing data that one could not justify its cost, discomfort, and slight danger. Had there been profuse diarrhea or blood in the motions, I would have employed colonoscopy but not large-bowel radiology.

The relative normality of the blood indices indicates that there was a relatively small area of ulcerated or inflamed gut. This suggests that the operative indications of subacute obstruction were more likely to be due to a fibrous stricture than to an acute exacerbation of florid Crohn's disease.

Some who prefer to withhold surgical intervention at any cost would argue that there should be an initial trial with steroids and antibiotics to reduce the inflammatory swelling of the bowel wall and thus reduce this element of obstruction. In this patient, I think that this course of action would be an unnecessary prevarication. I consider that the length of history and the absence of gross hematologic abnormalities, plus the impacted food particle seen on the x-ray film, show that this was a predominantly mechanical problem that needs a mechanical solution. So we decided to operate.

As she had diarrhea with an empty rectum and no fecal impaction shown on a plain x-ray film of the abdomen, no preoperative bowel preparation was given. Per-oral bowel preparation is not advised in patients with obstructive symptoms, and enemas are only employed in patients known to be constipated.

OPERATIVE FINDINGS

The only advantage of the preoperative "over-investigation" is that I was certain that we only had a terminal ileal problem, so this encouraged me to follow my preferences and perform a low transverse incision. I followed the "key-hole" appendectomy incision across in a suprapubic skinfold to give a generous laparotomy incision (Fig 52–2).

There were only a few adhesions behind the appendectomy scar and a number of matted loops of terminal ileum. Some of the loops were distended and food residue could be palpated through the wall of the gut. The whole matted mass appeared to constitute less than an eighth of the overall length of the small gut. The stomach, duodenum, gallbladder, jejunum, and colon—all looked and felt normal.

Question: What would you do?

Answer: Many would perform an en bloc excision with an end-to-end ileoascending colonic anastomosis; I would not quarrel with this decision, as there seems to be plenty of unaffected small gut. Furthermore, I think that the disease is already 20 years old, with little progression proximally or distally. Nevertheless, I am going to follow my principles of total dissection of the loops of gut in the inflamed mass to try to be as conservative as possible.

OPERATIVE PROCEDURE

A careful dissection of the matted loops was achieved without breaching the mucosa, although some muscular wall damage occurred. It was then clear that at least 100 cm of the gut was involved in the mass; to resect all of this could predispose to defects in bile acid and vitamin B_{12} absorption. The most severely affected area of the gut was the last 10 cm of the ileum, including the ileocecal valve. This was afflicted with the typical "hose-pipe thickening." Proximal to this was a series of distended areas of fairly thin-walled gut in some of which particulate matter could be palpated. These distended lengths were separated by very short segments (skip areas) less than 1 cm long. Apart from a little thickening of the mesentery just at the base of the skip area, there is relatively little thickening of the mesentery and minimal fat wrapping. However, the mesentery of the last 10 cm is grossly thickened with fat wrapping and large confluent nodes.

I elected to treat this lady by a terminal ileocecal resection, removing the cecal pole, the badly affected segment of the gut, and about 3 cm of the most distal of the distended loops of gut. Having cleaned out the lumen of the gut of the distended segment with an antiseptic, a balloon catheter on an introducer was passed up through the proximal stenotic areas, into what was obviously macroscopically normal bowel. The balloon catheter was then inflated with water until it had a diameter of 25 mm. The catheter with the balloon inflated was

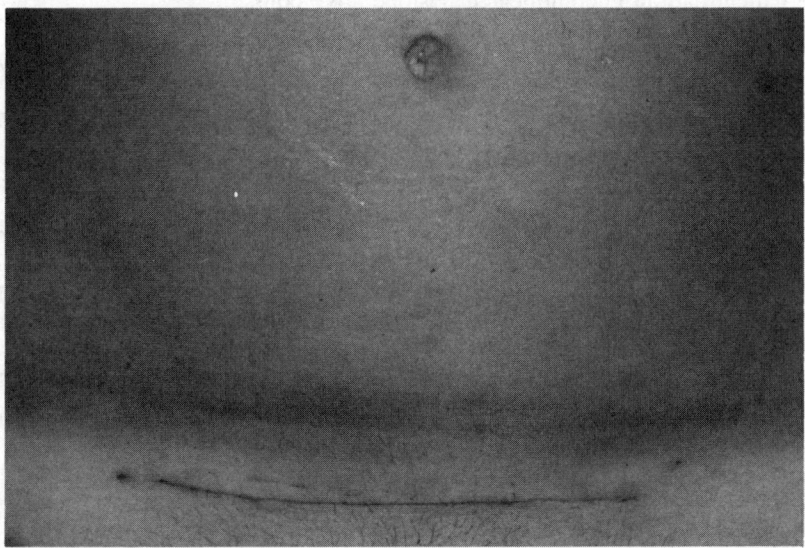

FIG 52–2.
A cosmetic suprapubic skin crease incision.

then drawn back through the gut, and any stricture sufficiently tight to prevent the passage of a 25-mm balloon was treated by stricturoplasty. Incising the bowel longitudinally from proximal to distal to the stricture, it was then sewn transversely with a continuous 3-0 absorbable suture. A total of four proximal strictures were so treated. The dilated bowel between the proximal three strictures contained much fibrous debris and undigested vegetable particles. The ileum was then anastomosed to the ascending colon in an end-to-end anastomosis with one layer of interrupted 3-0 absorbable sutures.

The anesthetist then inflated the stomach via a nasogastric tube with 3 to 4 L carbon dioxide. Within ten minutes this gas rapidly progressed down the gut with a little manual assistance by the surgeon. The distended gut was then checked to make sure there had been no unnoticed damage to the mucosa of the gut during the dissection and to make sure that the stricturoplasty sites and the anastomosis were gas-tight. As one small gas leak occurred at one stricturoplasty site, an extra suture was applied to correct the leak. I call this the bicycle-tire–puncture detection maneuver.

The peritoneal cavity was not drained. The transverse wound was closed with a continuous mass suture and the skin was closed with a subcuticular monofilament suture. Antibiotic cover was begun on induction of anesthesia and continued for five days thereafter, using metronidazole, 1 gm/day, and aminoglycoside, gentamicin, 80 mg three times a day, as we believe that a single dose of 24-hour cover is insufficient prophylaxis in patients with Crohn's disease. The patient had an uncomplicated postoperative course.

Question: What follow-up, medication, and surveillance are required?

Answer: Very little. Symptomatic treatment might be required for frequent stools, which are common in the first week or so. Loperamide is preferred.

There is no evidence that anti-inflammatory or immunoregulated drugs have any prophylactic value; they are unlikely to have any effect on the chance of recrudescence of the disease. Simple clinical and hematologic surveillance is all that is required. The hematologic indices are monitored to make sure there is no indication of deficiency of hemopoietics such as vitamin B_{12} or folic acid. The clinical indices worth monitoring are weight, stool frequency, and the presence or absence of abdominal pain. Radiologic surveillance is not indicated. Retrograde endoscopic review would almost invariably show the continuance of disease activity, as manifest by aphthous ulcer of the gut. This is simply an indication that no therapeutic modality alters the natural history of the disease.

The patient is given an optimistic but guarded prognosis.

BIBLIOGRAPHY

1. Alexander-Williams J, Fornaro M: Strictureplasty beim Morbus Crohn. *Der Chirurg* 1982; 53:799–801.

2. Allan RN: Crohn's disease: Treatment, in Bouchier IAD, Allan RN, Hodgson HJF, et al (eds): *Textbook of Gastroenterology*. London, Bailliere Tindall, 1984, pp 965–973.
3. Cooke WT, Mallas E, Prior P, et al: Crohn's disease: Course, treatment and long term prognosis. *Q J Med* 1980; 49:363–384.
4. Hares MM, Bentley S, Allan RN, et al: Clinical trials of the ethics and duration of anti-bacterial cover for elective resections in inflammatory bowel disease. *Br J Surg* 1982; 69:215–217.
5. Lee ECG, Papaionnou N: Minimal surgery for chronic obstruction in patients with extensive or universal Crohn's disease. *Ann R Coll Surg Engl* 1982; 64:229–233.

53

Chronic Fissure-in-ano

A 35-year-old man presented with complaints of bright red rectal bleeding and pain with defecation. This was the third time he had experienced these symptoms in several months. Previously, the patient had been receiving a regimen of stool softeners, local applications, and sitz baths. His symptoms had subsided with these treatments. Physical examination revealed a normal abdomen. Stool guaiac was negative. An anal fissure was noted in the posterior midline with an external tender fibrotic anal tag.

Consultant: Indru T. Khubchandani, M.D.

EXAMINATION AND DIAGNOSIS

The diagnosis of fissure-in-ano, also called anal ulcer, is best accomplished by careful inspection. Since most patients will present with severe discomfort, extreme gentleness and reassurance is necessary to facilitate the examination.

Usually less than three weeks in duration, an acute fissure generally presents as a breach in the anoderm, a crack with thin edges. As a rule, there is no external anal tag, although a small edematous skin fold may be evident distal to the fissure. Associated anal sphincter spasm makes the examination extremely painful. With adequate lubrication, following application of topical local anesthetic (such as 5% lidocaine cream), it is usually possible to insert an anoscope and a sigmoidoscope to rule out further pathology. The majority of these fissures heal spontaneously or with stool softeners, sitz baths, and local application of a soluble cream-based preparation of an emollient (my personal preference being a preparation of 1% benzocaine with 5% sulfathiazole) applied with a gloved finger. Since suppositories tend to migrate upward, their ingredients have minimal contact with the target area. Insertion of nozzles is traumatic and should also be avoided.

A chronic fissure that persists or recurs is evidenced by an area of ulceration in the anal canal below the dentate line, with visible transverse fibers of internal sphincter in the base. Classically, it would present as the "Triad of Brodie," with a proximal hypertrophic papilla at the dentate line and a distal external skin

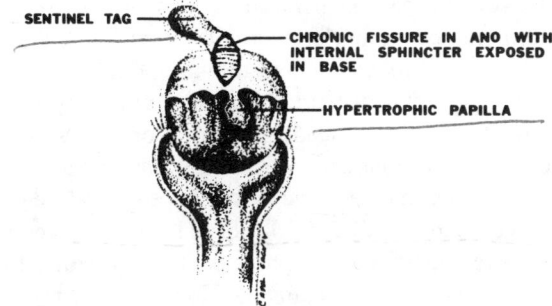

FIG 53–1.
Triad of Brodie with posterior chronic fissure-in-ano, sentinel tag, and hypertrophic papilla.

tag, also called a sentinel pile (Fig 53–1). The edges of the fissure are undermined and somewhat indurated, and there is absence of granulation tissue in the base.

The fissure mainly occurs in young adults and is somewhat more common in males. Over 80% of the fissures are located in the posterior midline. Anterior fissure is more common in females; only 1% has been recorded in males in most series. Infrequently, the fissure is found in both locations and, occasionally, in ectopic lateral situations. Multiple fissures or an ectopic fissure warrant consideration of an etiology other than idiopathic fissure-in-ano.

ETIOLOGY AND PATHOGENESIS

It is generally accepted that fissure-in-ano begins as an abrasion caused by the passage of a hard fecal bolus. The resultant spasm of the underlying internal sphincter causes a narrowing of the orifice that, in turn, causes stretching and more discomfort with the passage of each bowel movement. This vicious cycle prevents healing of the fissure. Occasionally the fissure may be caused by frequent diarrhea, which causes a tear in traumatized anoderm.

The common posterior midline location of the fissure is attributed to the anatomical lack of support in the region due to V-shaped divarication of the subcutaneous portion of the external sphincter muscle and the anorectal angulation. The unprotected anterior segment of lateral sphincter in the female results in the higher incidence of anterior fissures in women.

The anatomical features predisposing the anoderm to local trauma in the posterior quadrant are the presence of deep crypts in the region and the tethering of the anoderm by fibroelastic muscular extensions of the conjoined longitudinal muscle. These factors further contribute to the traction lateral drag on the midline during stretching.

Recent studies on manometric pressures of the anal sphincters in normal individuals and fissure patients demonstrate an underlying sphincter anomaly that results in the occurrence and persistence of anal fissure. Nothmann and Schuster recorded increased resting pressure of the internal sphincter in patients with anal fissure. Also, in these patients the abrupt relaxation of the internal sphincter in response to rectal distention does not gradually return to baseline pressure as it normally should. Instead, the period of relaxation is followed by a significant and prolonged contraction of the internal sphincter to higher than initial baseline levels. This characteristic "overshoot" response was seen in 90% of fissure patients compared with 26% of normal subjects. The overshoot phenomenon disappears temporarily after sphincter stretch treatment of fissure. The normal resting pressure is evidently maintained longer following surgical internal sphincterotomy. Another mechanism proposed for the formation of anal fissure is ischemia caused by elevated sphincter pressures.

Beware of fissures that are ectopic, multiple, indolent, moist, and/or discharging. A violaceous perianal discoloration or moist edematous skin tags with "bridging" may suggest the possibility of Crohn's disease. Anorectal disease may precede the gastrointestinal manifestation of Crohn's disease by several months or years. Crohn's disease is suspected in the patient whose fissure recurs after adequate surgical corrections. Tuberculosis, syphilis and other venereal diseases, leukoplakia, leukemia, reticulosis, squamous cell carcinoma of anal canal, and perianal Paget's disease may also present with a fissure-in-ano.

TREATMENT

It may be correctly assumed that this patient has a chronic posterior fissure-in-ano that failed to respond to conservative nonoperative therapy. Surgical treatments available for this condition are: (1) sphincter stretch, (2) posterior sphincterotomy with fissurectomy, and (3) lateral internal sphincterotomy using open or closed technique with local or general anesthesia. The author does not recommend injection of an oil-based local anesthetic solution.

Sphincter Stretch

Sphincter stretch is a time-honored modality of treatment for fissure-in-ano that has merit because of its simplicity. The procedure, popular in Great Britain, has been modified from the original uncontrolled sphincter divulsion with the patient under general anesthesia to a controlled insertion of four fingers for a period of four minutes. A higher incidence of disturbance of anal continence and an increased recurrence rate of 16% (reported by Hoffman and Goligher) have resulted in the unpopularity of this procedure on this side of the Atlantic.

Posterior Sphincterotomy With Fissurectomy

Sphincterotomy (or pectenotomy, as it was originally called) has been practiced for the treatment of anal fissure for many years. Eisenhammer's anatomical studies demonstrated the role of the internal sphincter in the etiology of the fissure and the salutary effect of its partial division.

The disadvantages of posterior midline sphincterotomy are a higher incidence of associated pain, an increased average length of time taken for the wound to heal, and considerable incidence of sphincter dysfunction due to formation of a gutter or "key-hole" deformity. Although still practiced in some centers, this technique has largely been supplanted by the lateral internal sphincterotomy.

Lateral Internal Sphincterotomy

Eisenhammer first recommended a lateral or posterolateral type of muscle division, noting that functional disturbance was less noticeable following the procedure. Anterior division weakens the sphincter most. Lateral wounds heal more readily than midline wounds.

Linear division of the internal sphincter should be performed distal to the dentate line. This represents the midpoint of the muscle and generally corrects the moderate stenosis or contracture. Three-quarter division is reserved for an extremely tonic sphincter. If the operation is performed with local anesthesia, the sphincterotomy should permit an easy passage of the large Hill-Ferguson anal retractor. Notaras described a technique of subcutaneous lateral internal sphincterotomy with the use of local anesthesia. With a large anal retractor slightly stretching the anal canal, the intersphincteric groove is readily palpated with a finger pushing away the subcutaneous external sphincter. A narrow blade (No. 11 Bard-Parker) scalpel is inserted through the perianal skin on the midlateral aspect and pushed cephalad with the flat of the blade sandwiched between the internal sphincter and anal skin until its point reaches the dentate line. The sharp edge of the blade is then turned toward the internal sphincter and, by incising outward and laterally for approximately 0.5 cm, the internal sphincterotomy is performed. The scalpel is withdrawn, and the bleeding at the puncture site is controlled by gentle pressure. The wound is left open.

Hoffman and Goligher modified the technique to the currently universally adopted mode of dividing the internal sphincter from the outer side (Fig 53–2), advancing the scalpel medially. Care is taken not to penetrate the mucosa (Fig 53–3). If the lining is punctured, the wound should be incised and a closure accomplished. Inserting a finger in the anal canal as a guide against the strokes of the advancing scalpel is a dangerous practice and should be avoided. A useful precaution to avoid mucosal penetration is to leave the innermost fibers of the sphincter muscle undivided, as they can later be easily ruptured by firm pressure with the finger.

Hoffman and Goligher compared the results of sphincter stretching, open posterior internal sphincterotomy, and lateral subcutaneous internal sphincterotomy. Of 90 patients cited in the study in which sphincter stretching was performed, impaired control for feces and flatus was reported in 2 and 12 patients, respectively, and fecal soiling in 20. In the group of 127 patients undergoing open posterior internal sphincterotomy, 11 and 24 patients had impaired control for feces and flatus, respectively, and 20 patients had fecal soiling. In the lateral subcutaneous internal sphincterotomy group of 99 patients, 1 patient had impaired control for feces, 6 for flatus, and 7 patients complained of fecal soiling. The recurrence rate of the fissure was only 3% in the lateral subcutaneous sphincterotomy group, compared to 7% after open posterior internal sphincterotomy and 16% after sphincter stretching. A definite advantage of subcutaneous lateral internal sphincterotomy was thus established.

In our series of 1,102 patients (642 females and 460 males), 1,046 (94.9%) reported the fissure to be completely healed, with an average healing time of

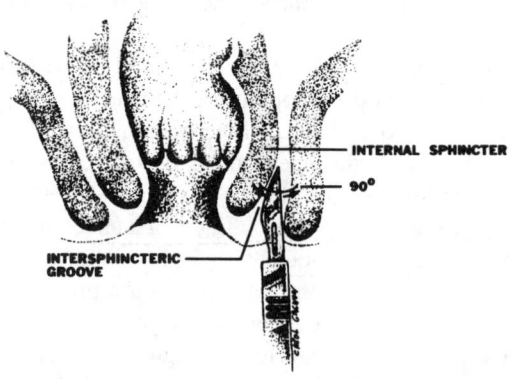

FIG 53–2.
A No. 11 scalpel inserted at the intermuscular plane and rotated counterclockwise by 90 degrees.

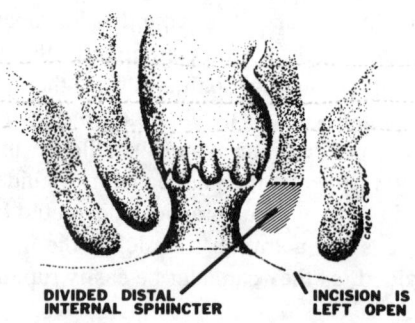

FIG 53–3.
Divided portion of distal internal sphincter with overlying mucosa and anoderm intact.

5.6 weeks, while 32 patients (2.9%) required reoperation. Frequent problems controlling flatus were reported by 72 patients (6.5%); 219 patients (19.9%) experienced occasional problems, and the remaining 538 patients (48.9%) rarely or never experienced lack of flatulence control. Only 3 patients (0.3%) reported incidents of accidental bowel movements, while 41 patients (3.7%) experienced this occasionally, and 785 patients (71.3%) reported that an accidental movement rarely or never occurred. Fecal soiling on a frequent basis was reported by 63 patients (5.7%), while 119 patients (10.8%) had this problem occasionally, and 647 patients (58.7%) responded that this rarely or never happened to them after the surgery. These questions were not responded to by 273 patients (24.8%).

Most patients with fissure-in-ano have associated anal pathology including hemorrhoidal disease. An open unilateral or, more frequently, bilateral internal anal sphincterotomy is therefore the preferred technique under these circumstances. The operation can be performed with such great facility with the patient under local anesthesia that administration of general anesthesia seems unwarranted. With the jackknife or left lateral position, the surgery may be performed in an ambulatory setting or with an overnight stay in the hospital.

SUMMARY

When an anal fissure has been established as chronic, such as in the present case, operative treatment is required for cure. The procedure of choice is partial lateral (unilateral or bilateral) internal sphincterotomy, employing the open or subcutaneous closed technique. My preferred technique is to perform an open partial distal lateral internal sphincterotomy following excision of associated hemorrhoidal pathology. The wound is closed completely with 5% polyglycolic acid sutures. If anal stenosis is still perceived, subcutaneous or open sphincterotomy is performed on the opposite side. The distal anal tag and the proximal hypertrophic papilla, if present, are excised. The fissure is not removed. The operation is performed in an ambulatory setting with the patient under local anesthesia.

Although it is possible to achieve a healing rate of 95% with the technique described here, the magnitude of incontinence is significant. Indeed, 1 in 5 patients admit to occasional lack of flatus control. Also, 3.7% of patients have accidental bowel movements and 10.8% complain of occasional fecal soiling. However, it is difficult to assess the preoperative integrity of the sphincter mechanism in these patients and, therefore, it is difficult to be totally accurate in assessing postoperative results.

BIBLIOGRAPHY

1. Eisenhammer S: The evolution of the internal anal sphincterotomy operation with special reference to anal fissure. *Surg Gynecol Obstet* 1959; 109:583–590.
2. Hoffman DC, Goligher JC: Lateral subcutaneous internal sphincterotomy in treatment of anal fissure. *Br Med J* 1973; 3:673–675.
3. Notaras MJ: The treatment of anal fissure by lateral subcutaneous internal sphincterotomy: A technique and results. *Br J Surg* 1971; 58:96–100.
4. Nothmann BJ, Schuster MM: Internal anal sphincter derangement with anal fissures. *Gastroenterology* 1974; 67:216–220.

54

Idiopathic Thrombocytopenic Purpura

A 41-year-old man notices an increased bleeding tendency while shaving. He also has a tendency to bruise easily. Examination reveals petechiae over the extremities, with a red hue surrounding the hemorrhage. The complete blood cell count (CBC) is normal, except for a platelet count of 20,000/cu mm. Therapy is initiated with bed rest. Following 100 mg/day of prednisone for two weeks, a prompt rise in platelet count from 20,000 to 125,000/cu mm is noted. When the steroid dose is tapered to 60 mg/day, a prompt fall in the platelet count to 35,000/cu mm occurs.

Consultant: George F. Sheldon, M.D.

DISCUSSION

The patient poses a problem in the differential diagnosis of thrombocytopenia and bleeding. Were the patient a female, the initial presentation would most likely be menorrhagia.

A 41-year-old man is an unusual candidate for idiopathic thrombocytopenic purpura. The usual patient is a woman in the third decade of life. In all cases, however, the team caring for the patient should consider the various illnesses that may cause thrombocytopenia and increased bleeding tendencies. These include the entire spectrum of leukemias, toxic exposures, occasionally hepatitis, and acquired immune deficiency syndrome (AIDS). The initial therapy is standard for all of these diagnoses and consists of attempting to raise the platelet count so that the most serious sequela of thrombocytopenia—intracranial hemorrhage—does not occur. While the patient is in the early diagnostic stages, steroids are recommended, as well as avoidance of activities that might be associated with trauma, especially head trauma. Bed rest with elevation of the head of the bed is used as an early temporizing measure while evaluation is completed.

The most important single test in the evaluation of patients with thrombocytopenia is the bone marrow examination. The bone marrow will establish a diagnosis of leukemia. If the patient has toxic suppression of the bone marrow, this will be reflected in the bone marrow examination as well. In patients with the idiopathic thrombocytopenic syndrome, increased megakaryocytes will be seen, with suggestion of hypertrophy of these megakaryocytes.

It is important to repeat platelet counts and ascertain that thrombocytopenia truly exists. In some patients, blood drawn in citrate anticoagulant will result in spurious levels of thrombocytopenia. If this is suspected, blood is drawn into tubes with heparin anticoagulation to avoid a spuriously low platelet count.

Idiopathic thrombocytopenia (ITP), sometimes called chronic idiopathic thrombocytopenic purpura or immune thrombocytopenic purpura, is a syndrome characterized by persistently low platelet count. The thrombocytopenia in most instances is secondary to a circulating antiplatelet factor that provides an immunoglobulin (IgG) antibody directed toward a platelet-associated antigen. It has been speculated that in some patients a circulating immune complex may have a causal role. It is not an autoimmune disease.

Platelet kinetics in patients with ITP are markedly altered, with an increased platelet production of four to five times normal and an increased megakaryocyte mass. These patients have a greatly shortened platelet survival because of sequestration of platelets in the spleen, liver, and other parts of the reticuloendothelial system. The amount of platelet-associated antibody usually reflects the severity of the disease. The antiplatelet factor is usually an IgG antibody, but in some instances may function in combination with IgM, IgA, or both.

The spleen is an important site of antibody production. The initial immune response to the platelet antigen probably occurs in the spleen and the bone marrow, where platelets and megakaryocytes may share antigenic determinants and trigger a response. Paradoxically, the spleen not only produces the immune response to the antigen, but also, in its role as a filter and phagocytic organ, it removes the sensitized platelets from the circulation, causing thrombocytopenia. With development and recirculation of memory cells (both B- and T-lymphocytes), the marrow then becomes a major site of antibody production. The liver and lymph nodes probably produce little antiplatelet antibody.

As 30% of the total circulating platelet mass is within the spleen at all times as an exchangeable platelet pool, and as the stagnant blood flow in the splenic microcirculation allows sensitized cells to be readily removed by phagocytic cells lining the reticular network of the pulp, the spleen is the major organ that removes platelets.

Most patients with idiopathic thrombocytopenic purpura are women aged 36. Clinical symptoms have usually occurred for six months prior to their seeking medical care. The average initial platelet count is usually 33,000/cu mm.

The diagnosis is suggested by spontaneous, easy bleeding, petechiae, and mucosal bleeding, as well as menorrhagia. Intracranial hemorrhage is a rare and usually fatal complication. The peripheral rash caused by idiopathic thrombo-

Only 15% of pts c̄ ITP respond to steroids.

cytopenic purpura appears to be partially due to serotonin released from platelets. The initial rash that occurs at the time of onset of clinical symptoms of the syndrome is a red-hued rash surrounded by cutaneous hemorrhage. As steroid treatment is initiated, the "allergic" feature disappears and the cutaneous hemorrhage remains as a manifestation. Eichner has suggested classifying patients into "dry purpura" that is associated with petechiae and ecchymosis, and those with "wet purpura" that is active bleeding from mucosal surfaces.

Patients with these symptoms should have a careful history with emphasis on determining the occurrence of recent exposure to quinine, quinidine, sulfonamides, thiazides, and most other drugs that can produce drug-dependent antibodies. Isoantibodies against transfusion products can also cause ITP. Collagen diseases such as systemic lupus erythematosus may produce a syndrome that is indistinguishable from ITP on initial presentation. Thrombocytopenia is also common in patients with chronic heroin use and with AIDS. Patients with ITP rarely have a palpable spleen (less than 2%) and, if a palpable spleen is present, the importance of the bone marrow studies increases, and the possibility of other diseases associated with thrombocytopenia is more likely.

TREATMENT

When ITP is diagnosed, the patient is usually hospitalized and bed rest is instituted. If actively bleeding, which is uncommon, the patient may receive blood and platelet transfusions. If platelets are transfused, they become coated with antibody and are destroyed. Platelet transfusions should be used if life-threatening bleeding is occurring. Patients are initially treated with prednisone (1 mg/kg/day) with the expectation of increasing the platelet count in three to seven days, with a maximum response expected within two to three weeks. Complete remission, however, with steroid treatment alone is usually less than 15%, although remission rates as high as 25% have been reported.

A rule of thumb is that only 15% of patients treated solely with steroids will achieve a permanent remission. However, with splenectomy, 85% of patients will have a normal platelet count within three months. Of the 15% who do not achieve this level of response after splenectomy, 10% will have markedly improved platelet counts and be able to have significant lowering of prednisone doses. Few of the 5% of patients who have minimal or no response to splenectomy will have a bleeding problem again, suggesting a positive response, even if increased platelet counts do not occur (Table 54–1).

In one large series reported by Eraklis and Filler, 88% of patients responded to splenectomy and developed normal platelet counts. Of those responding to splenectomy, 20% had platelet counts exceeding 100,000/cu mm by the third postoperative day, and 90% had normal platelet counts after one week. The remaining responders had normal platelet counts within one to six months. In

TABLE 54-1.

Results of Therapy in Chronic Idiopathic Thrombocytopenic Purpura*

Therapy	No. of Cases	Average Dose	Response Time (Days)	Response† (%)			
				Excellent	Good	Fair	Poor
Splenectomy	756	...	1–14	80	←—20—→		
Steroids	253	60–100 mg/day	14	19	←34→		47
Cyclophosphamide	61	50–200 mg/day	14–56	42	14	12	32
Vinblastine	20	10 mg/wk	10	5	←56→		39
Vincristine	21	2 mg/wk	10	←28→		48	24
Azathioprine	92	100–250 mg/day	60–120	8	18	26	48

*From McMillan R: *N Engl J Med* 1981; 304:1135. Used by permission.
†Response definitions are as follows: *excellent,* normal platelet count after therapy; *good,* normal platelet count during therapy; *fair,* improved platelet count during therapy; *poor,* no response. In some cases, details of the reports did not permit accurate placement, and in those cases percentages may apply to more than one response category (arrows).

three patients, thrombocytopenia recurred after a long interval and was attributed in one patient to an accessory spleen.

Other forms of therapy are other immunosuppressive agents such as cyclophosphamide and vincristine. Danazol is associated with a decrease in platelet-associated IgG also. These chemotherapeutic agents are occasionally helpful in allowing reduction of prednisone doses in resistant patients.

It is important to emphasize that children under the age of six often develop ITP following a viral upper respiratory infection. In contrast to the adult form of the disease, childhood ITP usually undergoes spontaneous remission. Although the patients usually receive a short course of prednisone, a clear benefit has not been demonstrated. In the occasional child, as well as adult, an intracranial hemorrhage is a life-threatening complication that occurs in 1% to 2% of all cases. If the patient develops intracranial hemorrhage, it usually occurs in the first month of the disease and may be spontaneous.

An additional therapeutic adjunct of great usefulness is intravenous gamma globulin, which reduces the effectiveness of platelet destruction temporarily by saturating macrophage Fc receptors, promoting a rise in the platelet count. Plasmapheresis also reduces antiplatelet antibody levels and can produce a temporary increase in the platelet count. Both of these methods will seldom produce long-term remission, but they are excellent preoperative treatment modalities. Gamma globulin administration in steroid treated nonresponders makes it possible to operate on most patients with idiopathic thrombocytopenic purpura without preoperative, intraoperative, or postoperative platelet transfusions.

SURGICAL APPROACH

Splenectomy is performed through a variety of abdominal incisions. The midline or subcostal incision is preferred. The spleen is usually of normal size and is assessed intraoperatively for firm ligamentous attachments. Unlike most other operative procedures, no general exploration of the abdomen is done until the spleen is removed, because the patient usually has a propensity for bruising of organs or intra-abdominal hemorrhage. The initial examination of the spleen includes evaluation of its attachments to the diaphragm in order to avoid tearing of the capsule during mobilization. It is preferable to incise the posterior splenic ligaments initially, allowing some mobilization of the spleen and tail of the pancreas. If the spleen is enlarged or if technical ease allows ligation of the splenic artery prior to any mobilization of the spleen, that is done early in the operation. (*Editor's note:* Agreed. The main splenic artery should always be ligated, preferably before the splenic hilum is dissected; however, if this is not possible, it should be ligated after the spleen is removed. I also make it a practice to oversew the greater curve area of the stomach where the short gastrics have been ligated; this may help prevent the occasional gastric perforation postoperatively.) In all instances, an attempt is made to ligate the splenic artery before the vein to allow the sequestered platelets, which account for up to 30% of the circulating platelet mass, to be returned to the circulation prior to ligating the splenic vein. When the spleen has been ligated, divided, and removed, a pack is placed in the left upper quadrant and a search for accessory spleens is undertaken. At that point in the operation, it usually is clear whether bleeding will occur from the abnormal platelets. Platelet transfusion, however, is rarely necessary. During the immediate postoperative period, steroid therapy is continued and the platelet count is monitored. It is usually possible for the steroid dose to be tapered immediately, and the patient can be discharged on a regimen of steroids with markedly lowered levels, that is discontinued over four to six weeks.

The mortality for splenectomy for ITP is less than 2% and is usually secondary to intracranial hemorrhage. In 80% of adult patients who have splenectomy for ITP, the platelet count will return to levels that are normal or above within the first six weeks following operation. In approximately 15% of patients, substantial improvement in platelet count occurs. In the 5% of patients who are platelet-count nonresponders, few develop significant bleeding.

Splenectomy is the primary therapy for ITP and should be done early in the disease before steroid-associated complications occur.

(*Editor's note:* There is a small, but finite, increased incidence of infection postsplenectomy, usually with encapsulated organisms. A pneumococcal vaccine (Pneumovax) should be given prior to operation. I usually have patients receive penicillin or erythromycin twice a day for one year, as this is when infections usually occur.)

BIBLIOGRAPHY

1. Eichner ER: Splenic function: Normal, too much and too little. *Am J Med* 1979; 66:311–320.
2. Eraklis AJ, Filler RM: Splenectomy in childhood: A review of 1413 cases. *J Pediatr Surg* 1972; 7:382–388.
3. McMillan R: Chronic idiopathic thrombocytopenic purpura. *N Engl J Med* 1981; 304:1135–1147.
4. Morgenstern L: The avoidable complications of splenectomy. *Surg Gynecol Obstet* 1977; 145:525–528.
5. Schwartz SI, Adams JT, Bauman AW: *Splenectomy for Hematologic Disorders.* Chicago, Year Book Medical Publishers, Inc, 1971.
6. Sheldon GF, Croom RD III, Meyer AA: The spleen, in Sabiston DC Jr (ed): *Textbook of Surgery*, ed 13. Philadelphia, WB Saunders Co, 1986, pp 1203–1230.
7. Traub AC, Perry JF Jr: Injuries associated with splenic trauma. *J Trauma* 1981; 21:840–847.

PART VI

Trauma and Intensive Care Unit

55

Duodenal Laceration

A 23-year-old man riding a motorcycle in rough country was thrown from his motorcycle, striking his right side on the handlebars before striking the ground. Initially it was thought to be a trivial injury; however, over the next 12 hours, increased right-sided abdominal pain became evident, as well as tachycardia, fever, faintness, malaise, and nausea. Upon admission to the hospital, there was a ground-glass appearance to the right upper quadrant on an abdominal radiograph (KUB) and a suggestion of air within the retroperitoneum. There was marked abdominal tenderness and rebound in the right upper quadrant, a fever of 103°F, and a white blood cell count of 22,000/cu mm.

Consultant: Donald D. Trunkey, M.D.

Although the mechanism of injury is strikingly different, this case is not too dissimilar from one that occurred almost 1,000 years ago. King William, the Conqueror of England, was also a victim of blunt abdominal trauma. In 1087, he was faced with a revolt of his son Robert and the treason of his half-brother Odo. King Philip of France, who was in open rebellion, had insulted King William by stating to his court that William was too fat to fight. William and his army crossed the channel and attacked the French with a viciousness that he had not previously displayed. With a large force, he harried the countryside up to Mantes and fell upon the city in a surprise attack during which terrible destruction ensued. The city was so completely burned that today it is hard to find traces of 11th century buildings in the town. As the King rode through the burning streets, his horse, frightened by burning embers, threw the corpulent King against the high pommel of the saddle with such force that he was lethally injured. He was taken initially to the Priory of Saint-Gervais where he lived an additional three weeks with great suffering and then died of intraabdominal sepsis on Sept 8, 1087. His body was removed to Caen, where the final insult occurred. The attendants, who were trying to force his body into the stone coffin, ruptured the abdomen and an incredible stench filled the church. The tomb was destroyed in 1562 by the Calvinists. Only a single thigh bone survived as a remnant of the King, but this too was lost during the revolutionary riots of 1793. Today, a simple stone slab is all that marks the grave of William the Conqueror. We will never know for sure what his injury was, but rupture to the duodenum would have to be high on the list since he lived for three weeks after his injury, which would almost be incompatible with rupture of the colon. The high pommel of the saddle in those days would certainly be consistent with an epigastric injury and rupture to the duodenum.

DIAGNOSIS

In this case presentation, the patient has clear-cut indications for immediate exploratory celiotomy. Diagnostic peritoneal lavage and computerized tomography (CT) scan in this particular case are not indicated. The patient has a fever, a white blood cell count of 22,000/cu mm and peritoneal irritation. It must be emphasized that these findings in and by themselves are indications for celiotomy.

In my experience, approximately 85% of all intra-abdominal injuries secondary to blunt trauma can be diagnosed by clinical findings. The exceptions are the pancreas and duodenum; these can be quite difficult because they are in a retroperitoneal position. History and physical examination can often lead the surgeon to make the diagnosis or, alternatively, to order special diagnostic studies such as diatrizoate (Gastrografin) swallow or CT scan. An equally acceptable approach is to admit the patient and do serial white blood cell counts, amylase determinations, hematocrit readings, and physical examination over a 12-hour period. Ideally, one should make the diagnosis before 24 hours, particularly if there is associated pancreatic injury. According to Northrup and Simmons, a missed pancreatic duct injury greater than 24 hours has a very high mortality.

In general, the rationale for special diagnostic studies includes head injury, paralysis, equivocal findings, hematuria, pelvic fractures, and presence of drugs and alcohol. The patient who has head injury or paralysis will be difficult to assess from a physical standpoint. If moderate or severe kinetic energy has been imparted to the body, special diagnostic studies are indicated on a routine basis. If the patient has equivocal findings on physical examination, this would be another indication for moving ahead with either diatrizoate (Gastrografin) swallow or CT scan. This is particularly true with duodenal or pancreatic injuries, since their retroperitoneal location often will not present with anterior peritoneal signs. Diagnostic peritoneal lavage is not a good test for picking up pancreas and duodenal injuries. At San Francisco General Hospital, three out of five major pancreatic injuries were missed by diagnostic peritoneal lavage. The CT scans are 80% accurate with pancreatic injuries, but in our experience CT scan is 100% accurate in duodenal injuries. Diatrizoate (Gastrografin) swallow is equally efficacious in making the diagnosis of duodenal injuries.

It must be emphasized that CT scan should not be overused or abused. During the past six years, we have performed 2,000 abdominal CT scans for abdominal injuries. These represented only 14% of all patients with abdominal trauma. Of these CT scans, 50% were positive; the other 86% of the patients were managed by clinical criteria.

The history can be extremely important in making the diagnosis of duodenal injury. If the paramedic had to extricate the patient from behind the steering column or if there is a history of blunt epigastric trauma, then duodenal injury should be suspect, and the minimum diagnostic study that will be considered is a diatrizoate (Gastrografin) swallow. In the present case, the mechanism of injury was highly suspect for causing epigastric injuries since the patient struck the handlebar and then the ground. Other aspects of the history that can be important, as demonstrated by this patient, are the gradual onset of abdominal pain and constitutional signs including fever, anorexia, and nausea.

In our experience, plain films of the abdomen are usually not very helpful, particularly immediately following injury. There will normally be some ileus present, but very few signs that will indicate rupture of the duodenum such as retroperitoneal air. Physical examination can again be notoriously misleading because of the absence of anterior peritoneal signs. If, however, the patient has involuntary guarding or rebound, such as in this particular patient, immediate celiotomy is indicated.

OPERATIVE MANAGEMENT

Essentially all celiotomies for trauma should be approached through a midline incision. The single exception would be for very small infants, who do better with transverse incisions. Once the abdomen has been entered, vascular injuries take priority, followed by control of hemorrhage from solid parenchymatous organs. Soilage should be cared for next, and then attention turned to exploration of central upper abdomen retroperitoneal hematomas. This implies a complete Kocher maneuver freeing up the lateral aspect of the duodenum, making sure that the posterior duodenum has not been injured, and carefully examining the pancreas. The lesser sac is also entered to complete the examination of the body and tail of the pancreas, making sure to examine the area near the hilum of the spleen. The ligament of Treitz is taken down, if necessary, to explore any hematoma involving the third or fourth portion of the duodenum.

In penetrating wounds of the duodenum, 80% to 85% can be managed with a two-layer closure. Judgment is used as to whether a tube duodenostomy is indicated. Usually it is not, but if there is any doubt as to the repair, tube duodenostomy is an excellent safety valve. If there are more extensive tears of the duodenum from penetrating trauma, segmental resection and end-to-end anastomosis with a two-layer closure can be performed safely. Injuries involving the duodenum and common duct may have to be approached differently. If the ampulla is injured, a Whipple operation may be necessary. If the common duct is primarily involved, ligation of the proximal end near the ampulla can be

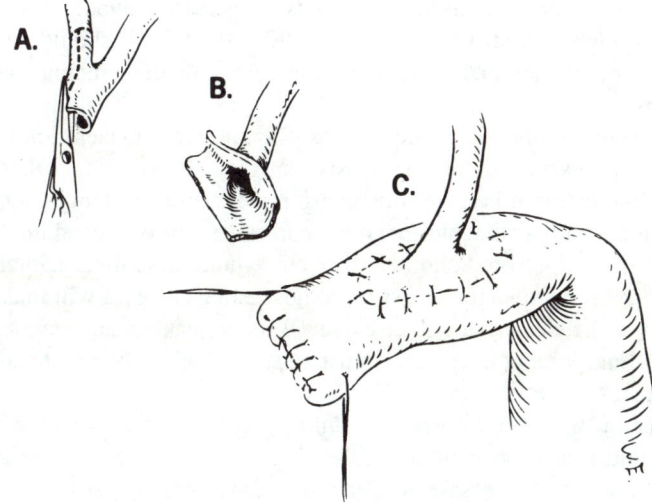

FIG 55–1.
Modified Carrel technique for normal common duct Roux-en-Y. The common duct is transected 1 cm proximal to bifurcation of cystic and common duct. The gallbladder is removed, preserving 1 cm of cystic duct. The common duct and cyst duct are opened, as shown in **A**, resulting in a "Carrel" patch, as shown in **B**. The final anastomosis is depicted in **C**.

performed and reimplantation of the common duct into a Roux-en-Y is carried out as shown in Figure 55–1. Invariably, the common duct is quite small (3 to 4 mm) in previously healthy patients, necessitating the modified Carrel approach. If there is segmental loss of the duodenum and/or associated injury to the pancreatic ducts, options include the diverticulization procedure as originally described by Berne or the modified technique performed by Jordan.

In the original technique proposed by Berne, gastric antrectomy was combined with gastrojejunostomy, tube duodenostomy, and extensive drainage of the area. Vagotomy and drainage of the bile duct were optional, depending on circumstances (Fig 55–2). Gastrostomy and needle catheter or other feeding jejunostomy were optional. The modified version, suggested by Jordan and coworkers and by Vaughan and associates, is more commonly employed and omits the antrectomy, but instead it sutures or staples the pylorus closed and involves gastrojejunostomy, duodenostomy, and wide sump drainage of the right upper quadrant (Fig 55–3). Vagotomy, gastrostomy, and needle catheter jejunostomy or other feeding jejunostomy are optional. (*Editor's note:* Our own practice is to aggressively employ gastrostomy for comfort and/or ultimate feeding and jejunostomy for early utilization of gut feeding.)

Both of these techniques put the duodenum at rest while it heals. Devitalizing injuries of the duodenum may require pancreaticoduodenectomy (Whipple) with anastomosis of the common duct and pancreas to a Roux-en-Y of jejunum.

(*Editor's note:* Even in experienced hands, pancreatico/duodenectomy in this setting has a high mortality, ranging from 20% to 30%. It should be reserved, in my opinion, for hemorrhage and injuries not capable of being managed by other means.)

Blunt trauma more commonly causes circumferential laceration to the duodenum, thus necessitating more extensive surgery. Often, simple lateral repair is not possible or there is a tenuous anastomosis. In all instances such as this, a tube duodenostomy is the minimal decompressive type of procedure that should be performed. My personal choice, however, would be to diverticulize the duodenum and put it completely at rest. In almost all instances, I will make an extra effort to save the duodenum if possible. Blunt injury causing combined pancreatic-duodenal injuries invariably must be treated with diverticulization and in a few instances resection.

A question that often comes up during exploration is whether or not the pancreatic ducts have been injured. The Seattle group of Berni and colleagues has now shown that it is safe to perform duodenotomy and to cannulate the pancreatic duct and perform a pancreaticogram. If there is associated duodenal injury, morbidity from a pancreaticogram does not appear to be increased. It is imperative to rule out pancreatic ductal injury because this may influence operative management. In almost all instances in which pancreatic ducts have been involved, drains are indicated. If, however, there is isolated duodenal injury,

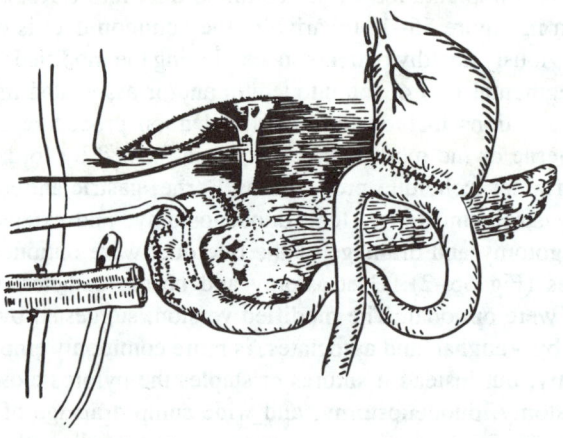

FIG 55–2.
The original proposal for duodenal diverticulization for duodenal and pancreatic injury by Berne. This method of diverticulization involves an antrectomy and vagotomy, and complete separation of the duodenum, a maneuver that some authorities find inappropriate in the view of the severe pancreatic injury and the undoubted shock and sepsis that follows. An alternative is given in Figure 55–3. (From Berne CJ, Donovan AJ, White EJ, et al: *Am J Surg* 1974; 127:504. Used by permission.)

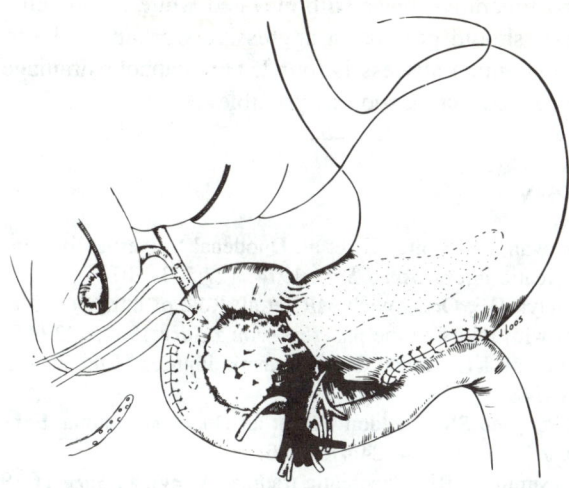

FIG 55–3.
An alternative method of duodenal diverticulization as proposed by Jordan and colleagues and Vaughan and colleagues. The pancreas, which had been lacerated, is widely drained by sump drains; a lateral tube duodenostomy is placed, in this case, *above* the area of duodenal laceration, and a T-tube placed in the common duct. Not shown is the pyloric exclusion suture that is placed through the gastrojejunostomy. Alternatively, other authors have used staplers across the pylorus. Either method is efficacious. Mortality in this injury is due to the severity of the injury and not necessarily to the means used to exclude the duodenum.

drains are not necessary unless the injury has been extensive and there are associated organs injured.

ADJUNCTIVE MEASURES

Any patient with suspected duodenal injuries should have antibiotics given during the perioperative period. Ideally, the first dose should have been given in the emergency room and continued for 72 hours postoperatively. If the surgeon can anticipate that there will be a nutrition problem, another adjunctive measure that can be performed at the time of the original celiotomy is tube jejunostomy. In general, I favor enteral feeding over parenteral. A nutritional plan must be instituted within 48 hours of injury. Tube duodenostomies should be removed between the 9th and 11th postoperative day. Drains should be removed on the fourth or fifth day postoperatively unless there is copious drainage, at which time an amylase determination is made; if there is a high amylase level in the drainage, the tube should be left in for a minimum of 14 days and even longer to establish a good drain tract or until the fistula dries up.

Persistent postoperative fever with elevated white blood cell counts or any evidence of sepsis should prompt an aggressive workup, including CT examination. If intra-abdominal abscess is found, percutaneous drainage or reexploration should be carried out as soon as possible.

BIBLIOGRAPHY

1. Berne LJ, Donovan AJ, White HJ, et al: Duodenal "diverticulization" for duodenal and pancreatic injury. *Am J Surg* 1974; 127:503–507.
2. Berni GA, Bandyk DF, Oreskovich MR, et al: Role of intraoperative pancreatography in patients with injury to the pancreas. *Am J Surg* 1982; 143:602–605.
3. Graham JM, Mattox KL, Jordan GL: Traumatic injuries of the pancreas. *Am J Surg* 1978; 136:744–748.
4. Levison MA, Petersen SR, Sheldon GF, et al: Duodenal trauma: Experience of a trauma center. *J Trauma* 1984; 24:475–480.
5. Northrup WF, Simmons RL: Pancreatic trauma: A review. *Surgery* 1972; 71:27–43.
6. Vaughan GD, Frazier OH, Graham DY, et al: The use of pyloric exclusion in the management of severe duodenal injuries. *Am J Surg* 1977; 134:785–790.

56

Inferior Vena Caval Laceration

A 24-year-old man, with alcohol on his breath, was found in an alley, apparently stabbed in the epigastrium. He was hypotensive and tachycardic, with a 3-cm knife wound to the left of the midline in the epigastrium. MAST trousers were applied but, despite the infusion of 2 L of crystalloid, he remained hypotensive. He was taken immediately for laparotomy. At laparotomy, there were 200 cc of blood within the peritoneal cavity and a severed vessel in the gastric omentum. On further exploration, however, above the pancreas in the retroperitoneum, there was a rather large hematoma containing dark venous blood. This lesion appeared to be expanding.

Consultant: Kenneth Davis, Jr., M.D.

DISCUSSION

Because this patient presents in shock, refractory to initial resuscitation efforts, a major intra-abdominal vascular injury is presumed. Intravenous lines, 14-gauge or larger, are inserted in the upper extremities. The lower extremities are avoided, if possible, because of the possibility of an inferior vena caval injury. Central venous lines are avoided because of the time required for their insertion and potential difficulty involved with insertion, associated complications, and the smaller diameter of the catheters (16-gauge). Blood is withdrawn at the time of line insertion for type and crossmatch. Type-specific blood should be available in less than ten minutes should the clinical situation demand its use. In extreme situations, low titer O-negative blood (or O-positive in patients other than women of child-bearing age) can be used. A nasogastric tube and Foley catheter are promptly inserted and the patient is quickly transported to the operating room.

The entire chest and abdomen are sterilely prepped, as are the thighs, if possible, in preparation for any and all possibilities. The presence of MAST trousers may limit the area that may be prepped initially. A generous midline incision is performed for maximal exposure. Free blood and clots are evacuated with dry lap pads and each of the four quadrants packed with dry lap pads. The small bowel is eviscerated to identify rapidly any obvious source of hemorrhage.

The lacerated omental vessel is promptly clamped and ligated with a 3-0 silk tie. The expanding retroperitoneal hematoma is approached by mobilizing the right side of the colon from its lateral peritoneal reflection, and Kocher maneuver is performed on the duodenum. Proximal and distal control of the inferior vena cava is obtained by direct pressure, using sponge sticks at the levels of the caudate lobe and the renal veins. A 3-cm longitudinal laceration of the anterior wall of the suprarenal vena cava is identified. The edges are gently separated so that the posterior wall can be inspected through the lumen. A curved vascular clamp is then applied over the laceration, partially occluding the cava. A lateral venorrhaphy can then be performed, using a continuous 4-0 Polypropylene suture. The vascular clamp is removed, and no further bleeding is noted. The rest of the peritoneal cavity is explored, and no other injuries are found.

MANAGEMENT OF ABDOMINAL STAB WOUNDS

As with all trauma patients, an initial assessment of injuries is performed and treatment priorities established, as advocated by the American College of Surgeons Advanced Trauma Life Support Course. This consists of a primary survey looking for and treating life-threatening conditions, incorporating the ABCs (airway, breathing, circulation) of cardiopulmonary resuscitation and complete exposure of the patient. This is followed by a resuscitation phase in which the management of shock is begun by the insertion of large-bore peripheral intravenous (IV) lines and rapid infusion of crystalloid and/or blood. Intubation of the stomach and urinary bladder is carried out. A secondary survey consists of a head-to-toe evaluation and any indicated diagnostic procedures. The final phase is the definitive care phase that encompasses the management of fractures, operation, or stabilization for transfer.

Management of abdominal stab wounds has evolved over the years from mandatory exploration of all wounds entering the peritoneal cavity to a more selective approach, ranging from selective observation in the absence of peritoneal signs or hypotension to local wound exploration and/or peritoneal lavage for wounds penetrating the posterior fascia or peritoneum. For patients presenting with shock, peritoneal signs or evisceration of peritoneal contents, exploratory laparotomy is mandatory. Preoperative diagnostic studies are governed by the patient's condition and the clinician's index of suspicion. Blood is generally drawn for type and crossmatching, complete blood cell count (CBC), electrolyte determination, and coagulation studies. Urine is dipsticked for blood and sent for urinalysis. A stool sample from the rectal examination should be tested for occult blood. A chest x-ray film is helpful in looking for a pneumothorax in patients with upper abdominal stab wounds. An upright view is generally not necessary and may provoke postural hypotension. Abdominal x-ray films are usually of no benefit and are not routinely obtained. An intravenous pyelogram

(IVP) may be obtained if hematuria is present or if a wound is judged to be in close proximity to the kidney.

For impalement injuries, or if the weapon was not withdrawn at the time of injury, the object is left in place to avoid the release of any possible tamponade. The weapon may be shortened (if necessary) for transport or to complete the preparation; it is prepped into the field and can usually be covered with a sterile glove. Removal is accomplished only after the identification of injuries and after proximal and distal control of injuries has been obtained.

Retroperitoneal hematomas resulting from penetrating trauma warrant exploration. This especially applies to centrally located hematomas because of the number of vital structures located in this area, namely the aorta, inferior vena cava, pancreas, and duodenum. When faced with a patient in shock with a tense, distended abdomen, consideration should be given to performing a left thoracotomy and cross-clamping the descending aorta near the diaphragm. This can maintain perfusion to the heart and brain while restoring blood pressure prior to releasing the tamponade by opening the abdomen.

INFERIOR VENA CAVAL INJURIES

The mortality rate for inferior vena caval injuries has decreased from 100% to 30% to 50% over the last 30 years. The mortality associated with isolated stab wounds is 9%. Survival is influenced by a number of factors, the key factor being the presence of shock, especially refractory shock. Blunt trauma and shotgun wounds have the worst prognosis. The level of injury plays a role in determining mortality, with infrarenal injuries having the most favorable prognosis and retrohepatic injuries the worst (with a mortality of 60% to 80%). Associated injuries, especially concomitant vascular injuries, can also influence outcome. Of the patients who survive to reach the hospital, early deaths are due to exsanguination or coagulopathy. Late deaths are generally due to sepsis or multisystem organ failure.

The two most important points in management are generous exposure and proximal and distal control of the cava prior to exploring a hematoma or attempting repair. Exposure is best achieved by mobilization of the right part of the colon medially by incising the lateral peritoneal reflection and the hepatic flexure. Additional exposure may be gained by reflecting the duodenum and head of the pancreas by performing a generous Kocher maneuver. Initially, proximal and distal control is best achieved by direct pressure using sponge sticks. Noncrushing vascular clamps may be applied; however, sponge sticks are less likely to injure the cava further. Straight clamps are preferable because mobilization along the posterior aspect of the vena cava can easily lead to avulsion of a lumbar vein, especially in the infrarenal area. Distal control is equally important as proximal control in venous injuries because of back bleeding and collateral blood flow.

Injuries of the retrohepatic vena cava often require insertion of an atrial-caval shunt in order to isolate the liver and better control blood loss. Occlusion of the vena cava at this level or ligation above the level of the renal veins will result in a loss of venous return to the heart and may result in cardiac arrest. Heaney and associates, in 1966, described a method of vascular isolation of the liver that included occlusion of the infrarenal and suprahepatic vena cava, a Pringle maneuver, and occlusion of the aorta at the level of the diaphragm to increase afterload and maintain cardiac output. Schrock and associates, in 1968, described the use of an atrial-caval shunt. A median sternotomy can be easily performed by extending the laparotomy incision. This is preferable to a right thoracotomy or thoracoabdominal incision because it provides better exposure of both lobes of the liver (especially the left lobe) and is less damaging to the diaphragm and its innervation. The pericardium is opened and the cava can be easily encircled with a vessel loop intrapericardially. A purse-string suture is then placed in the right atrial appendage and snared. A large-diameter chest tube or endotracheal tube can then be passed through an atriotomy made in the center of the purse-string suture. The shunt is then positioned just above the renal veins and the cava occluded by a vessel loop or inflation of the endotracheal tube balloon. Prior to insertion, a side hole should be fashioned corresponding to the level of the right atrium. The end of the tube remains outside of the atrium and is clamped to prevent back-bleeding or air embolization, and the intrapericardial vessel loop is tightened around the proximal or suprahepatic portion of the inferior vena cava. A Pringle maneuver must be done in conjunction with this for complete vascular isolation of the liver. Alternative methods of shunting include the insertion of the shunt from the femoral vein through the infrarenal vena cava. This approach can be technically more difficult and carries the risk of lumbar vein injury. This infrarenal approach also requires ligation of the vena cava at this level. A third method of shunting involves a specially designed intracaval occlusion and shunting catheter. This is inserted through the femoral vein and provides balloon tamponade intraluminally at the level of the retrohepatic cava. When faced with an injury in this area, the decision to insert a shunt is best made very early, prior to massive blood loss, hypothermia, and coagulopathy.

TECHNIQUES FOR REPAIRING VENA CAVAL INJURIES

The current interest in repairing venous injuries was renewed during the Vietnam War and has been well documented by Rich. Morbidity and mortality have been low; however, long-term patency rates are as yet unknown. Since veins are capacitance vessels, flow rates and pressure are much lower; thus, stasis and thrombosis are more likely to occur. Antigravitational flow and compression by intra-abdominal contents are also problems when dealing with the inferior vena cava. The thin-walled veins tear easily when handled; therefore, technique must be meticulous and handling very delicate. The presence of a suture line makes veins even more susceptible to thrombosis. Other problems, such as tension and twisting, may also work against a successful repair. Some protection against thrombosis can be afforded by the use of low-molecular-weight dextran or heparinization in the postoperative period. Temporary creation of a distal arteriovenous fistula to increase blood flow and pressure has been described as a means to maintain patency. Case reports describe good results; however, there are no large series, and this technique has therefore not gained widespread popularity. Closure can be performed in two to four weeks after the formation of a neointima, with long-term patency demonstrated by venogram.

Most injuries can be successfully managed by lateral venorrhaphy. After proximal and distal control has been obtained as described above, a Satinsky clamp can be applied, isolating the laceration by partial occlusion. The laceration can then be closed with a continuous 3-0 or 4-0 Polypropylene suture. Care must be taken to ensure that the edges are everted and that no adventitia is exposed in the lumen; this can lead to thrombosis and/or embolization. Residual oozing can be controlled with interrupted sutures or the temporary application of Gelfoam. For through-and-through injuries, the posterior wall is best repaired intraluminally. The anterior laceration can be enlarged, if necessary, for better exposure. Posterior dissection and rolling the vein over to expose the posterior surface can be extremely dangerous, especially in the infrarenal area, because of the risk of avulsing a lumbar vein. Narrowing of the lumen has not been a significant problem postoperatively. The risk of thrombosis and pulmonary embolization following venous repair has been very low.

Ligation of the inferior vena cava is being used much less frequently. Ligation of the suprarenal vena cava can cause dysrhythmias and cardiac arrest secondary to decreasing the venous return to the heart; this has proved to be almost uniformly fatal. Venous hypertension of the renal veins with renal infarction can also occur. Ligation of the infrarenal vena cava is reserved for complex injuries that cannot be reconstructed because of the size of the defect or for use in the unstable patient with concomitant injuries. Lower extremity edema can be a significant problem in the postoperative period.

Resection and primary anastomosis may be attempted when lateral venorrhaphy would result in unacceptable stenosis. The anastomosis must be completely free of any tension. When primary anastomosis is not feasible, reconstruction can be attempted by interposition grafting. Autogenous saphenous vein is the most suitable material. A patch graft can be used to repair large tangential defects. To replace a large segmental defect, a long segment of saphenous vein can be harvested, opened longitudinally, and either divided into panels and sewn together or wrapped in a spiral fashion around a large-diameter chest tube and the edges sewn together. Both measures serve to create a graft of comparable diameter to the inferior vena cava. However, these procedures can be time-consuming and the long suture lines increase the risk of thrombosis. When saphenous vein is not available, synthetic material such as polytetrafluoroethylene (PTFE) may be used. However, patency rates are not as good and, in the face of contamination, the possibility of graft infection must be taken into account. Interposition grafts should be longer than the segment to be replaced in order to minimize tension.

SUMMARY

Injuries of the inferior vena cava continue to carry a high mortality based on the location and the etiology of injury as well as on the presence of shock. Most injuries can be successfully managed by lateral venorrhaphy with minimal morbidity. Wide exposure, in conjunction with proximal and distal control, is essential for successful management.

BIBLIOGRAPHY

1. *Committee on Trauma: Advanced Trauma Life Support Course.* Chicago, American College of Surgeons, 1984.
2. Buscaglia LC, Blaisdell W, Lim RC: Penetrating abdominal vascular injuries. *Arch Surg* 1969; 99:764–769.
3. Conti S: Abdominal venous trauma, in Blaisdell FW, Trunkey DD (eds): *Abdominal Trauma.* New York, Thieme-Stratton, 1982, vol 1, pp 253–278.
4. Graham JM, Mattox KL, Beall AC, et al: Traumatic injuries of the inferior vena cava. *Arch Surg* 1978; 113:413–418.
5. Heaney JD, Stanton WK, Halbert DS, et al: An improved technique for vascular isolation of the liver: Experimental study and case reports. *Ann Surg* 1966; 163:237–241.
6. Kashuk JL, Moore EE, Millikan JS, et al: Major abdominal vascular trauma: A unified approach. *J Trauma* 1982; 22:672–679.
7. Kudsk KE, Bongard F, Lim RC: Determinants of survival after vena caval injury. *Arch Surg* 1984; 119:1009–1012.
8. Mattox KL: Abdominal venous injuries. *Surgery* 1982; 91:497–501.
9. Millikan JS, Moore EE, Coghill TH, et al: Inferior vena cava injuries. *J Trauma* 1983; 23:207–212.
10. Rich NM, Spencer FC: *Vascular Trauma.* Philadelphia, WB Saunders Co., 1978.
11. Rich NM: Principles and indications for primary venous repair. *Surgery* 1982; 91:492–496.
12. Schrock T, Blaisdell FW, Mathewson C: Management of blunt trauma to the liver and hepatic veins. *Arch Surg* 1968; 96:698–704.
13. Stewart MT, Stone HH: Injuries of the inferior vena cava. *Am Surg* 1986; 52:9–13.

57

Central Hepatic Laceration

A 22-year-old man was removed with difficulty from an automobile wreck in which he was the driver. He was hypotensive at the scene, placed in MAST trousers, and infused with 2 L of crystalloid in transit because of a distended abdomen, tachycardia, and hypotension. On admission to the emergency room, the abdomen was obviously distended and the patient was hypotensive; abdominal paracentesis revealed large amounts of nonclotting blood. Upon exploration, there was a large stellate laceration of the right lobe of an otherwise normal-appearing liver; the laceration measured 9 cm in its greatest diameter and approximately 6 cm deep. The liver appeared viable, but there was significant bleeding from this area of laceration.

Consultant: David V. Feliciano, M.D.

The operative approach to major hepatic parenchymal injuries has changed in the past five to ten years. This has primarily been due to the recognition that classic approaches have often failed to control hemorrhage from large lobar lacerations and have been associated with an unacceptable morbidity and mortality.

CLASSIC APPROACH

During the 30-year period after World War II, the approach to hepatic injuries remained relatively constant. Clamping of the hepatoduodenal ligament for occlusion of vascular inflow (Pringle maneuver) was restricted to 10- to 15-minute periods, deep mattress sutures were used to control moderate parenchymal hemorrhage, major resection was performed for large or deep lacerations with significant hemorrhage, and open Penrose drainage was used after most types of repair. In the 1970s, selective hepatic artery ligation became a popular form of treatment as well.

A review of the operations performed and results obtained with the classic approach reveals many pitfalls. For example, it is not practical to release the Pringle maneuver every 10 to 15 minutes during the repair of a major hepatic injury. Many surgeons routinely extended the Pringle clamp-time during this period and recognized that the liver continued to bleed and appear viable. Mattress sutures, while certainly effective in compressing small vessels and coapting the

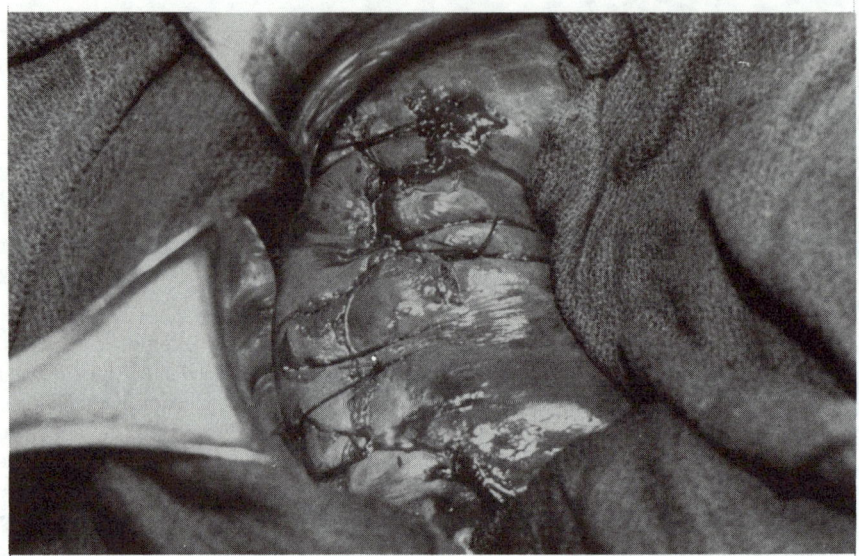

FIG 57–1.
Extensive hepatic necrosis results when mattress sutures are used to control parenchymal hemorrhage.

edges of moderate-sized lacerations, are clearly ineffective in controlling hemorrhage from deeply placed parenchymal vessels such as the intrahepatic veins. Also, reoperations for continuing postoperative hemorrhage have often revealed the presence of necrosis of *all* hepatic tissue under mattress sutures (Fig 57–1). This has been a likely cause of the postoperative "liver fever" noted in many patients in the past. Lobar resection around deep parenchymal lacerations has had an operative mortality of 25% to 30% when performed in the presence of hypothermia, acidosis, and transfusion-induced coagulopathies. Selective hepatic artery ligation has been very effective in controlling hemorrhage from intrahepatic branches of a lobar artery, but it will not control venous hemorrhage and has often led to further necrosis of parenchyma if mattress sutures have been used. Finally, when open Penrose drainage was used routinely as part of the treatment of hepatic injuries, a perihepatic abscess rate of 4% to 20% resulted. This suggests that other forms of drainage should be tried.

CURRENT APPROACH

Incision/Adjuncts

The midline celiotomy incision is commonly used for all patients with abdominal trauma. It is especially useful for patients with major hepatic injuries, as extension to a median sternotomy may be necessary on rare occasions to control associated hemorrhage from the posterior hepatic veins or retrohepatic vena cava.

In the patient described here, the first intraoperative maneuvers would be to ligate and divide the falciform ligament, insert an upper hand retractor, evacuate all blood and clot from the peritoneal cavity, and rapidly assess the extent of the hepatic injury. With a large stellate laceration in the right lobe associated with active hemorrhage, an angled Glover clamp or other vascular clamp should be applied to the hepatoduodenal ligament. No attempt should be made to separate the common bile duct from the vascular structures in the ligament prior to application of the clamp. Laparotomy pads are then placed directly onto the laceration, and bimanual compression above and below the right lobe is applied by the first assistant.

At this point the surgeon should inform the operating room nurses, anesthesia team, and blood bank that he/she is dealing with a complex or major hepatic injury. The nurses are instructed to obtain metallic clips and applicators in various sizes, narrow retractors to hold the laceration open, a sternal saw, and an autotransfusion apparatus. The anesthesia team turns on the warming blanket under the patient and obtains warm crystalloid solutions for further infusion. The blood bank is informed that extra blood may be necessary and that fresh frozen plasma should be thawed.

Pringle Maneuver

The Pringle maneuver is left in place as control of hemorrhage from the stellate laceration is obtained. All of the experimental studies on use of the hepatoduodenal clamp in the past 100 years have been performed in laboratory animals, many of which have portal bacteremia and a low tolerance for hepatic ischemia. It is of interest, however, that the first four dogs studied by Pringle in the early 1900s all tolerated over one hour of vascular inflow occlusion to the liver; hence, Pringle has been misquoted for the past 80 years. Trauma surgeons such as Pachter and associates, elective hepatic surgeons such as Huguet, and surgeons involved with hepatic transplantation have all recently and carefully documented that Pringle clamp-times greater than one hour are readily tolerated by the human liver. While laboratory data suggest that topical cooling of the liver and intravenous steroids may improve hepatic tolerance to ischemia, no controlled clinical data are available at this time.

The Pringle maneuver is released when the surgeon has controlled hemorrhage from the laceration. Release precipitates further hemorrhage, although it can usually be controlled by the routine measures described below.

Hepatotomy With Selective Vascular Ligation

With a Pringle maneuver in place, the right triangular and anterior and posterior coronary ligaments are sharply divided and the right lobe manually elevated into the wound. Much as with repair of the spleen, the extent of injuries to either hepatic lobe can only be visualized by full mobilization into the midline wound. It is often useful to place multiple laparotomy pads behind the mobilized lobe to keep it elevated. An alternative approach is to have the first assistant use his/her left hand to keep the lobe elevated; however, this severely restricts his/her ability to aid the surgeon during successive steps of the operation.

The edges of the stellate laceration are then separated by placing narrow Deavor retractors into the depths of the wound, if necessary. When the laceration is deep but very narrow (as in the tract of a missile or knife wound), the liver substance may actually have to be opened further in line with the laceration or by connecting entrance and exit sites. This is called a *hepatotomy* and is usually performed using the finger fracture technique through hepatic parenchyma with selective clipping and division of palpable vessels and biliary ducts, as reported by Pachter et al. To control hemorrhage from the depths of a stellate laceration, *selective vascular ligation* (clipping) is performed when small intrahepatic arteries and veins are the cause. If a major intrahepatic vein is lacerated, lateral venorrhaphy with a 5-0 or 6-0 Polypropylene suture should be attempted. Exposure must be ideal for this to be accomplished, as any traction on such repairs before completion inevitably extends the tear or avulses further small venous branches.

When diffuse hemorrhage is coming from all sides of a friable stellate laceration, clipping or selective ligation is often best accomplished by going beyond the disrupted hepatic parenchyma. In essence, new edges of the laceration are created by the finger fracture technique and all feeding vessels into the laceration are controlled where they can be easily visualized in intact parenchyma.

On occasion, hemorrhage will rapidly and continuously fill the stellate laceration faster than allows for proper inspection. Injury to deep intrahepatic veins, a hepatic vein outside the liver, or the retrohepatic vena cava may be present, and an extra suction apparatus (preferably attached to the autotransfusion machine) should be made available. If further inspection confirms injury to a hepatic vein or the retrohepatic vena cava behind the liver, the surgeon must make a decision as to the next technical maneuver. The classic approach to such major vascular injuries has been to extend the midline celiotomy incision to a median sternotomy. The heart is then exposed and an atriocaval shunt (No. 36 chest tube with an extra hole cut 20 cm from the most proximal hole and a clamp occluding the end opposite the holes) is inserted through the right atrial appendage into the retrohepatic and infrahepatic vena cava. After positioning the regular holes of the chest tube below the renal veins and the additional hole at the level of the right atrium, umbilical tapes previously placed around the suprarenal vena cava and intrapericardial inferior vena cava are pulled tight. This diverts blood flow from the lower one half of the body through the shunt, decreases free bleeding from the hepatic vein or retrohepatic vena cava, and often allows the surgeon to perform a venous repair. Insertion of the shunt is, of course, time-consuming and requires some technical finesse. For this reason, Pachter and associates have championed the use of further finger fracture through the base of a stellate laceration or missile tract until the laceration in the posterior hepatic veins or retrohepatic vena cava can be directly visualized and repaired. This alternative approach appears to have excellent results, but it is probably best utilized by surgeons with extensive experience in hepatic trauma.

Resectional Debridement With Selective Vascular Ligation

When either penetrating or blunt injuries devascularize hepatic tissue at the periphery of a lobe, *resectional debridement* is performed. With a Pringle maneuver in place, the surgeon uses finger fracture just beyond the ragged devascularized area. As with a hepatotomy, the goal is to ligate selectively vessels and biliary ducts where they can be readily seen. As the injured area is debrided away, control of hemorrhage is simultaneously performed. Any areas of hemorrhage on the raw edge of the liver after completion of the resectional debridement can be suture ligated with absorbable chromic suture or silk suture, if so desired.

Resectional debridement is preferred to formal hepatic lobectomy as it is almost always quicker, associated with less blood loss, and is safer for the patient who has transfusion-induced coagulopathies. If the surgeon is able to avoid placing large crushing mattress sutures on the edge of the liver, there should be less necrosis of hepatic tissue after surgery and, hence, less drainage and fever.

Use of the Omentum

When a surgeon has performed hepatotomy with selective vascular ligation as was recommended in the patient described, a large cavity remains in the injured hepatic lobe. This cavity should no longer be a source of hemorrhage if appropriate clipping and ligation have been performed. As the surgeon has avoided placing deep mattress sutures to control hemorrhage, it is now certainly inappropriate to use such sutures to close the cavity. Various authors have recommended that the greater omentum be mobilized on an intact vascular pedicle and loosely placed into a hepatotomy site or lobar laceration *after* hemostasis has been obtained. This living omental pack is then fixed in place, with a few loose chromic sutures connecting the two sides of the hepatotomy site or laceration (Fig 57–2). The pack presumably seals small leaking vessels and biliary ducts, absorbs drainage from the raw areas of the cavity, and fills in an area of dead space that might otherwise be a site for postoperative infection. While formal data on use of the living omental pack are limited at this time, centers using this adjunct believe that it decreases postoperative drainage and infection as compared to closure of hepatic cavities with mattress sutures.

When resectional debridement on the edge of the liver has been performed, a raw surface remains, much as with the use of a hepatotomy in the middle of the lobe. It has been suggested that a living omental pedicle be applied to this surface as well, for the reasons noted above. In order to cover a large raw surface, the omental pedicle has to be opened up so that only one thin layer of omentum may cover much of the debrided edge. Personal experience has shown that this thin layer tends to trap fluid collections under it adjacent to the liver, rather than absorb them. Therefore, the use of a thinned-out omental pack on a large raw edge of the liver is *not* recommended at this time.

Perihepatic Packing

In patients with complex hepatic injuries, control of parenchymal hemorrhage is compromised by the rapid infusion of cold red blood cells, metabolic acidosis of shock, and hepatic dysfunction. All of these may lead to so-called nonmechanical hemorrhage from hepatotomy sites, debrided parenchyma, or ruptured subcapsular hematomas. One adjunct to help control nonmechanical hemorrhage is the insertion of *perihepatic packing with laparotomy pads* prior to closure of the abdomen.

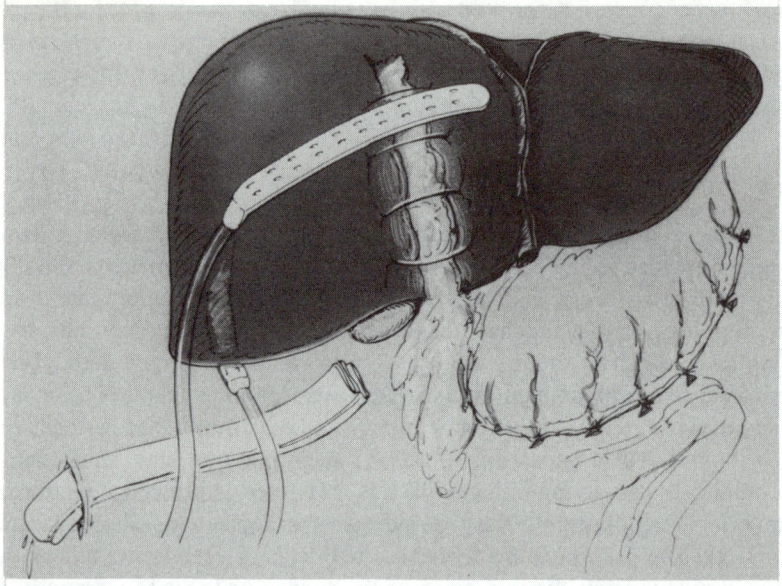

FIG 57–2.
A living omental pack is fixed into a hepatotomy site with several loose chromic sutures. Closed and open drainage may be necessary after treatment of complex hepatic injuries.

While the exact time at which further attempts at control of hepatic hemorrhage should stop and packs be inserted is a matter of personal preference, some general guidelines may be helpful. The patient who develops failure to clot during repair of hepatic injuries is most commonly one who has received 10 units of bank blood, has a body temperature under 32°C, and maintains an arterial pH in the 7.2 to 7.3 range. In patients in this group or in the group with extensive subcapsular hematomas, the insertion of perihepatic packs should be considered.

It is helpful to place a small nonadherent piece of Steri-Drape over any raw hepatic surface prior to inserting folded dry laparotomy pads between the diaphragm and the injured lobe. This will prevent the laparotomy pads from sticking to exposed hepatic parenchyma at the time of pack removal. On occasion, increased tamponade can be obtained by packing both above and below the injured lobe.

In the postoperative period, the sudden appearance of oliguria suggests that the packs are creating too much pressure in the suprarenal vena cava. Intraabdominal pressure can be measured by the Foley catheter technique described by Kron et al. in 1984. If it is greater than 20 to 25 mm Hg, the patient should be returned to the operating room for evacuation of perihepatic clot and some laparotomy pads.

In the experience at Ben Taub General Hospital, with over 80 patients with hepatic injuries packed since 1978, packs have most commonly been removed at reoperation three to four days following the original operation. At this time the trauma surgeon confirms or completes hepatic hemostasis, debrides necrotic hepatic tissue, irrigates clot and bile out of the abdomen, and changes drain sites.

The selective use of perihepatic packing in 5% of all patients with hepatic injuries appears to be a valuable adjunct when nonmechanical hemorrhage or subcapsular hematomas are present. Using these techniques, a survival rate of 60% to 90% has been obtained in patients with complex hepatic injuries.

Drainage

The need for and type of drainage used after repair of hepatic injuries remains controversial. Several retrospective studies have confirmed that perihepatic abscesses are actually more common when drainage is used and only minor or modest hepatic injuries were present. Yet it is clear that drainage is mandatory after treatment of complex injuries, as some leakage of bile and blood is inevitable. Many surgeons use closed drainage systems only; others add some open Penrose drains to allow for evacuation of thick clot or hepatic tissue that has sloughed. Using no drains for minor or modest hepatic injuries and a combination of both open and closed drainage systems for complex hepatic injuries, the postoperative perihepatic abscess rate for all patients with hepatic injuries should average 3% to 5% (as reported by Moore).

MORTALITY AND MORBIDITY

Approximately 75% to 80% of deaths in patients with hepatic injuries occur in the perioperative period from shock or transfusion-related coagulopathies. The remaining 20% to 25% of patients who die succumb to single- or multiple-organ failure that is usually associated with the original magnitude of injury and state of shock. The overall mortality recently reported in our series of 1,000 patients with hepatic injuries was 10.5%.

In patients surviving the immediate perioperative period, the most common major complications were perihepatic abscesses, recurrent bleeding, sepsis, pneumonia, and renal failure. Perihepatic abscesses can often be managed by reopening old drain tracts or via percutaneous methods in the radiology department. Recurrent bleeding may be amenable to reoperation, frequently with packing, after the patient has been warmed and coagulopathies corrected. Sepsis, pneumonia, and renal failure are all manifestations of immune failure and shock and are common causes of late deaths.

CONCLUSION

The liver remains the most commonly injured organ in all patients with abdominal trauma. Parenchymal hemorrhage is best controlled by use of new techniques such as hepatotomy with selective vascular ligation, resectional debridement with selective vascular ligation, or selective use of perihepatic packing. Viable omental packs placed into hepatotomy sites or lobar lacerations in which hemorrhage has previously been controlled are helpful in decreasing postoperative drainage and fever. Overall mortality for all patients with hepatic injuries is 10%, while perihepatic abscesses continue to be the most common major postoperative complication.

ACKNOWLEDGMENT

The author acknowledges the technical assistance of Mary LeJeune.

BIBLIOGRAPHY

1. Feliciano DV, Mattox KL, Burch JM, et al: Packing for control of hepatic hemorrhage, *J Trauma* 1986; 26:738–743.

2. Feliciano DV, Mattox KL, Jordan GL Jr, et al: Management of 1000 consecutive cases of hepatic trauma (1979–1984). *Ann Surg* 1986; 204:438–445.
3. Kron IL, Harman PK, Nolan SP: The measurement of intra-abdominal pressure as a criterion for abdominal re-exploration. *Ann Surg* 1984; 199:28–30.
4. Moore EE: Critical decisions in the management of hepatic trauma. *Am J Surg* 1984; 148:712–716.
5. Pachter HL, Spencer FC, Hofstetter SR, et al: Experience with finger fracture technique to achieve intra-hepatic hemostasis in 75 patients with severe injuries to the liver. *Ann Surg* 1983; 197:771–778.
6. Pachter HL, Spencer FC, Hofstetter SR, et al: The management of juxtahepatic venous injuries without an atriocaval shunt: Preliminary clinical observations. *Surgery* 1986; 99:569–575.

58

Stab Wound

A patient was brought to the Emergency Department by friends one-half hour after being stabbed in the left lower quadrant of the abdomen. The patient appeared drunk but coherent; there was an alcohol-like odor to his breath, and he did not know his assailant. On physical examination he was afebrile and slightly tachycardic, with a pulse rate of 100 beats per minute but normal blood pressure of 110/68 mm Hg. There was a 2-cm stab wound of the left lower quadrant. The patient complained of pain in the immediate vicinity of the wound, and there was local tenderness on palpation. Physical examination of the abdomen was otherwise normal, with bowel sounds present and normally active. Hematocrit reading was 44% and white blood cell count 9,500/cu mm.

Consultant: Gerald W. Shaftan, M.D.

This patient is prototypical, as close to a "garden variety" penetrating abdominal trauma as one is likely to see. The manner of abdominal wounding may vary according to the region of the country, the ethnic distribution, the combatants, the time of day, season, ambient atmospheric temperature, or even the touted phases of the moon. Wounds that have penetrated the integument of the torso must be considered as possible penetration into the peritoneal cavity (coelom), but mere penetration into the peritoneal cavity from any penetrating wound no longer is sufficient indication for exploratory celiotomy. (Exploration of the peritoneal cavity or coelom [celom] is an exploratory celiotomy. Since the *laparos* is the flank area between the costal margin and the iliac crest, a standard extraperitoneal exploration of the kidney may be the only entymologically correct use of "exploratory laparotomy.") Injury to intraperitoneal and retroperitoneal structures requiring repair, or a reasonable presumption of such injury, is the only proper indication for peritoneal exploratory operation. It is always surprising to see surgeons who are scrupulous about the indications for other emergency general surgical operations run unthinkingly to the operating room because a patient has a "penetrating" wound of the abdomen. A knife wound of the abdomen, as in the patient presented here, may or may not enter the peritoneal cavity and, even if it does penetrate, it can do so without significant damage to intraperitoneal structures. Stab wounds, therefore, are the usual starting point for surgeons learning to apply their diagnostic skills of patient and abdominal examination to assessing the need for exploratory celiotomy, a technique that we dubbed "selective conservatism."

Let us look at our prototypical patient. He is a young man, slightly inebriated, so that his signs and symptomatology may be unreliable. While he is normotensive, he also often is mildly tachycardic and tachypneic, usually secondary to anxiety and apprehension. We must presume that the usual AMPLE trauma history has been taken. Allergy, Medications, Past medical history, and Last meal are of primary importance for the anesthesiologist who may need to put the patient to sleep. The Events, while interesting, often are vague, consciously or unconsciously inaccurate, and in any event add little, except possibly time-sequencing, to our diagnostic ability. The physical examination must begin with the patient completely undressed, and it should be a systematic examination. Even in the sober, well-oriented patient following an assault, only the major insult stands out and other significant injuries may be forgotten and must not be overlooked. Rapid, *routine* sequential physical examination will include the head, neck, thorax, upper extremities, abdomen, pelvis, and lower extremities. The patient must be turned to examine the back and buttocks. A rectal examination and stool for blood should be as much a part of the trauma assessment as they would be for an elective preoperative examination; the presence of blood in the rectum of a trauma patient must be considered evidence of injury to the gastrointestinal system unless otherwise explained.

Examination of the abdomen, after visual inspection for wounds, begins with gentle palpation away from the wound to determine if the abdominal wall is tender, spastic, or whether a peritoneal irritation sign can be elicited. Percussion tenderness to look for parietal peritoneal irritation frequently is easier and more accurate than the classic rebound maneuver in the patient with abdominal wall wounding. After all abdominal quadrants and the flanks have been palpated, listen for bowel sounds. While normally active intestinal sounds do not give us assurance of a lack of injury to intraperitoneal structures, the absence of bowel sounds, or when they are markedly hypoactive, *in the patient who is not in shock*, usually signifies that the peritoneal cavity has been contaminated with some noxious substance, such as intestinal contents, bile, or blood, producing a reflex ileus. *The silent abdomen is an unusually reliable sign indicating the need for exploratory celiotomy*.

Each step in this evaluation process is a branching algorithm; a positive finding indicating the need for celiotomy should end the algorithm and the investigation. Rarely are corroborative studies of the need for operation required. This is an especially important point that is so often overlooked by younger surgeons in training who fail to recognize that the purpose of the evaluative process is to determine a presumptive, *not* a certain, indication for operation in patients with penetrating and blunt abdominal trauma. Thus, unless acting under an investigative protocol, physical findings on abdominal examination that are suspicious of peritoneal irritation require operative, *not* radiographic or laboratory, exploration.

If our patient, however, does not have the classic physical stigmata of a surgical abdomen, I believe that the next logical investigation is the examination of intraperitoneal fluid. The peritoneal tap, or exploratory paracentesis, for evaluation of intraperitoneal injury classically was described in 1926 by Neuhoff and Cohen in the *Annals of Surgery*. During the succeeding four decades, investigators attempted to improve the accuracy of simple tap by increasing the number of abdominal quadrants perforated or the frequency of peritoneal aspiration. There even were descriptions of the placement of a polyethylene catheter for intermittent aspiration with the hope that eventually sufficient fluid would present at its terminal opening for aspiration. Simple aspiration is rapid and accurate for positive findings, but the failure to obtain fluid has *no* diagnostic or prognostic importance. This has not been appreciated by some surgeons who interpret a nonproductive tap as a negative tap. Thus, diagnostic peritoneal tap (DPT) was reported to have a high incidence of false-negative results and was believed to be unreliable.

In 1965, Root and his associates demonstrated that diagnostic peritoneal lavage (DPL) had a high degree of accuracy. Since fluid was placed into the coelom, fluid always had to be returned. Certainly, no one to date has suggested that the failure to return any fluid through the peritoneal dialysis cannula was a "negative lavage." Used at first only with blunt trauma, DPL gradually has been adopted for the evaluation of patients who had sustained possible penetrating injuries of the abdomen. Thal, who advocated its use in stab wounds of the abdominal wall, prefaces DPL by an exploration of the wound. If the wound track does not perforate the peritoneum, the patient can be sent home from the Emergency Department. (*Editor's note:* It should be pointed out that patients are rarely in the position during wound exploration that they were in while being stabbed; consequently, movement of the abdominal wall layers complicates this approach.) If there is evidence of perforation, or it cannot be ruled out, the peritoneal lavage is indicated.

I prefer a simpler and more direct approach. If the physical examination and ancillary studies do not mandate exploratory celiotomy, all patients should have a percutaneous peritoneal tap/lavage. We use a 14-gauge, 3 1/4-in. Angiocath that has been modified by Deseret with four additional side holes close to the terminal opening. It is advanced into the peritoneal cavity through a tiny skin nick in the infraumbilical midline after infiltration with 2% lidocaine with epinephrine. As soon as the peritoneum is perforated, the needle obturator is withdrawn, permitting the catheter to be advanced safely and repositioned within the peritoneal cavity. If fluid does not spontaneously rise within the translucent cannula, a syringe is attached to the cannula and gently aspirated. Fluid obtained, whether blood, intestinal contents, or even pus, is a positive diagnostic peritoneal tap, and exploratory operation is the further evaluative study indicated. If the aspiration is nonproductive, however, a liter of 1.5% dialysis solution is instilled through the cannula into the peritoneal cavity, gently agitated within the coelom by "jellying the belly" and then allowed to flow from the hub of the cannula into collection tubes in a fashion similar to spinal fluid sampling. Grossly bloody, feculent, or purulent fluid again is an indication for operation although, as a routine, a red and white blood cell count of the aspirate is done. Additionally, we still do routine amylase determinations on the lavage effluent.

I prefer not to perform wound exploration, but to presume that every penetrating-type injury has entered the peritoneal cavity. The only advantage to the Parkland technique is that a number of patients following a limited abdominal wall exploration in the emergency department can be spared the rigors of hospital admission, since all patients undergoing peritoneal tap and lavage should be observed.

We use a 20,000/ml red blood cell count as our lower level of significance indicating the need for operation. Other centers use different levels of significance, ranging from 100,000 or 50,000 red blood cells, down to 1,000 red blood cells per ml. (*Editor's note:* In general, the lower the number of red blood cells considered a "positive tap," the higher the percentage of negative explorations. On the other hand, fewer patients requiring exploration will be missed.) Our criterion has given us a negative or unnecessary exploration rate of 8% when operation was based upon lavage effluent counts alone. In addition, a white blood cell count greater than 500/ml or the presence of vegetable or other foreign fibers also is considered a positive lavage indicating the need for celiotomy.

The precise role of the imaging department in evaluating the patient with penetrating abdominal trauma is still under evaluation. Certainly every patient should have an upright chest film or a lateral decubitus film of the abdomen to look for the presence of free air, as well as an abdominal flat film. We have been disappointed in this radiographic sign because of its scarcity even if perforation of the stomach or colon is found at operation. Nevertheless, the presence of free subdiaphragmatic or subparietal air may occasionally be an early indication of hollow visceral injury.

Contrast studies of the gastrointestinal tract and the genitourinary system may have value in detecting injuries to these viscera, especially with the extraperitoneal portions of these systems. For example, diatrizoate (Gastrografin) studies of the upper gastrointestinal tract may disclose esophageal or duodenal perforations that, because of their extraperitoneal position, may not produce signs of peritoneal irritation or a positive lavage effluent until late in the patient's management course. Similarly, retroperitoneal injuries of the colon from back or flank penetrating wounds are notorious for late septic, often fatal complications. Perforations of the large bowel may be more readily detected by radiographic studies than at the operating table. Injuries to the kidney, ureter, and bladder may be seen by adequate intravenous pyelography and cystourethrography that find traumatic lesions that might be overlooked during routine operative exploration.

When extraperitoneal or intraparenchymal injury is suspected, the computerized tomographic (CT) scan is an umbrella study enabling the surgeon, with his skilled trauma-radiologic colleague, to assess these injuries accurately. For that reason, in patients with possible extraperitoneal injuries, not only do we use oral and intravenous contrast but add a diatrizoate (Gastrografin) enema for assessment of the retroperitoneal colon and the flexures. In general, of course, a CT scan is not indicated in the evaluation of the patient with penetrating-type trauma, especially anterior abdominal penetrating wounds. Positive findings are rare; we have just found our first descending colon retroperitoneal injury after three years of this study, but that patient had benign clinical signs and a negative tap and lavage.

There can be no denying that early necessary operation is the "motherhood" in the management of penetrating abdominal trauma, just as unnecessary celiotomy is the "sin."

"The application of trained surgical judgment rather than dogma is the more rational and intelligent approach to the management of abdominal injury." Certainly, with the diagnostic facilities that we have today, that statement is more true than when I first wrote it in 1960. As Jarvis stated 42 years ago, "With thorough diagnostic consideration, negative exploration should become less frequently necessary as the experience of any given surgeon increases with this type of injury."

Index

A

Abdomen: stab wounds, management, 422–423
Abscess
  pancreatic, wide sump drainage of, 224
  pericolic, CT of, 359
Adenocarcinoma (*see* Gastric, adenocarcinoma)
Adenoma of rectum, extensive villous, 328–335
  biopsy in, 330
  carcinoma in, 330
  case review, 332–334
  clinical features, 329–330
  location, 328–329
  surgical management, options of, 331–332
Adrenal
  carcinoma
    extending into kidney and pancreas, 276
    extending into liver and vena cava, 275
  cortex tumor, 271–277
    clinical presentation, 271–272
    diagnosis, 272–274
    surgical approach, 274–276
Alcoholic pancreatitis (*see* Pancreatitis, alcoholic)
Alkaline (*see* Gastritis, alkaline reflux)
Allen's method: to control gastroduodenal artery bleeding, 107, 108–109
Anastomosis

biliary-enteric, in Klatskin tumor surgery, 162–164
with colostomy in diverticulitis with intramesenteric perforation, 361
ileo-anal, 349
ileosigmoid, with colectomy in splenic flexure obstruction, 319–322
with resection in splenic flexure obstruction, 322-324
in splenic flexure cancer, 320
two-layer, in benign gastric ulcer, 101
Angiography: mesenteric, 368–369
Antibiotics: and Crohn's disease, 305–306
Antigen: carcinoembryonic, in medullary thyroid carcinoma, 258
Antrectomy: in pyloric channel ulcer, 121
Anus
  ileal-anal anastomosis, 349
  ileoanal operative technique in familial polyposis coli, 348–350
  reconstruction, 333–334
Appendicitis: treatment in carcinoid, 312
Arteries
  gastroduodenal, Allen's method to control bleeding from, 107, 108–109
  mesenteric (*see* Mesenteric artery)
Aspiration: fine-needle, in breast mass, 61–62

B

Babcock clamp, 100

Barium
  follow-through exam of terminal ileum, 395
  study of paraesophageal hernia, incarcerated, 42
Barrett's esophagus
  Chicago experience with, 24
  with dysplasia and reflux, 23–28
    cancer risk in, 26–27
    complications, 25
    diagnosis, 26
    discussion, 23–24
    etiology, 25
    incidence, 24–25
    treatment, 27–28
Bile duct(s)
  common
    in alcoholic pancreatitis, 192
    divided, 233–238
    divided, diagnosis, 234–235
    divided, presentation, 233–234
    divided, treatment, 235–238
    stone in, 152
  dilated, in postcholecystectomy syndrome, 180
  stenosis and beading of, 156
  transection in Klatskin tumor surgery, 162
Biliary, 143–250
  enteric
    anastomoses in Klatskin tumor surgery, 162–164
    bypass: in sclerosing cholangitis, 154
Billroth I gastroduodenostomy: in pyloric channel ulcer, 121
Biopsy: in adenoma of rectum, extensive villous, 330
Bleeding (*see* Hemorrhage)
Bowel preparation
  for Crohn's disease surgery, 306
  in diverticulitis, acute perforated, 388
Breast
  carcinoma in situ, bilateral, 67–75
    diagnosis, 68–69
    intraductal, 69
    invasion, risks of, 72
    invasion, route of preinvasion to, 71
    lobular, 68, 70
    multicentricity, 70–71
    recurrence, 72–73
    surgical approach, 73–74
    terminology, 67–68
    treatment, 69–72
  mass, 59–66
    adjuvant therapy, systemic, 65
    aspiration, fine-needle, 61–62
    diagnosis, 59–62
    history, pertinent, 59–60
    mammography of, 62
    physical examination, 60–61
    surgical procedure, decision-making relative to, 62–64
    technical considerations, 64–65
Bypass: biliary enteric, in sclerosing cholangitis, 154

C

Calcitonin: in medullary thyroid carcinoma, 256
Cancer
  gallbladder, 184–188
    extended operations for, 186
  risk in Barrett's esophagus with dysplasia and reflux, 26–27
  splenic flexure, resection with anastomosis in, 320
Carcinoembryonic antigen: in medullary thyroid carcinoma, 258
Carcinoid, 311–317
  appendicitis in, treatment, 312
  care, objectives in proper, 311–315
  diagnosis, 311
    establishing the pathologic, 312
  histology, 313
  localization of, 316
  metastases of, monitoring the treatment, 314–315
  presentation, 311
  resection, 314
  spread of, determining extent of, 312–314
  treatment, 315–317
Carcinoma
  in adenoma of rectum, extensive villous, 330

adrenal (*see* Adrenal, carcinoma)
breast (*see* Breast, carcinoma)
stomach fundus, reconstruction after total gastrectomy, 90
thyroid (*see* Thyroid, carcinoma)
Cardia: manometry of, in gastroesophageal reflux, 34–35
Carrel technique: modified for common duct Roux-en-Y, 417
Catheters: Ring, in Klatskin tumor surgery, 163
Cecostomy: for splenic flexure obstruction, 324–325
Cecum: ectasia in, 369
Chest
  pain due to strangulated stomach, 38
  radiography of solitary pulmonary nodule, 54
Cholangiography
  during cholecystectomy, 236
  endoscopic retrograde, in sclerosing cholangitis, 151
  operative, in acute cholecystitis, 177
  in pancreatitis, gallstone, 203
  T-tube
    of bile duct stenosis and beading, 156
    of gallstones, 147
Cholangiopancreatography: endoscopic retrograde, 152
Cholangitis, sclerosing, 145–158
  biliary enteric bypass in, 154
  clinical features, 148–150
  clinical manifestations, 149
  diagnosis, 150–153
    differential, 151–153
  discussion, 145–147
  incidence, 148
  liver transplant in, 157
  pathology, 148
  role of interventional radiologist in, 154–157
  treatment, 153–157
Cholecystectomy
  cholangiography during, 236
  jaundice after, 237
  postcholecystectomy syndrome (*see* Postcholecystectomy syndrome)
Cholecystitis, acute, 171–178
  diagnosis, 172–173

DISIDA imaging in, 174
medical therapy, 172–173
operation for, timing of, 174–175
operative cholangiography in, 177
operative procedure, 175–177
postoperative course, 177–178
ultrasound in, 173
Clamp
  Babcock, 100
  Payr, 100
Colectomy: subtotal, with ileosigmoid anastomosis in splenic flexure obstruction, 319–322
Colitis: ulcerative, 342–345
Collis procedure: with GIA stapler, 7
Colon
  bleeding, causes of, 366
  reconstruction, 333–334
  tumors, benign and malignant, 330–331
Colonic endoscopy: in acute perforated diverticulitis, 388
Colostomy: with anastomosis in diverticulitis with intramesenteric perforation, 361
Corticosteroids: and Crohn's disease, 305
Cricopharyngeal myotomy: technique, 21
Crohn's disease, 303–310
  antibiotics in, 305–306
  corticosteroids and, 305
  diagnostic procedures, 304
  parenteral nutrition in, 306–307
  postoperative care, 310
  presentation, 303–304
  resection in, 152
  surgery
    bowel preparation for, 306
    performance of, 307
    preparation for, 305–307
    procedure, 307–310
    timing of, 307

D

DISIDA imaging: in acute cholecystitis, 174
Diverticular bleeding, 363–370
  assessment, 363–365

Diverticular bleeding *(cont.)*
  diagnosis, 365–367
  discussion, 363
  resuscitation, 363–365
  treatment, 367–370
Diverticulectomy: pharyngoesophageal, with myotomy, 19
Diverticulitis
  (*See also* Fistula, sigmoid vesical)
  acute perforated, 386–393
    abdominal closure, 392–393
    bowel preparation, 388
    drains in, 392
    endoscopy of, colonic, 388
    incision, 388
    overview, 386–387
    peritoneal toilet, 392
    position of patient, 388
    preoperative approach, 387–388
    radiography of, 387
    stoma marking, 388
    surgery, choice of, 388–390
    surgery, conduct of, 390–392
    surgery, historical note, 388–390
    surgery, late, 393
    wound closure, 392–393
  with intramesenteric perforation, 353–361
    contrast studies in, 355–356
    CT in, 356
    diagnosis, differential, 354–355
    diagnostic studies, 355–357
    discussion, 353–354
    endoscopy in, 357
    exteriorization of proximal and distal limbs, 359
    Hartmann procedure in, 360
    radiography in, 355
    surgery, 357–361
    ultrasound in, real-time, 355
  sigmoid, surgery of, 360
Diverticulization (*see* Duodenum, diverticulization)
Diverticulum
  pharyngoesophageal (*see* Zenker's *below*)
  Zenker's, 16–22
    management, 16–17
    surgical approach, 17–21
Drains
  in diverticulitis, acute perforated, 392
  in liver laceration, central, 433–434
Duodenal ulcer
  bleeding, 104–111
    initial approach, 104–106
    prognosis, 111
    surgical approach, 106–110
    surgical approach, alternative, 111
  giant, 130–135
    case scenario, 133–134
    clinical presentation, 131
    investigation, 131–133
    obstruction in, 134
    pylorus in, patulous, 133
    spasm in, 134
    standing out as duodenum empties barium, 132
    treatment, 134–135
  obstructing, 112–116
    decompression, 113–114
    diagnosis, 112–113
    electrolytes in, 114–115
    fluid in, 114–115
    nonoperative treatment, preparation and trial of, 113–115
    nutrition in, 114–115
    surgery of, selection of, 115–116
  perforated, 78–85
    definitive surgery, 82–83
    discussion, 78–80
    parietal cell vagotomy with omental patch closure for, 84
    simple closure, 81–82
    simple closure vs. definitive surgery, 81
    treatment options, 80–81
Duodenum
  diverticulization, 418
    method of Jordan, 419
    method of Vaughan, 419
  laceration, 414–420
    adjunctive measures, 419–420
    diagnosis, 415–416
    operative management, 416–419
    Roux-en-Y, common duct, Carrel modification, 417
  ulcer (*see* Duodenal ulcer)
Dysplasia (*see* Barrett's esophagus with dysplasia)
Dyspnea: due to strangulated stomach, 38

E

Ectasia: in cecum, 369
Edema: sigmoid, CT of, 358
Electrolytes: and obstructing duodenal ulcer, 114–115
Endocrine, 251–278
  for ulcer recurrence, 126
Endoscopic
  retrograde cholangiography in sclerosing cholangitis, 151
  retrograde cholangiopancreatography, 152
  stenting after sphincteroplasty, 151
Endoscopy: in diverticulitis with intramesenteric perforation, 357
Enteritis, regional, with stricture, 394–399
  comments, 394–396
  incision, cosmetic suprapubic skin, 397
  operative findings, 396
  operative procedure, 397–398
Esophagitis: reflux, with hiatus hernia, 29–36
Esophagocardiomyotomy, 8
Esophagojejunostomy: end-to-side, technical steps, 89
Esophagus, 1–75
  acid exposure in gastroesophageal reflux, 35
  Barrett's (*see* Barrett's esophagus)
  gastroesophageal (*see* Gastroesophageal)
  paraesophageal hernia (*see* Hernia, paraesophageal)
  perforation, linear, 12
  stricture, 2–9
    diagnosis, 2–6
    with perforation after dilatation, 10–15
    with perforation after dilatation, diagnostic approach, 10–11
    with perforation after dilatation, surgical approach, 11–14
Extrasphincteric (*see* Fistula, extrasphincteric)

F

Fissurectomy: in fissure-in-ano, 402–403
Fissure-in-ano, chronic, 400–406
  diagnosis, 400–401
  etiology, 401–402
  examination, 400–401
  fissurectomy in, 402–403
  pathogenesis, 401–402
  sphincter stretch in, 402
  sphincterotomy in, 402–405
  treatment, 402–405
  triad of Brodie and, 401
Fistula
  extrasphincteric
    relationship of fistula tract to sphincter mechanism in, 383
    secondary to transphincteric fistula, 383–384
    secondary to trauma, 384
  ileal, 289–297
    approach to patient, 289–297
    decision, 294
    healing phase, 295–297
    investigation, 292–294
    overview, 289
Fistula
  ileal
    stabilization, 290–292
    therapy, definitive, 295
  -in-ano, high, 379–385
    postoperative care, 384
    preoperative evaluation, 380
    surgery, approaches to, 380–384
    surgery, preparation for, 380
  intersphincteric, 381
    relationship of fistula tract to sphincter mechanism in, 382
  sigmoid vesical, 336–341
    (*See also* Diverticulitis)
    diagnosis, 336–339
    prognosis, 340
    treatment, 339–340
  surgery of, various operations, 296
  transsphincteric
    extrasphincteric fistula secondary to, 383–384
    with high intersphincteric component, 382–383

Fistula *(cont.)*
  ultrasound of, 293
Fluid: and obstructing duodenal ulcer, 114–115

G

Gallbladder
  cancer, 184–188
    extended operations for, 186
    mobilization in Klatskin tumor surgery, 162
    specimen in gallstone pancreatitis, 201
  asymptomatic, 167–170
  cholangiography of, 147
  pancreatitis *(see* Pancreatitis, gallstone)
Gastrectomy
  gastric emptying after, 139
  reflux values after, 139
  total, for carcinoma of fundus of stomach, reconstruction after, 90
Gastric, 77–142
  (See also Stomach)
  adenocarcinoma, 86–92
    operative management, 87–91
    overview, 86
    postoperative management, 91–92
    preoperative management, 87
  emptying after gastrectomy, 139
  ulcer, benign, 93–103
    diagnosis, 95–96
    etiology, 94–95
    incidence, 93–94
    surgery of, 98–101
    suture line, 102
    treatment, 96
    treatment, medical, 96–98
  vagotomy, selective, in pyloric channel ulcer, 121
Gastrin: in Zollinger-Ellison syndrome, 269
Gastrinoma: management, 266
Gastritis
  alkaline reflux, 136–142
    diagnostic evaluation, 138–140
    nonoperative therapy, 140
    operative approach, 140–142
    overview, 136–137

  prognosis, 142
Gastroduodenal artery: Allen's method to control bleeding from, 107, 108–109
Gastroduodenostomy: Billroth I, in pyloric channel ulcer, 121
Gastroesophageal reflux
  combined upright and supine reflux, 34
  complications, 33–34
  diagnosis, 29–32
  mechanism of, 32–33
  mild reflux only in upright position, 34
  treatment, 34–35
GIA stapler: in Collis procedure, 7

H

Hartmann procedure: in diverticulitis with intramesenteric perforation, 360
Hemorrhage
  colon, causes of, 366
  diverticular *(see* Diverticular bleeding)
  duodenal ulcer *(see* Duodenal ulcer, bleeding)
  of gastroduodenal artery, Allen's method for, 107, 108–109
  of pseudocyst, 214–215
  variceal *(see* Varices, bleeding)
Hepatic *(see* Liver)
Hepaticojejunostomy: latex tube stents for, 155
Hepatotomy: with vascular ligation, 429–431
Hernia
  hiatus, with reflux esophagitis, 29–36
  paraesophageal, symptomatic, 37–45
    anatomical classification, 39
    barium study of, 42
    clinical features, 39–40
    overview, 37–38
    treatment, 40–44
Hiatus hernia: with reflux esophagitis, 29–36
Hyperparathyroidism, asymptomatic, 261–264
  clinical assessment, 261–264
  discussion, 261

Hypotension: due to strangulated stomach, 38

I

Ileal
 -anal anastomosis, 349
 fistula (see Fistula, ileal)
Ileitis: acute, 298–302
Ileoanal operative technique: in familial polyposis coli, 348–350
Ileosigmoid anastomosis: with colectomy in splenic flexure obstruction, 319–322
Ileostomy: loop, in splenic flexure obstruction, 325
Ileum: terminal, barium follow-through examination, 395
Imaging: DISIDA, in acute cholecystitis, 174
Intensive care unit: and trauma, 413–440
Intersphincteric fistula, 381
 relationship of fistula tract to sphincter mechanism in, 382
Intestine
 large, 279–412
 small, 279–412

J

Jaundice: after cholecystectomy, 237
Jejunal loops: Roux-en-Y, in Klatskin tumor surgery, 164

K

Kidney: adrenal carcinoma extending into, 276
Klatskin tumor, 159–166
 biliary enteric anastomoses, 162–164
 clinical presentation, 159–160
 diagnosis, 160–161
 dissection for, 161
 operative management, 161–164

bile duct transection, 162
gallbladder mobilization, 162
Ring catheters in, 163
Roux-en-Y jejunal loop in, 164
Silastic stents in, 163
options for unresectable tumors, 165
postoperative care, 164–165
radiotherapy of, 164–165
results, 165–166
stent insertion, 161–162

L

Latex tube stents: for hepaticojejunostomy, 155
Liver
 adrenal carcinoma extending into, 275
 laceration, central, 427–435
  classic approach, 427–428
  current approach, 428–434
  drainage, 433–434
  hepatotomy with vascular ligation, 429–431
  incision, 428–429
  morbidity in, 434
  mortality in, 434
  omentum in, 431–432
  perihepatic packing, 432–433
  Pringle maneuver, 429
  resectional debridement with vascular ligation, 431
 necrosis, 428
 transplant (see Transplantation, liver)

M

Malignancy (see Cancer)
Mammography: of breast mass, 62
Manometry of cardia: in gastroesophageal reflux, 34–35
Mesenteric angiography, 368–369
Mesenteric artery
 superior, divided into four zones, 283
 thrombosis, acute, 281–288
  clinical features, 282

Mesenteric artery *(cont.)*
  diagnosis, 283
  results, 287
  second-look operation, 286
  surgical treatment, 284–287
Mesentery *(see* Diverticulitis, with intramesenteric perforation)
Metastases: in carcinoid, monitoring the treatment, 314–315
Monitoring: pH, in gastroesophageal reflux, 34–35
Morbidity: in liver laceration, central, 434
Mortality: in liver laceration, central, 434
Myasthenia gravis, 46–52
  dissection extent, 49
  incision for, 48
  operative procedure, 48–50
  overview, 46–47
  preoperative preparation, 47–48
  prognosis, 50–51
  cricopharyngeal, technique, 21
  with pharyngoesophageal diverticulectomy, 19

N

Necrosis: hepatic, 428
Neoplasms *(see* Tumors)
Neorectal reservoir, 343
Nutrition
  duodenal ulcer and, obstructing, 114–115
  parenteral, in Crohn's disease, 306–307

O

Omental
  pack, 432
  patch closure: for perforated duodenal ulcer, 84
Omentum: in liver laceration, 431–432

P

Pain: chest, due to strangulated stomach, 38

Pancreas, 143–250
  abscess, wide sump drainage of, 224
  adrenal carcinoma extending into, 276
  divisum and postcholecystectomy syndrome, 180–181
  tumors, incisions for, 267
Pancreaticojejunostomy: Roux-en-Y, in alcoholic pancreatitis, 197
Pancreatitis
  acute, 217–225
    diagnostic assessment, 217–219
    prognostic evaluation, 219–220
    treatment, 220–224
  alcoholic, with chain of lakes, 189–199
    bile duct in, common, 192
    duodenal-preserving resection of pancreatic head, 197
    hospital course, 189–191
    pancreatic duct dilatation, 195
    pancreatic duct stricture, 194
    Roux-en-Y pancreaticojejunostomy in, 197
    surgeon in, commitment of, 192–193
    surgeon in, qualifications of, 193
    surgeon in, role of, 191–192
    surgery for, selection of most appropriate, 193–198
  gallstone, 200–206
    cholangiography in, 203
    clinical approach, 201–202
    diagnostic approach, 202–203
    gallbladder specimen in, 201
    historical approach, 201
    operative approach, 203–205
    preoperative approach, 202–203
  severity, early objective signs used to classify, 220
Paraesophageal *(see* Hernia, paraesophageal)
Parenteral nutrition: in Crohn's disease, 306–307
Parietal cell vagotomy: for perforated duodenal ulcer, 84
Payr clamp, 100
Pericolic
  (See also Diverticulitis, with intramesenteric perforation)
  abscess, CT of, 359

Index 449

Perineal rectosigmoidectomy, 376
Peritoneal toilet: in acute perforated diverticulitis surgery, 392
pH monitoring: in gastroesophageal reflux, 34–35
Pharyngoesophageal
 diverticulectomy with myotomy, one-stage, 19
 diverticulum (see Diverticulum, Zenker's)
Polyposis coli, familial, 346–352
 diagnosis, 346–347
 follow-up, long-term, 351
 ileoanal operative technique, 348–350
 postoperative course, early, 350–351
 surgery
  choice of operation, 347–348
  need for, 347
  results, 351
Postcholecystectomy syndrome, 179–183
 diagnostic considerations, 179–181
 dilated bile ducts in, 180
 evocative tests, 181–182
 operative approach, 182–183
 pancreas divisum and, 180–181
 postoperative course, 183
 sphincteroplasty in, results, 182
Pringle maneuver: in liver laceration, 429
Pseudocyst, 207–216
 acute, 208–209
 case report, 209–210
 chronic, 209
 complications, 214–215
 drainage
  external, 211–212
  internal, 212–214
 follow-up, long-term, 215–216
 hemorrhage of, 214–215
 with infection, 215
 with obstruction, 215
 overview, 207
 pathophysiology, 207–208
 resection, 212
 rupture of, 214
 surgical procedures, 210–214
  general, 210–211
Pulmonary nodule, solitary, 53–58
 diagnosis, 53–56
  differential, 54–55
  historical factors, 55

 prognosis, 57
 radiography of, 55–56
 chest, 54
 treatment, 56–57
Purpura, idiopathic thrombocytopenic, 407–412
 discussion, 407–409
 surgery
  approach, 410–411
  results, 410
 treatment, 409–410
Pyloric ulcer, channel, 117–123
 anatomy, 118–119
 antrectomy in, 121
 Billroth I gastroduodenostomy in, 121
 discussion, 117
 incidence, 118
 surgery for, recommended, 121
 treatment, 119–121
 vagotomy in, selective gastric, 121
Pylorus: patulous, in giant duodenal ulcer, 133

R

Radiography
 of diverticulitis
  acute perforated, 387
  with intramesenteric perforation, 355
 of pulmonary nodule, solitary, 54, 55–56
Radiologist: interventional, in sclerosing cholangitis, 154–157
Radiotherapy: of Klatskin tumor, 164–165
Reconstruction
 coloanal, 333–334
 after gastrectomy, total, for carcinoma of fundus of stomach, 90
Rectopexy: presacral, and sigmoid resection, 375
Rectosigmoidectomy: perineal, 376
Rectum
 adenoma (see Adenoma of rectum)
 neorectal reservoir, 343
 prolapse, 371–378
  examination, 372–373
  overview, 371–372

Rectum *(cont.)*
  postoperative course, 377
  surgical procedures, 373–377
Reflux
  in Barrett's esophagus *(see* Barrett's esophagus, with dysplasia and reflux)
  esophagitis with hiatus hernia, 29–36
  gastritis *(see* Gastritis, alkaline reflux)
  gastroesophageal *(see* Gastroesophageal reflux)
  values after gastrectomy, 139
Ring catheters: in Klatskin tumor surgery, 163
Roux-en-Y
  common duct, modified Carrel technique for, 417
  jejunal loop in Klatskin tumor surgery, 164
  pancreaticojejunostomy in alcoholic pancreatitis, 197
Rupture: of pseudocyst, 214

S

Sclerosing *(see* Cholangitis, sclerosing)
Sigmoid
  CT of, 357
  diverticulitis, surgery of, 360
  edema, CT of, 358
  fistula *(see* Fistula, sigmoid)
  resection with presacral rectopexy, 375
Silastic stents: in Klatskin tumor surgery, 163
Sonography *(see* Ultrasound)
Spasm: of giant duodenal ulcer, 134
Sphincter stretch: in fissure-in-ano, 402
Sphincteroplasty
  in postcholecystectomy syndrome, results, 182
  transduodenal, in sclerosing cholangitis, 151
Sphincterotomy: in fissure-in-ano, 402–405
Splenic flexure
  cancer, resection with anastomosis in, 320
  obstruction, 318–327

  cecostomy in, 324–325
  colectomy with ileosigmoid anastomosis in, 319–312
  ileostomy in, loop, 325
  operation, choice of, 319–325
  prognosis, 326–327
  resection, one-stage segmental, with anastomosis, 322–324
  resection, primary, 325
  resection, three-stage, 322
  surgery of, principles of, 325–326
Stab wounds, 436–440
  of abdomen, management, 422–423
Stapler: GIA, in Collis procedure, 7
Stenosis: of bile ducts, 156
Stent(s)
  insertion for Klatskin tumor, 161–162
  latex tube, for hepaticojejunostomy, 155
  Silastic, in Klatskin tumor surgery, 163
Stenting: endoscopic, after sphincteroplasty, 151
Stomach
  (See also Gastric)
  fundus carcinoma, reconstruction after total gastrectomy, 90
  strangulated, causing chest pain, dyspnea and hypotension, 38
Stone: in bile duct, 152
Sump drainage: wide, of pancreatic abscess, 224

T

Thorax, 1–75
Thrombocytopenic *(see* Purpura, idiopathic thrombocytopenic)
Thrombosis *(see* Mesenteric artery thrombosis)
Thyroid carcinoma, medullary, 253–260
  calcitonin and tumor size, 256
  carcinoembryonic antigen in, 258
  discussion, 253–258
  treatment, 259–260
Tomography, computed
  in diverticulitis with intramesenteric perforation, 356
  of pericolic abscess, 359

of sigmoid, 357
  edema, 358
Transplantation of liver, 239–250
  in cholangitis, sclerosing, 157
  comments, general, 239–240
  donor procedure, 244–245
  operative considerations, 244–248
  postoperative considerations, 248–249
  preoperative considerations, 241–244
  preoperative evaluation, 241–244
  recipient procedure, 245–248
Transsphincteric fistula
  extrasphincteric fistula secondary to, 383–384
  with high intersphincteric component, 382–383
Trauma
  extrasphincteric fistula secondary to, 384
  intensive care unit and, 413–440
Triad of Brodie: with fissure-in-ano, 401
T-tube (*see* Cholangiography, T-tube)
Tumors
  adrenal cortex (*see* Adrenal, cortex tumor)
  carcinoid (see Carcinoid)
  colon, benign and malignant, 330–331
  Klatskin (see Klatskin tumor)
  pancreas, incisions for, 267

U

Ulcer
  duodenal (*see* Duodenal ulcer)
  gastric (*see* Gastric, ulcer)
  pyloric (*see* Pyloric ulcer)
  recurrent, 124–129
    causes, 125–126
    endocrine basis for, 126
    inadequate surgery in, 125–126
    investigation, 127
    marginal, 124–129
    treatment, 127–128

Ulcerative colitis, 342–345
Ultrasound
  in cholecystitis, acute, 173
  of fistula, 293
  real-time, in diverticulitis with intramesenteric perforation, 355

V

Vagotomy
  gastric, selective, in pyloric channel ulcer, 121
  parietal cell, for perforated duodenal ulcer, 84
Varices, bleeding, 226–232
  decision-making in, clinical, 230–231
  diagnosis, 226–229
  discussion, 226
  surgical options, 231
  treatment, 229–230
    algorithm for, 227
Vena cava
  adrenal carcinoma extending into, 275
  laceration, inferior, 421–426
    discussion, 421–422
    management of abdominal stab wounds, 422-423
    repair techniques, 424–426
Vesical (*see* Fistula, sigmoid vesical)
Vessels: ligation with hepatotomy, 429–431

Z

Zenker's diverticulum (*see* Diverticulum, Zenker's)
Zollinger-Ellison syndrome, 265–270
  diagnostic approach, 265–266
  gastrin levels in, postoperative, 269
  gastrinoma management, 266
  postoperative course, 268–269